T-Lymphocyte and Inflammatory Cell Research in Asthma

T-Lymphocyte and Inflammatory Cell Research in Asthma

edited by

G. JOLLES
Rhône-Poulenc Rorer
Antony
France

J.-A. KARLSSON
Rhône-Poulenc Rorer
Dagenham
UK

and

J. TAYLOR
Rhône-Poulenc Rorer
Dagenham
UK

ACADEMIC PRESS
Harcourt Brace & Company
London San Diego New York
Boston Sydney Tokyo Toronto

ACADEMIC PRESS LIMITED
24/28 Oval Road,
London NW1 7DX

United States Edition published by
ACADEMIC PRESS INC.
San Diego, CA 92101

This book is printed on acid-free paper

A catalogue record for this book is
available from the British Library

ISBN 0-12-388170-6

Based on the Proceedings of the Seventh International Round Table of the
Rhône-Poulenc Rorer Foundation. Les Pensières 1992

Typeset by Photo·graphics, Honiton, Devon
and printed in Great Britain by
T J Press, Padstow, Cornwall

Contributors

Alexander, A.G. Department of Allergy and Clinical Immunology, National Heart and Lung Institute, London SW3 6ZY, UK.

Ashton, M. Rhône-Poulenc Rorer, Rainham Road South, Dagenham, Essex RM10 7XS, UK.

Barnes, N.C. The London Chest Hospital, Bonner Road, London E2 9JX, UK.

Bousquet, J. Clinique des Maladies Respiratoires, Hôpital Arnaud de Villeneuve, 555, Route de Ganges, 34059 Montepellier, France.

Brzezinska-Blaszczyk, E. Department of Immunology, Medical University of Łódź, ul Mazowiecka 11, 92-215 Łódź, Poland.

Bureau, M. Unité de Pharmacologie Cellulaire, Unité Associée Institut Pasteur-INSERM 285, 25 rue du Dr Roux, 75015 Paris, France.

Burke, L. Department of Allergy and Allied Respiratory Disorders, Hunt's House, Guy's Hospital, London SE1 9RT, UK.

Campa, J.S. Biochemistry Unit, Department of Thoracic Medicine, National Heart and Lung Institute, University of London, Manresa Road, London SW3 6LR, UK.

Capron, A. Centre d'Immunologie et de Biologie Parasitaire, Unité Mixte INSERM U 16-CNRS 624, Institut Pasteur, 59029 Lille, France.

Capron, M. Centre d'Immunologie et de Biologie Parasitaire, Unité Mixte INSERM U 16-CNRS 624, Institut Pasteur, 59029 Lille, France.

Chanez, P. Clinique des Maladies Respiratoires, Hôpital Arnaud de Villeneuve, 555, Route de Ganges, 34059 Montpellier, France.

Chihara, J. Centre d'Immunologie et de Biologie Parasitaire, Unité Mixte INSERM U 16-CNRS 624, Institut Pasteur, 59029 Lille, France.

Church, M.K. Clinical Pharmacology, Centre Block, Southampton General Hospital, Tremona Road, Southampton SO9 4XY, UK.

Coëffier, E. Unité de Pharmacologie Cellulaire, Unité Associée Institut Pasteur-INSERM 285, 25, rue du Dr Roux, 75015 Paris, France.

Corrigan, C.J. Department of Allergy and Clinical Immunology, National Heart and Lung Institute, Dovehouse Street, London SW3 6LY, UK.

Damon, M. INSERM U 58, Avenue de Navacelle, 34100 Montpellier, France.

De Brito, F.B. Rhône-Poulenc Rorer, Rainham Road South, Dagenham, Essex RM10 7XS, UK.

De Carli, M. Division of Clinical Immunology and Allergology, Istituto di Clinical Medica 3, University of Florence, Florence, Italy.

Del Prete, G.F. Division of Clinical Immunology and Allergology, Istituto di Clinical Medica 3, University of Florence, Florence, Italy.

Demoly, P. Clinique des Maladies Respiratoires, Hôpital Arnaud de Villeneuve, 555, Route de Ganges, 34059 Montpellier, France.

Desquand, S. Unité de Pharmacologie Cellulaire, Unité Associée Institut Pasteur-INSERM 285, 25, rue du Dr Roux, 75015 Paris, France.

Desreumaux, P. Centre d'Immunologie et de Biologie Parasitaire, Unité Mixte INSERM U 16-CNRS 624, Institut Pasteur, 59029 Lille, France.

Gant, V. Department of Allergy and Allied Respiratory Disorders, Hunt's House, Guy's Hospital, London SE1 9RT, UK.

Godard, P. Clinique des Maladies Respiratoires, Hôpital Arnaud de Villeneuve, 555, Route de Ganges, 34059 Montpellier, France.

Hallsworth, M. Department of Allergy and Allied Respiratory Disorders, Hunt's House, Guy's Hospital, London SE1 9RT, UK.

Harrison, N.K. Biochemistry Unit, Department of Thoracic Medicine, National Heart and Lung Institute, University of London, Manresa Road, London SW3 6LR, UK.

Higgins, J.A. Department of Immunology, St. Mary's Hospital Medical School, Imperial College of Science, Technology and Medicine, Norfolk Place, London W2 1PG, UK.

Hitoshi, Y. Department of Biology, Institute for Medical Immunology, Kumamoto University, Medical School, 2-2-1 Honjo, Kumamoto 860, Japan and Department of Immunology, Institute of Medical Science, University of Tokyo, 4-6-1 Shiroganedai, Minato-ku, Tokyo 108, Japan.

Holgate, S.T. Immunopharmacology Group, Centre Block, Southampton General Hospital, Tremona Road, Southampton SO9 4XY, UK.

Howell, C. Department of Allergy and Allied Respiratory Disorders, Hunt's House, Guy's Hospital, London SE1 9RT, UK.

Jarman, E.R. Department of Immunology, St. Mary's Hospital Medical School, Imperial College of Science, Technology and Medicine, Norfolk Place, London W2 1PG, UK.

Karlsson, J.-A. Rhône-Poulenc Rorer, Rainham Road South, Dagenham, Essex RM10 7XS, UK.

Kay, A.B. Department of Allergy and Clinical Immunology, National Heart and Lung Institute, Dovehouse Street, London SW3 6LY, UK.

Lamb, J.R. Department of Immunology, St. Mary's Hospital Medical School, Imperial College of Science, Technology and Medicine, Norfolk Place, London W2 1PG, UK.

Lane, S.J. Department of Allergy and Allied Respiratory Disorders, Hunt's House, Guy's Hospital, London SE1 9RT, UK.

Laurent, G.J. Biochemistry Unit, Department of Thoracic Medicine, National Heart and Lung Institute, University of London, Manresa Road, London SW3 6LR, UK.

Lawrence, C.E. Rhône-Poulenc Rorer, Rainham Road South, Dagenham, Essex RM10 7XS, UK.

Lee, T.H. Department of Allergy and Allied Respiratory Disorders, Hunt's House, Guy's Hospital, London SE1 9RT, UK.

Leff, A.R. Department of Medicine MC6076, Section of Pulmonary and Critical Care Medicine, The University of Chicago, 5841 S. Maryland Avenue, Chicago, IL 60637, USA.

Lefort, J. Unité de Pharmacologie Cellulaire, Unité Associée Institut Pasteur-INSERM 285, 25, rue du Dr Roux, 75015 Paris, France.

Maggi, E. Divisio of Clinical Immunology and Allergology, Istituto di Clinica Medica 3, University of Florence, Florence, Italy.

Manetti, R. Division of Clinical Immunology and Allergology, Istituto di Clinica Medica 3, University of Florence, Florence, Italy.

Martins, M.A. Fiocruz, Rio de Janeiro, Brazil.

Michel, F.B. Clinique des Maladies Respiratoires, Hôpital Arnaud de Villeneuve, 555, Route de Ganges, 34059 Montpellier, France.

Mosmann, T. Department of Immunology, University of Alberta, Edmonton, Alberta T6G 2H7, Canada.

O'Hehir, R.E. Department of Immunology, St. Mary's Hospital Medical School, Imperial College of Science, Technology and Medicine, Norfolk Place, London W2 1PG, UK.

Palfreyman, M. Rhône-Poulenc Rorer, Rainham Road South, Dagenham, Essex RM10 7XS, UK.

Parronchi, P. Division of Clinical Immunology and Allergology, Istituto di Clinica Medica 3, University of Florence, Florence, Italy.

Piccini, M.P. Division of Clinical Immunology and Allergology, Istituto di Clinica Medica 3, University of Florence, Florence, Italy.

Plumas, J. Centre d'Immunologie et de Biologie Parasitaire, Unité Mixte INSERM U 16-CNRS 624, Institut Pasteur, 59029 Lille, France.

Pretolani, M. Unité de Pharmacologie Cellulaire, Unité Associée Institut Pasteur-INSERM 285, 25, rue du Dr Roux, 75015 Paris, France.

Raeburn, D. Rhône-Poulenc Rorer, Rainham Road South, Dagenham, Essex RM10 7XS, UK.

Romagnani, S. Division of Clinical Immunology and Allergology, Istituto di Clinica Medica 3, University of Florence, Florence, Italy.

Silva, P. Fiocruz, Rio de Janeiro, Brazil.

Soh, C. Department of Allergy and Allied Respiratory Disorders, Hunt's House, Guy's Hospital, London SE1 9RT, UK.

Souness, J. Rhône-Poulenc Rorer, Rainham Road South, Dagenham, Essex RM10 7XS, UK.

Takatsu, K. Department of Biology, Institute for Medical Immunology, Kumamoto University, Medical School, 2-2-1 Honjo, Kumamoto 860, Japan and Department of Immunology, Institute of Medical Science, University of Tokyo, 4-6-1 Shiroganedai, Minato-ku, Tokyo 108, Japan.

Tavernier, J. Roche Research Ghent, Ghent, Belgium.

Tominaga, A. Department of Biology, Institute for Medical Immunology, Kumamoto University, Medical School, 2-2-1 Honjo, Kumamoto 860, Japan.

Vargaftig, B.B. Unité de Pharmacologie Cellulaire, Unité Associée Institut Pasteur-INSERM 285, 25, rue du Dr Roux, 75017 Paris, France.

Venge, P. Laboratory for Inflammation Research, Department of Clinical Chemistry, University Hospital, S-751 85 Uppsala, Sweden.

Vincent, D. Unité de Pharmacologie Cellulaire, Unité Associée Institut Pasteur-INSERM 285, 25, rue du Dr Roux, 75015 Paris, France.

Weller, P.F. Beth Israel Hospital, DA 617, 330 Brookline Avenue, Boston, MA 02215, USA.

Participants

Advenier, C. Institut Biomédical des Cordeliers, 15 rue de l'Ecole de Medecine, 75270 Paris Cedex 06, France.

Ashton, M.J. Rhône-Poulenc Rorer, Dagenham Research Centre, Rainham Road South, Dagenham, Essex RM10 7XS, UK.

Bost, P.E. Rhône-Poulenc Rorer, Central Research, 20 Avenue Raymond Aron, 92165 Antony Cedex, France.

Bousseau, A. Rhône-Poulenc Rorer, Centre de Recherches de Vitry, 13 Quai Jules Guesde, BP 14-94403 Vitry-sur-Seine Cedex, France.

Brefort, G. Rhône-Poulenc Rorer, Scientific Direction, 20 Avenue Raymond Aron, 92165 Antony Cedex, France.

Brochet, M.F. Rhône-Poulenc Rorer, Clinical Department, 20 Avenue Raymond Aron, 92165 Antony Cedex, France.

Campbell, H. Rhône-Poulenc Rorer, Central Research, 640 Allendale Road, King of Prussia, PA 19406, USA.

Chang, M. Rhône-Poulenc Rorer, Central Research, 640 Allendale Road, King of Prussia, PA 19406, USA.

Dahl, R. University Hospital of Aarhus, Department of Respiratory Diseases, DK 8000 Aarhus C, Denmark.

Deregnaucourt, J. Rhône-Poulenc Rorer, Project Management, 20 Avenue Raymond Aron, 92165 Antony Cedex, France.

Drazen, J.M. Brigham & Women's Hospital, Harvard Medical School, 75 Francis Street, Boston, MA 02115, USA.

Floch, A. Rhône-Poulenc Rorer, Centre de Recherches de Vitry, 13 Quai Jules Guesde, BP 14-94403 Vitry-sur-Seine Cedex, France.

Garaud, J.-J. Rhône-Poulenc Rorer, Clinical Development, 20 Avenue Raymond Aron, 92165 Antony Cedex, France.

Gimbol, M.J. Rhône-Poulenc Rorer, Central Research, 500 Virginia Drive, Fort Washington, PA 19034, USA.

Haslett, C. City Hospital, Greenbank Drive, Edinburgh EH10 5SB, UK.

Jolles, G. Rhône-Poulenc Rorer, Scientific Direction, 20 Avenue Raymond Aron, 92165 Antony Cedex, France.

Moqbel, R. National Heart & Lung Institute, Dovehouse Street, London SW3 6LY, UK.

Nijkamp, F.P. University of Utrecht, Catharijnesingel 60, 3511 GH Utrecht, Holland.

Osborn, C. Rhône-Poulenc Rorer, Rainham Road South, Dagenham, Essex RM10 7XS, UK.

Page, C. King's College London, Biomedical Sciences Division, Manresa Road, London SW3 6LX, UK.

Reilly, J. Rhône-Poulenc Rorer, 500 Virginia Drive, Fort Washington, PA 19034, USA.

Rumfitt, I. Rhône-Poulenc Rorer, Rainham Road South, Dagenham, Essex RM10 7XS, UK.

Saetta, M. Universita Di Padova, Istituto di Medicina de Lavoro, 1-35127 Padova, Via Facciolati 71, Italy.

Schreiber, A.B. Rhône-Poulenc Rorer, Central Research, 640 Allendale Road, King of Prussia, PA 19406, USA.

Skoogh, B.-E. Renströmska Sjukhuset, Department of Pulmonary Diseases, Box 17301, 40264 Göteborg, Sweden.

Smith, J.A. Rhône-Poulenc Rorer, Central Research, 800 Business Center Drive, Horsham, PA 19044, USA.

Souness, J. Rhône-Poulenc Rorer, Dagenham Research Centre, Rainham Road South, Dagenham, Essex RM10 7XS, UK.

Taylor, J.B. Rhône-Poulenc Rorer, Dagenham Research Centre, Rainham Road South, Dagenham, Essex RM10 7XS, UK.

Terlain, B. Rhône-Poulenc Rorer, Centre de Recherches de Vitry, 13 Quai Jules Guesde, BP 14-94403 Vitry-sur-Seine Cedex, France.

Tobey, R. Rhône-Poulenc Rorer, Central Research, 800 Business Center Drive, Horsham, PA 19044, USA.

Walters, E.H. General Hospital, Chest Unit, Newcastle upon Tyne NE4 6BE, UK.

Warne, P.J. Rhône-Poulenc Rorer, Dagenham Research Centre, Rainham Road South, Dagenham, Essex RM10 7XS, UK.

Withnall, M.T. Rhône-Poulenc Rorer, Dagenham Research Centre, Rainham Road South, Dagenham, Essex RM10 7XS, UK.

Wood-Raines, D. Rhône-Poulenc Rorer, Central Research, 800 Business Center Drive, Horsham, PA 29044, USA.

Preface

It is well established that asthma is an inflammatory disease of the airway mucosa, and drugs like inhaled glucocorticoids are now commonly introduced early in therapy. A characteristic feature of this disease is the vast number of eosinophils in airway tissue, although many other migratory and resident inflammatory cells with the capacity to synthesize and release cytokines and putative asthma mediators are present in the inflamed mucosa. The cross-talk between lymphocytes and these cells and the roles of cytokines in complex biological networks are currently areas of intense research.

The conference which gave rise to this book was organized in Turnberry, Scotland, in November 1991 and was sponsored by a grant from the Rhône-Poulenc Rorer Foundation. It brought together researchers from three continents to debate, during two days, the latest developments in select areas of inflammatory research. The lectures were grouped into three sessions in which the biology of immunocompetent and inflammatory cells was introduced; a few contributions were further devoted to a more general overview focused on new perspectives in asthma. The lively discussions that followed many of the presentations formed an excellent basis for the exchange of views on cellular interplay and communication and on the relative importance of cells/mediators in disease. We believe that this volume, specially edited to provide all those interested in asthma research with the data and reviews presented during the conference, will contribute to further insights into the pathology of asthma and to the development of novel efficacious drugs for the treatment of asthma and related respiratory disorders.

Finally, we hope that this volume will convey to the reader some of the thought-provoking discussions that resulted from the excellent presentations and a participative audience mediated by skilful chairmen in a splendid Scottish environment.

G. Jolles, J.-A. Karlsson and J. Taylor

Acknowledgements

It is our pleasure to thank sincerely all the contributors as well as all the participants who agreed to come to Scotland to attend the International Round Table on "New Perspectives in Asthma": their active cooperation made this conference a highly successful scientific event and enabled the preparation of the present volume.

We are especially grateful to Professor S.T. Holgate for his generous advice during the preparation of the Round Table and also to the moderators of the sessions who stimulated and organized the discussions: Professors Church, Leff, Nijkamp, Page and Romagnani.

We wish to acknowledge the financial support of the Rhône-Poulenc Rorer Foundation who acted as the full sponsor of the Round Table according to its objective to foster exchanges on scientific topics of current interest between experts from academia and industry and to provide the International Scientific Community with the results of these conferences.

We want further to express our gratitude to Mrs Raindle and Mrs Sommet: both assisted us most diligently in the organization of the meeting and Mrs Sommet contributed afterwards very efficiently to the final preparation of the manuscripts. Tape transcription of the discussions was performed by Dr Mary Firth and her professionalism and competence were highly appreciated.

Finally we wish to thank Dr Carey Chapman and the staff of Academic Press Ltd (London) for their expert and kind assistance in producing this volume.

Contents

Part I

Lymphocytes as Orchestrators of Airway Inflammation

1

T-Lymphocytes in Allergic Asthma

C.J. CORRIGAN and A.B. KAY

Department of Allergy and Clinical Immunology, National Heart and Lung Institute, Dovehouse Street, London SW3 6LY, UK

Introduction

It is now widely accepted that chronic mucosal inflammation plays an important role in the pathogenesis of asthma, despite the fact that the precise relationship of this inflammation to symptoms or objective measures of disease severity remain unclear. This was not always the case: in the early part of this century, following the discovery of histamine and its link with allergy and anaphylaxis, asthma was regarded essentially as intermittent spasm of bronchial smooth muscle, although "vascular turgescence" of the bronchial mucosa and increased secretion of mucous glands were also acknowledged. With the discovery of glucocorticoid therapy, it became clear that the bronchi were not normal between attacks, in the sense that glucocorticoids could often "open up" the airways even in ostensibly well-controlled patients. It was realized that, for many patients, asthma is a chronic disease with intermittent acute exacerbations. This new concept of asthma as a chronic inflammatory disease with intermittent acute exacerbations has had very important implications for therapeutic management. It is the aim of this article to describe certain aspects of the immunobiology of CD4 T-lymphocytes which are relevant to the asthma process and to discuss how these cells and their products may contribute to the observed pathological features. It should be borne in mind that these cells do not act in isolation but

T-Lymphocyte and Inflammatory Cell Research in Asthma
ISBN 0-12-388170-6

interact both with other inflammatory leukocytes and with resident tissue cells and local neural networks. Indeed, it is likely that this interaction is responsible for the unique and characteristic eosinophil-rich inflammatory response observed in the asthmatic bronchial mucosa.

Evidence for Mucosal Inflammation in Asthma

The classical studies of bronchial histopathology in patients having died of asthma (Houston *et al.*, 1953; Dunnill, 1960; Dunnill *et al.*, 1969) showed an intense invasion of the bronchial mucosa with inflammatory cells, particularly eosinophils, macrophages and lymphocytes. Neutrophils were present but in fewer numbers. Deposition of eosinophil products in and around the bronchial epithelium was a particularly prominent feature (Filley *et al.*, 1982). Other features noted in these studies which appear to be typical of asthma include loss of surface lining epithelium, thickening of the reticular layer beneath the basement membrane of the epithelium, dilatation of blood vessels, mucosal oedema and hypertrophy of both submucosal glands and bronchial smooth muscle.

More recent studies have concentrated on living asthmatics with milder disease, utilizing the techniques of bronchoalveolar lavage (BAL) and bronchial biopsy through the fibreoptic bronchoscope. These studies have shown that many of the inflammatory changes observed in asthma deaths are also a feature of milder, apparently well-controlled disease. Elevated numbers of eosinophils, both in the bronchial mucosa and in BAL fluid, were constant features of mild asthma (Kirby *et al.*, 1987; Wardlaw *et al.*, 1988; Azzawi *et al.*, 1990). Similarly, increased numbers of activated lymphocytes, identified either as irregular, atypical lymphocytes by transmission electron microscopy (Jeffery *et al.*, 1989) or as interleukin-2 (IL-2) receptor bearing cells as shown by immunocytochemistry (Azzawi *et al.*, 1990) were also invariably seen. There exists evidence that activation of T-lymphocytes and subsequent eosinophil recruitment and secretion may contribute to epithelial damage and possibly also to bronchial hyperresponsiveness in asthma (Glynn and Michaels, 1960; Salvato, 1968; Laitinen *et al.*, 1985; Beasley *et al.*, 1989). In contrast, recent studies of the bronchial mucosa in patients with mild asthma associated with atopy demonstrated no significant changes in the numbers of mast cells or of their subtypes in the bronchial mucosa (Bradley *et al.*, 1991; Jeffery *et al.*, 1992). Similarly, bronchial mucosal neutrophils were not increased in number in these patients (Jeffery *et al.*, 1989, 1992; Beasley *et al.*, 1989).

Asthma has been traditionally subdivided clinically according to its apparent aetiology (intrinsic, extrinsic and occupational), implying possible variability in its pathogenesis. One important question therefore relates to whether these clinical distinctions are apparent in histopathological terms. Preliminary studies addressing this question would suggest that they are not: an autopsy study of the bronchial mucosa of a patient who had died with severe occupational asthma showed histological changes similar to those seen in fatal non-occupational asthma (Fabbri *et al.*, 1988), while a recent immunocytochemical study (Bentley *et al.*, 1992) comparing bronchial biopsies from extrinsic and occupational asthmatics showed that these were indistinguishable in terms of their inflammatory cell infiltrate: in both cases the biopsies showed increased numbers of activated eosinophils and T-lymphocytes, but not neutrophils and monocyte/macrophages, as compared with biopsies from normal control subjects. Similarly, examination of BAL fluid obtained from a group of "intrinsic" asthmatics (Mattoli *et al.*, 1991) showed increased numbers of activated T-lymphocytes, eosinophils and neutrophils as compared with normal controls. These observations suggest that the bronchial response in patients with asthma is uniform, regardless of the nature of the provoking agent, and lend support to the hypothesis that the pathogenesis of asthma is independent of coexisting atopy.

Human Experimental Models of Asthma

The majority of studies which have so far been performed on asthmatic inflammation have concentrated on the possible pro-inflammatory roles of granulocytic leukocytes, particularly eosinophils and mast cells. Furthermore, many of these investigations have been based on comparisons of the numbers and activation status of these cells and the concentrations of their mediators before and after experimental allergen challenge, although a few studies have compared diseased patients with normal controls. The clinical response (bronchoconstriction) to acute allergen challenge in some allergic asthmatics is biphasic, consisting of an early and late phase response. The early phase response develops within 10 min and usually resolves within 1–3 h, and is generally attributed to degranulation of cells sensitized by binding of allergen-specific immunoglobulin E (IgE) (principally mast cells). The late phase response begins as the early phase response resolves, reaches a maximum within 6–10 h and can last for 24 h or more if untreated. It is associated with an influx of various inflammatory cells into the challenged mucosa. The traditional view has been that late phase responses occur as an "all or nothing" event in a given individual. Recent studies, however, indicated that the development of late asthmatic responses could occur as a continuous spectrum of severity depending on the dose of allergen administered (Crimi *et al.*, 1986; Durham *et al.*, 1988). It seems likely, therefore, that all sensitive subjects would develop late responses if it were possible to administer a sufficiently high dose of allergen.

It has been argued by many that the late phase response to allergen challenge represents a valid clinical model of the expression and severity of "real" atopic asthma. Experimental observations which have been cited to justify this conclusion include the following:

1) The development of late phase responses in children was associated with a higher frequency of asthmatic attacks in the preceding year (Warner, 1976).
2) In patients with occupational asthma, the development of exposure-related symptoms was unusual unless the patient also developed late phase responses following laboratory challenge (Chan-Yeung and Lam, 1986).
3) Successful abrogation of asthmatic symptoms after immunotherapy in house dust mite-sensitive children was associated with suppression of the late asthmatic response following repeated allergen challenge (Warner *et al.*, 1978).
4) An increase in non-specific bronchial hyperresponsiveness was observed to occur 3 h after allergen challenge, just prior to the development of the late phase response (Durham *et al.*, 1988) and was shown to persist for several days (Cartier *et al.*, 1982). This early increase in responsiveness correlated with the magnitude of the subsequent late phase fall in FEV_1 (forced expiratory volume in 1 s).
5) Glucocorticoids, which reduce bronchial hyperresponsiveness in "real" asthma, were shown to inhibit development of the late phase response whereas bronchodilators, including β_2-agonists and theophylline, with no effect on hyperresponsiveness, did not (Burge *et al.*, 1982; Cockcroft and Murdock, 1987; Cockcroft *et al.*, 1989).

There exists, therefore, clear evidence that the late phase bronchoconstrictor response following laboratory allergen challenge is accompanied by increased bronchial responsiveness, thereby ostensibly fulfilling the criteria for the definition of "real" asthma. Nevertheless, some doubts must remain concerning the validity of this model. One major problem is the uncertainty as to how far events associated with the late phase reaction are dependent on the IgE-mediated events of the preceding immediate reaction. On the one hand, the modest correlation between the magnitudes of the two reactions, at least in the skin (Frew and Kay, 1988a), and their differential susceptibility to inhibition by drugs such as glucocorticoids suggest that different mechanisms may be operating in their pathogenesis. On the other hand, late asthmatic responses were observed in some cases to follow challenge with non-specific stimuli such as exercise (Lee *et al.*, 1983). Furthermore, passive cutaneous sensitization with allergen-specific IgE-containing serum conferred the ability to mount late phase reactions to subsequent challenge with the same allergen or with anti-IgE (Dolovich *et al.*, 1973; Solley *et al.*, 1976). These observations raise the possibility that events such as cell activation and recruitment observed in association with the late phase reaction in various tissues are no more than a non-specific consequence of the local release of mast cell and other mediators. In other words, the late phase response may be a model for the exacerbation, rather than the pathogenesis of asthma, and then only in atopic individuals.

Immunobiology of CD4 T-Lymphocytes and Evidence for Their Involvement in Asthma

General Comments

The basic strategies used to implicate particular leukocytes in the pathogenesis of allergic diseases are based on demonstrating increases in the numbers and/or the activation status of these cells, or increased concentrations of their mediators in patients with disease as compared to controls. These studies may be static and observational, but more commonly address changes in cell numbers and activation after experimental allergen challenge. The possible relevance of experimental allergen challenge studies particularly to the pathogenesis of asthma has already been discussed.

In the case of asthma, cell numbers and function are often related to bronchial hyperresponsiveness. Notwithstanding the fact that its precise cause is unknown, bronchial hyperresponsiveness is widely regarded as a useful measurement of asthma severity since it is invariably observed in asthmatics and its degree can be correlated with both the severity of symptoms and the amount of anti-asthma therapy required for disease control (Hargreave *et al.*, 1981; Juniper *et al.*, 1981). Nevertheless, because the precise cause of bronchial hyperresponsiveness is unknown, observations linking cell numbers and their activation status with the degree of bronchial hyperresponsiveness in asthmatics can never provide better than circumstantial evidence for the involvement of these cells or their products.

Pro-inflammatory Role of CD4 T-Lymphocytes

CD4 T-lymphocytes have a central role to play in any antigen-driven inflammatory process (cell- or antibody-mediated), since they are the only cells capable of recognizing "foreign" antigenic material after processing by antigen presenting cells. It is now clear that CD4 T-lymphocytes, after activation by antigen, have the capacity to elaborate a wide variety of protein mediators called lymphokines. These lymphokines have the capacity to orchestrate that differentiation, recruitment, accumulation and activation of specific granulocyte effector cells at mucosal surfaces. A full description of the properties of individual lymphokines is beyond the scope of this article, but the general properties of these mediators which are responsible for their pro-inflammatory actions may be summarized as follows:

1) They can increase the production of specific granulocytes from precursor cells both in the bone marrow and at sites of inflammation.
2) They can prolong the survival of specific granulocytes, thereby bringing about their accumulation in tissues.
3) Some lymphokines are directly chemotactic for specific granulocytes and can cause preferential adherence of specific granulocytes to vascular endothelium.
4) They can prime specific granulocytes for an enhanced response to physiological activating stimuli.
5) They influence the activation of B-lymphocytes and the classes of antibodies which they produce in immune responses.

To take as an example the case of eosinophils, CD4 T-lymphocytes are a major source of interleukin-5 (IL-5) which was demonstrated to act in the following ways:

1) It promotes the differentiation of mature eosinophils from precursor cells (Sanderson *et al.*, 1985; Campbell *et al.*, 1987).
2) It prolongs the survival of eosinophils *in vitro* from days to weeks, especially in the presence of fibroblasts or endothelial cells (Rothenberg *et al.*, 1987, 1989).
3) It exhibits chemotactic activity for eosinophils but not neutrophils *in vivo*, although this effect was weak and requires further confirmation (Wang *et al.*, 1989).
4) It enhances the adhesion of eosinophils, but not neutrophils to vascular endothelial cells, a vital initial step in tissue emigration (Walsh *et al.*, 1990). This selective adhesion may be mediated at least partly through very late antigen-4 (VLA-4), which is a ligand for vascular cell adhesion molecule-1 (VCAM-1) on the surface of stimulated endothelial cells and which is expressed by eosinophils but not neutrophils (Walsh *et al.*, 1991).
5) It primes eosinophils for increased activity in a number of subsequent effector responses, including antibody-mediated killing of parasitic larvae, elaboration of lipid mediators and activation by PAF (Lopez *et al.*, 1988; Rothenberg *et al.*, 1989).

These mechanisms offer the first explanations as to how eosinophils accumulate preferentially in the bronchial mucosa in asthma. The important role of lymphokines, particularly IL-5, is self-evident.

Similar effects on eosinophils were exhibited by IL-3 (Rothenberg *et al.*, 1988) and granulocyte–macrophage colony-stimulating factor (GM-

CSF) (Silberstein *et al.*, 1986; Lopez *et al.*, 1986), although unlike IL-5 these lymphokines are not eosinophil specific. Interferon-γ was shown to enhance eosinophil cytotoxicity (Valerius *et al.*, 1990). The observations that T-lymphocyte clones from patients with the hypereosinophilic syndrome demonstrated IL-5-like activity (Raghavachar *et al.*, 1987) and that cultured T-lymphocytes from patients with asthma spontaneously secreted lymphokines which could prolong eosinophil survival (Walker *et al.*, 1991) directly support the hypothesis that eosinophil numbers and function may be regulated by T-lymphocytes *in vivo*.

Similarly, expansion and differentiation of mast cells in tissues was shown to be dependent on IL-3 and IL-4 (Stevens and Austen, 1989). A deficiency of mucosal mast cells was demonstrated in the gastrointestinal tract of humans with defective T-lymphocyte function (Irani *et al.*, 1987). In nude mice, IL-3 restored the intestinal mucosal mast cell response to *Strongyloides* infection and facilitated worm expulsion (Abe and Nawa, 1988).

These experiments emphasize the facts that activated CD4 T-lymphocytes have the propensity to bring about selective accumulation and activation of specific granulocytes in tissues, and that T-lymphocyte-mediated granulocyte accumulation and activation need not be dependent on the presence of antibodies, including IgE. CD4 T-lymphocytes are therefore pro-inflammatory cells in their own right and can no longer be regarded simply as "helper" cells for the production of antibody.

T-Lymphocytes and the Regulation of IgE Synthesis

Individuals are said to be "atopic" if they synthesize inappropriately elevated quantities of IgE. Some of this IgE may be specific for certain environmental antigens or "allergens". Whilst IgE-mediated mechanisms may not be indispensable for the development of asthma (not all asthmatics are demonstrably atopic), there seems little doubt that they are responsible for the acute exacerbation of symptoms sometimes observed in asthmatics after allergen exposure. To this extent at least the regulation of IgE synthesis is of relevance to the pathogenesis of asthma.

Early observations showed that certain T-lymphocyte clones derived from both atopic and non-atopic individuals by non-specific activation with phytohaemagglutinin, when added to autologous or allogeneic B-lymphocytes, could enhance the synthesis of IgE (as compared to that of IgG) by the B-lymphocytes (Romagnani *et al.*, 1987). It was later discovered that the amount of preferential IgE synthesis induced by T-lymphocyte clones was related to the amount of IL-4 secreted by the clones, and inversely related to the amount of interferon-γ secreted (Del Prete *et al.*, 1988; Maggi *et al.*, 1988). Physical contact between the T- and B-lymphocytes is also essential, since exogenous IL-4 alone did not increase IgE synthesis by pure B-lymphocyte populations. The fact that T-lymphocyte contact and IL-4 can induce preferential IgE synthesis in B-lymphocytes regardless of their antigen specificity (Parronchi *et al.*, 1990) may partly explain why polyclonal as well as allergen-specific IgE synthesis occurs in atopic individuals. Other lymphokines, including low molecular weight B cell growth factor ($BCGF_{low}$) and IL-2 further enhanced IL-4-induced IgE synthesis in these *in vitro* systems (De Kruyff *et al.*, 1989), probably through their non-specific enhancement of B-lymphocyte proliferation.

Despite these observations, it is still not clear why certain individuals synthesize allergen-specific IgE and others do not. At the population level, atopy shows a strong tendency to be inherited, and recent data suggest that it may be inherited as an autosomal dominant trait with a high degree of penetrance (Cookson and Hopkin, 1988; Cookson *et al.*, 1989). For this reason, researchers have looked for global differences in the regulation of IgE synthesis between atopic and non-atopic individuals, in particular an increased synthesis of IL-4 by T-lymphocytes derived from atopic individuals. Such differences have proven hard to find: only one of three patients with atopic dermatitis demonstrated T lymphocyte clones which were deficient in interferon-γ production (Romagnani *et al.*, 1989), whilst a study of T-lymphocyte clones derived from a patient with the hyper-IgE syndrome failed to show distinct patterns of lymphokine secretion (Quint *et al.*, 1989).

An alternative possibility is that only allergen-specific T-lymphocytes in atopic individuals show abnormalities of lymphokine synthesis. This has been regarded as unlikely, since allergens apparently show no particular structural features which allow them to be distinguished from other antigens. Nevertheless, it was recently shown that *Dermatophagoides pteronyssinus*-specific T-lymphocyte clones from two atopic patients secreted large amounts of IL-4 and small amounts of interferon-γ on exposure to specific allergen, whereas stimulation of *D. pteronyssinus*-specific clones from an HLA-matched non-atopic donor resulted in the secretion of large amounts of interferon-γ and little IL-4 (Wierenga *et al.*, 1990). Furthermore, T-lymphocyte clones from the same atopic patients specific for non-allergen antigens (*Candida albicans* or tetanus toxoid) produced small amounts of IL-4 and large amounts of interferon-γ. These observations, if found to be generally applicable in larger numbers of patients and with a wide variety of allergens, would support the hypothesis that atopic patients have regulatory abnormalities confined to T-lymphocytes specific for allergens.

In summary, it is clear that CD4 T-lymphocytes have an important role to play in the regulation of IgE synthesis. Although there exists some preliminary evidence that T-lymphocyte dysfunction contributes to inappropriate IgE synthesis, there is no reason as yet to suppose that this accounts for the strong heritable element of atopy. In fact, it seems more likely that the heritability of atopy operates at the level of the mucosal environment where allergen exposure occurs, rather than at the level of allergen-specific T-lymphocytes.

TH_1 and TH_2 CD4 T-Lymphocytes

At the present time not all lymphokines have been implicated in the pathogenesis of asthmatic inflammation. IL-3, IL-5 and GM-CSF are strongly implicated in that they can selectively recruit and activate mast cells and eosinophils, and IL-4 is implicated in the sense that it is responsible for the promotion of inappropriate IgE synthesis and the consequences thereof. The genes encoding these lymphokines are located relatively close together in the human genome, on the long arm of chromosome 5, raising the possibility that their expression may be at least in part coordinately regulated. There is already good evidence that this is the case in mouse T-lymphocytes. Antigen-activated murine CD4 T-lymphocyte clones can be divided into two broad types, called TH_1 and TH_2, according to the pattern of lymphokines they secrete (Mosmann and Coffman, 1989). TH_1 cells secrete IL-2, interferon-γ and TNF-β, but not IL-4, IL-5 and IL-6. TH_2 cells secrete IL-4, IL-5 and IL-6 but not IL-2, interferon-γ and TNF-β. Other lymphokines, including IL-3 and GM-CSF are secreted by both cell types. The mechanisms which determine expression of TH_1 or TH_2 phenotypes are not completely understood. Interferon-γ, when added to antigen-stimulated cultures of mouse CD4 T-lymphocytes favoured the expression of the TH_1 phenotype (Gajewski *et al.*, 1989), whilst another lymphokine secreted by TH_2 cells, called "cytokine synthesis inhibitory factor" or IL-10, inhibited TH_1 clone proliferation through an effect on antigen-presenting cells (Fiorentino *et al.*, 1989, 1991). Thus, products of TH_1 clones have the capacity to inhibit the growth of TH_2 clones, and vice versa.

The functional capacities of TH_1 and TH_2 CD4 T-lymphocyte clones differ in a manner which reflects their respective patterns of lymphokine synthesis. TH_2 clones, through their secretion of IL-4 and IL-5, serve as excellent helper cells for the synthesis of immunoglobulins including IgE by B-lymphocytes *in vitro* (Stevens *et al.*, 1988), since both these lymphokines non-specifically enhance B-lymphocyte activation. In addition, by their secretion of IL-3, IL-4 and IL-5, TH_2 clones could activate mast cells and eosinophils, and are therefore strongly implicated in the pathogenesis of allergic and asthmatic inflammation.

TH_1 clones have been shown to provide help for B-lymphocyte IgG synthesis in some, but not all *in vitro* systems (Coffman *et al.*, 1988). TH_1 clones strongly suppress IgE production through their release of interferon-γ which also suppresses B-lymphocyte proliferation in a non-specific fashion (Reynolds *et al.*, 1987). TH_1 cells, but not TH_2 cells were also shown to have the capacity to elicit delayed type hypersensitivity (DTH) reactions *in vivo*. In an experimental system where T-lymphocytes and antigen were injected directly into mouse footpads, only TH_1 clones were able to elicit antigen-specific swelling (Cher and Mosmann, 1987). It is not clear why TH_2 cells cannot elicit DTH reactions, but one obvious possibility is that the lymphokines produced by these cells are irrelevant to the pathogenesis of DTH.

In contrast to murine cells, human CD4 T-lymphocyte clones stimulated at random using lectins do not fall cleanly into TH_1 and TH_2 patterns, and there are many examples of clones which secrete a mixture of lymphokines characteristic of both categories (Quint *et al.*, 1989; Paliard *et al.*, 1988). Nevertheless, T-lymphocytes with TH_1- and TH_2-type patterns of lymphokine secretion do appear to exist *in vivo* (see below). These data can be reconciled with those from mice if it is assumed that precursors of TH_1 and TH_2 cells (TH_0 cells) exist which secrete a mixture of TH_1 and TH_2 type lymphokines, and that these TH_0 cells develop into TH_1 or TH_2 cells under the influence of extraneous factors such as their antigen specificity, the site of antigen presentation and the nature of the antigen presenting cells.

This discovery of a functional dichotomy of activated CD4 T-lymphocytes, which have the propensity either to mediate DTH reactions and suppress IgE synthesis (TH_1) or to mediate allergic and asthmatic inflammation and promote IgE synthesis (TH_2) is likely to have a profound impact on our future understanding of allergic inflammation and inappropriate IgE synthesis.

Experimental Observations Implicating Activated CD4 T-Lymphocytes in the Pathogenesis of Asthma

In two recent studies of bronchial biopsies obtained from mild atopic asthmatics (Azzawi *et al.*, 1990; Bradley *et al.*, 1991), the numbers and activation status of mucosal T-lymphocytes were assessed by immunostaining with monoclonal antibodies directed against T-lymphocyte phenotypic and activation markers. Interestingly, the total numbers of both CD4 and CD8 T-lymphocytes in the bronchial mucosa of these mild asthmatics were not significantly elevated as compared to normal controls; CD4 cells predominated over CD8 in both cases. In contrast, only cells in the biopsies from asthmatics showed evidence of IL-2 receptor expression, suggesting activation. Furthermore, in the biopsies from asthmatics, the numbers of activated T-lymphocytes could be correlated with both the total numbers of eosinophils and the numbers of activated eosinophils. Finally, the degree of activation could be correlated with disease severity, as assessed by measurement of bronchial hyperresponsiveness. These observations provide circumstantial evidence supporting the hypothesis that activated CD4 T-lymphocytes control the numbers and activation status of eosinophils in asthmatic bronchial inflammation, and that the degree of activation is one factor which determines disease severity. Using immunostaining and flow cytometry, it was shown that a proportion of CD4 T-lymphocytes, but not CD8 cells, in the peripheral blood of patients with acute severe asthma are activated, as assessed by expression of IL-2 receptor, HLA-DR and VLA-1 (Corrigan *et al.*, 1988). The degree of activation of these cells decreased after therapy to an extent that could be correlated with the degree of clinical improvement (Corrigan and Kay, 1990).

Some studies demonstrated an increase in the relative numbers of lymphocytes found in BAL fluid obtained from patients with mild, stable asthma (Graham *et al.*, 1985), whereas others showed similar numbers in asthmatics and normal controls (Wardlaw *et al.*, 1988). Studies on the activation status and the production of lymphokines by these cells are eagerly awaited. In a further study employing allergen bronchial challenge of sensitized atopic asthmatics (Metzger *et al.*, 1987), a selective increase in CD4 cells in BAL fluid was observed 48 h after allergen challenge in those subjects who had previously been shown to develop a late phase reaction. These findings complement those of a decrease in CD4 T-lymphocyte numbers in the peripheral blood following allergen inhalation by atopic asthmatics (Gerblich *et al.*, 1984), and together suggest that a process of selective recruitment of CD4 T-lymphocytes to the lung may occur in association with the late phase asthmatic reaction to allergen bronchial challenge. The possible relevance (or otherwise) of this model to the pathogenesis of "real" asthma has already been discussed. Similarly, in a study employing cutaneous allergen challenge of atopic subjects (Frew and Kay, 1988b), activated CD4 T-lymphocytes were selectively recruited during the course of the late phase reaction.

Despite the fact that sensitive enzyme-linked immunoadsorbent assays

(ELISA) and radioimmunoassays for many lymphokines are now available, measurement of lymphokine secretion *in vivo* is very difficult owing to their low concentrations and rapid metabolism. Furthermore, the concentrations of lymphokines in the peripheral blood and BAL fluid of asthmatics may only dimly reflect those concentrations released locally in the inflamed mucosa. In a study referred to above (Corrigan and Kay, 1990), serum concentrations of interferon-γ were shown to be elevated in a group of acute severe asthmatics as compared to mild asthmatics and normal controls. Interferon-γ secretion is characteristic of a "TH_1-type" response, but since "TH_2-type" lymphokines were not measured in this study it is impossible to assess the relative contributions of each type of response. Furthermore, TH_1-type CD4 T-lymphocyte activation might be a superimposed phenomenon in acute severe asthma, owing to intercurrent infection, for example.

One useful alternative to the direct measurement of lymphokine concentrations is the detection of the synthesis of their mRNA using the technique of *in situ* hybridization with lymphokine-specific cDNA probes or riboprobes. Although this is not a strictly quantitative technique, it does have the advantage that it can localize the secretion of lymphokines within cells and tissues. Using this technique it was recently demonstrated that IL-5 mRNA was elaborated by cells in the bronchial mucosa of a majority of mild asthmatics but not normal controls (Hamid *et al.*, 1991). The amount of mRNA detected correlated broadly with the numbers of activated CD4 T-lymphocytes and eosinophils in biopsies from the same subjects, providing direct evidence supporting the hypothesis that activated CD4 T-lymphocytes secrete IL-5 within the asthmatic bronchial mucosa which regulates the numbers and activation status of eosinophils. In a further study using *in situ* hybridization, the cutaneous inflammatory responses to challenge with allergen in atopic subjects and tuberculin in non-atopic subjects were compared (Kay *et al.*, 1991). Both types of response (late phase allergic and DTH) were associated with an influx of activated CD4 T-lymphocytes, but whereas mRNA molecules encoding IL-2 and interferon-γ were abundant within the tuberculin reactions, very little mRNA encoding these lymphokines was observed in the late phase allergic reactions. Conversely, mRNA encoding IL-4 and IL-5 was abundant in the late phase allergic but not the tuberculin reactions. In effect, the profiles of lymphokine secretion in the allergic and tuberculin reactions closely paralleled those of TH_2 and TH_1 CD4 T-lymphocytes, respectively. Furthermore, the relative numbers and types of granulocytes infiltrating these reactions reflected the different patterns of lymphokine release (Gaga *et al.*, 1991). The detection of mRNA does not necessarily equate with protein synthesis and it will need to be shown that translation and secretion of these lymphokines also occurs. Furthermore, as discussed above, T-lymphocytes are not the only potential sources of these lymphokines. Finally, it must be borne in mind that the antigen specificity of the recruited T-lymphocytes is unknown, and since the tuberculin response was elicited in non-atopic subjects, it is not certain whether the TH_1-type response observed in the DTH reaction was antigen-specific or atopy-specific. Nevertheless, these observations provide direct evidence in support of the hypothesis that activated T-lymphocytes, through their patterns of lymphokine secretion, regulate the types of granulocyte which participate in inflammatory reactions. Furthermore, they demonstrate that TH_1 and TH_2 CD4 T-lymphocyte responses can be detected in humans under physiological conditions, and that the antigen specificity of the T-lymphocytes might be one factor which determines which type of response is initiated.

Summary and Conclusions

The Nature of Allergic and Asthmatic Inflammation

Evidence is accumulating that chronic asthmatic and allergic inflammation represent a specialized form of cell-mediated immunity, in which secretion of specific lymphokines principally by activated T-lymphocytes bring about the accumulation and activation of specific granulocytes, particularly eosinophils, locally in the mucosa. The release of inflammatory mediators from these granulocytes subsequently results in tissue damage and may contribute to further inflammatory cell recruitment. This scheme does not envisage an indispensable role for antibody-dependent inflammatory mechanisms, including those mediated by IgE. There is little doubt, on the other hand, that IgE-mediated mechanisms may exacerbate asthma and allergic diseases. Inhaled allergens in sensitized atopic individuals have been shown to increase bronchial hyperresponsiveness both in an experimental setting and on natural exposure (Cartier *et al.*, 1982; Boulet *et al.*, 1983). Furthermore, there is increasing evidence that allergen load is important for the development of symptoms both of atopy and asthma and that removal of patients from allergens decreases the severity of clinical asthma and bronchial hyperresponsiveness (Platts-Mills and Chapman, 1987; Platts-Mills *et al.*, 1982). Nevertheless, the simple observations that the synthesis of allergen-specific IgE in some individuals does not necessarily result in allergic disease and that not all patients with asthma and rhinitis are demonstrably atopic would support the argument that allergen-specific IgE synthesis is neither necessary nor sufficient for the development of these diseases. It is possible to hypothesize that asthma and rhinitis result from an inherited defect in the local mucosal environment (such as a defect in epithelial integrity or a dysregulation of local immune tolerance to environmental allergens) which facilitates the development of chronic cell-mediated inflammation accompanied in some individuals by inappropriate IgE synthesis. It will be of vital importance in the future to delineate the relative importance of cell-mediated and IgE-mediated mechanisms in these diseases in order to plan effective therapeutic strategies.

The precise aetiology of asthma remains unknown. It is clearly too simplistic to suppose that the question is simply one of the presence or absence of allergen-specific IgE (although it was of interest that the prevalence of asthma was closely related to the serum IgE level standardized for age and sex (Burrows *et al.*, 1989)). Nevertheless, it is not unreasonable to suppose that asthmatic inflammation is antigen driven. The resident inflammatory cells of the mucosa, after inappropriate antigen recognition might become misdirected, forsaking their probable defensive role for one of tissue damage. The nature of the putative activating antigen(s) is unclear. Whilst inhaled aeroallergens are obvious candidates in "atopic" asthma, it seems unlikely that they can be implicated in every case; indeed, even in atopic asthmatics exacerbating factors other than allergens (such as viral infections) may be more prominent clinically. A further possibility is that asthma is an "autoimmune" disease, the driving antigens being normal antigens within the bronchial mucosa inappropriately recognized by local T-lymphocytes.

The Way Ahead

Further studies on the temporal course and natural history of asthmatic inflammation are needed. In view of the emerging importance of T-lymphocyte-mediated chronic inflammatory reactions in this disease, it would undoubtedly be of value to ascertain the antigen specificity and profiles of lymphokine secretion of T-lymphocytes within the inflamed mucosa. This might lead to the discovery of pathogenetic subdivisions of the disease which are as yet unrecognized, and point the way to new therapeutic strategies involving the inhibition of accumulation or activation of particular granulocytes at the mucosal surface either directly or indirectly through inhibition of lymphokine secretion.

References

Abe, T. and Nawa, Y. (1988). Worm expulsion and mucosal mast cell response induced by repetitive IL-3 administration in *Strongyloides ratti* infected nude mice. *Immunology* **63**, 181–185.

Azzawi, M., Bradley, B., Jeffery, P.K., Frew, A.J., Wardlaw, A.J., Knowles, G., Assoufi, B., Collins, J.V., Durham, S.R. and Kay, A.B. (1990). Identification of activated T lymphocytes and eosinophils in bronchial biopsies in stable atopic asthma. *Am. Rev. Respir. Dis.* **142**, 1410–1413.

Beasley, R., Roche, W., Roberts, J.A. and Holgate, S.T. (1989). Cellular events in the bronchi in mild asthma and after bronchial provocation. *Am. Rev. Respir. Dis.* **139**, 806–817.

Bentley, A.M., Maestrelli, P., Fabbri, L.M., Robinson, D.R., Bradley, B.L., Jeffery, P.K., Durham, S.R. and Kay, A.B. (1993). Activated T-lymphocytes and eosinophils in the bronchial mucosa in occupational asthma. *J. Allergy Clin. Immunol.* **89**, 821–829.

Boulet, L.-P., Cartier, A., Thomson, N.C., Roberts, R.S., Dolovich, J. and Hargreave, F.E. (1983). Asthma and increases in nonallergic bronchial responsiveness from seasonal allergen exposure. *J. Allergy Clin. Immunol.* **71**, 399–406.

Bradley, B.L., Azzawi, M., Assoufi, B., Jacobson, M., Collins, J.V., Irani, A., Schwartz, L.B., Durham, S.R., Jeffery, P.K. and Kay, A.B. (1991). Eosinophils, T-lymphocytes, mast cells, neutrophils and macrophages in bronchial biopsies from atopic asthmatics: comparison with atopic non-asthma and normal controls and relationship to bronchial hyperresponsiveness. *J. Allergy Clin. Immunol.* **88**, 661–674.

Burge, P.S., Efthimiou, J., Turner-Warwick, M. and Nelman, P.T. (1982). Double blind trials of inhaled beclomethasone dipropionate and fluocortin dibutyl ester in allergen-induced immediate and late asthmatic reactions. *Clin. Allergy* **12**, 523–531.

Burrows, B., Martinez, F.D., Halonen, M., Barbee, R.A. and Cline, M.G. (1989). Association of asthma with serum IgE levels and skin-test reactivity to allergens. *New Engl. J. Med.* **320**, 271–277.

Campbell, H.D., Tucker, W.Q.J., Hort, Y., Martinson, M.E., Mayo, G., Clutterbuck, E.J., Sanderson, C.J. and Young, I.G. (1987). Molecular cloning, nucleotide sequence and expression of the gene encoding human eosinophil differentiation factor (interleukin-5). *Proc. Natl. Acad. Sci. U.S.A.* **84**, 6629–6633.

Cartier, A., Thomson, N.C., Frith, P.A., Roberts, R. and Hargreave, F.E. (1982). Allergen-induced increase in bronchial responsiveness to histamine: relationship to the late asthmatic response and change in airway calibre. *J. Allergy Clin. Immunol.* **70**, 170–177.

Chan-Yeung, M. and Lam, S. (1986). State of the art: occupational asthma. *Am. Rev. Respir. Dis.* **133**, 686–703.

Cher, D.J. and Mosmann, T.R. (1987). Two types of murine helper T-cell clone. II. Delayed-type hypersensitivity is mediated by TH_1 clones. *J. Immunol.* **138**, 3688–3694.

Cockcroft, D.W. and Murdock, K.Y. (1987). Protective effect of inhaled albuterol, cromolyn, beclomethasone and placebo on allergen-induced early asthmatic responses, late asthmatic responses and allergen-induced increases in bronchial responsiveness to inhaled histamine. *J. Allergy Clin. Immunol.* **79**, 734–740.

Cockcroft, D.W., Murdock, K.Y., Gore, P.B., O'Byrne, P.M. and Manning, P. (1989). Theophylline does not inhibit allergen-induced increase in airway responsiveness to methacholine. *J. Allergy Clin. Immunol.* **83**, 913–920.

Coffman, R.L., Seymour, B.W., Lebman, D.A., Kiraki, D.D., Christiansen, J.A., Shrader, B., Cherwinski, H.M., Sarelkoul, H.F.J., Finkelman, F.D., Bond, M.W. and Mosmann, T.R. (1988) The role of helper T-cell products in mouse B-cell differentiation and isotype regulation. *Immunol. Rev.* **102**, 5–28.

Cookson, W.O.C.M. and Hopkin, J.M. (1988). Dominant inheritance of atopic IgE responsiveness. *Lancet* **i**, 86–88.

Cookson, W.O.C.M., Sharp, P.A., Faux, J.A. and Hopkin, J.M. (1989). Linkage between IgE responses underlying asthma and rhinitis and chromosome 11q. *Lancet* **i**, 1292–1295.

Corrigan, C.J. and Kay, A.B. (1990). CD4 T-lymphocyte activation in acute severe asthma. Relationship to disease severity and atopic status. *Am. Rev. Respir. Dis.* **141**, 970–977.

Corrigan, C.J., Hartnell, A. and Kay, A.B. (1988). T-lymphocyte activation in acute severe asthma. *Lancet* **i**, 1129–1131.

Crimi, E., Brusaco, V., Losurdo, E. and Crimi, P. (1986). Predicative accuracy of late asthmatic reaction to *Dermatophagoides pteronyssinus*. *J. Allergy Clin. Immunol.* **78**, 908–913.

De Kruyff, R.H., Turner, T., Abrams, J.S., Palladino, M.A. and Umetsu, D.T. (1989). Induction of human IgE synthesis by $CD4^+$ T-cell clones. Requirement for interleukin-4 and low molecular weight B-cell growth factor. *J. Exp. Med.* **170**, 1477–1493.

Del Prete, G.F., Maggi, E., Parronchi, P., Chretien, I., Tiri, A., Macchia, D., Ricci, M., Bancherau, J., de Vries, J. and Romagnani, S. (1988). IL-4 is an essential factor for the IgE synthesis induced *in vitro* by human T-cell clones and their supernatants. *J. Immunol.* **140**, 4193–4198.

Dolovich, J., Hargreave, F.E., Chalmers, R., Shierk, J., Gauldie, J. and Bienenstock, J. (1973). Late cutaneous allergic responses in isolated IgE-dependent reactions. *J. Allergy Clin. Immunol.* **52**, 38–46.

Dunnill, M.S. (1960). The pathology of asthma with special reference to changes in the bronchial mucosa. *J. Clin. Path.* **13**, 27–33.

Dunnill, M.S., Massarella, G.R. and Anderson, J.A. (1969). A comparison of the quantitative anatomy of the bronchi in normal subjects, in status asthmaticus, in chronic bronchitis and in emphysema. *Thorax* **24**, 176–179.

Durham, S.R., Craddock, C.F., Cookson, W.O. and Benson, M.K. (1988). Increases in airway responsiveness to histamine precede allergen-induced late asthmatic responses. *J. Allergy Clin. Immunol.* **82**, 764–770.

Fabbri, L.M., Danielli, D., Crescioli, S., Bevilaqua, P., Meli, S., Saetta, M. and Mapp, C.E. (1988). Fatal asthma in a subject sensitised to toluene diisocyanate. *Am. Rev. Respir. Dis.* **137**, 1494–1498.

Filley, W.V., Holley, K.E., Kephart, G.M. and Gleich, G.J. (1982). Identification by immunofluorescence of eosinophil granule major basic protein in lung tissues of patients with bronchial asthma. *Lancet* **ii**, 11–16.

Fiorentino, D., Bond, H.W. and Mosmann, T.R. (1989). Two types of mouse

T helper cells. IV. TH_2 clones secrete a factor that inhibits cytokine production by TH_1 clones. *J. Exp. Med.* **170**, 65–80.

Fiorentino, D.F., Zlotnik, A., Vieira, P., Mosmann, T.R., Howard, M., Moore, K.W. and O'Garra, A. (1991). IL-10 acts on the antigen-presenting cell to inhibit cytokine production by TH_1 cells. *J. Immunol.* **146**, 3444–3451.

Frew, A.J. and Kay, A.B. (1988a). The pattern of human late-phase skin reactions to extracts of aeroallergens. *J. Allergy Clin. Immunol.* **81**, 1117–1121.

Frew, A.J. and Kay, A.B. (1988b). The relationship between infiltrating $CD4^+$ T-lymphocytes, activated eosinophils and the magnitude of the allergen-induced late phase cutaneous reaction. *J. Immunol.* **141**, 4158–4164.

Gaga, M., Frew, A.J., Varney, V.A. and Kay, A.B. (1991). Eosinophil activation and T-lymphocyte infiltration in allergen-induced late phase skin reactions and classical delayed-type hypersensitivity. *J. Immunol.* **147**, 816–822.

Gajewski, T.F., Joyce, J. and Fitch, F.W. (1989). Antiproliferative effect of interferon-γ in immune regulation. III. Differential selection of TH_1 and TH_2 murine helper T-lymphocyte clones using recombinant IL-2 and recombinant interferon-γ. *J. Immunol.* **143**, 15–20.

Gerblich, A.A., Campbell, A.E. and Schuyler, M.R. (1984). Changes in T-lymphocyte subpopulations after antigenic bronchial provaction in asthmatics. *New Engl. J. Med.* **310**, 1349–1352.

Glynn, A.A. and Michaels, L. (1960). Bronchial biopsy in chronic bronchitis and asthma. *Thorax* **15**, 142–153.

Graham, D.R., Luksza, A.R. and Evans, C.C. (1985). Bronchoalveolar lavage in asthma. *Thorax* **40**, 717.

Hamid, Q., Azzawi, M., Ying, S., Moqbel, R., Wardlaw, A.J., Corrigan, C.J., Bradley, B., Durham, S.R., Collins, J.V., Jeffery, P.K., Quint, D.J. and Kay, A.B. (1991). Expression of mRNA for interleukin-5 in mucosal bronchial biopsies from asthma. *J. Clin. Invest.* **87**, 1541–1546.

Hargreave, F.E., Ryan, G., Thomson, N.C., O'Byrne, P.M., Latimer, K., Juniper, E.F. and Dolovich, J. (1981). Bronchial responsiveness to histamine or methacholine in asthma: measurement and clinical significance. *J. Allergy Clin. Immunol.* **68**, 347–355.

Houston, J.C., De Navasquez, S. and Trounce, J.R. (1953). A clinical and pathological study of fatal cases of status asthmaticus. *Thorax* **8**, 207–213.

Irani, A.A., Craig, S.S., De Blois, G., Elson, C.O., Schechter, N.M. and Schwartz, L.B. (1987). Deficiency of tryptase-positive, chymase-negative mast cell type in gastrointestinal mucosa of patients with defective T-lymphocyte function. *J. Immunol.* **138**, 4381–4386.

Jeffery, P.K., Wardlaw, A.J., Nelson, F.C., Collins, J.V. and Kay, A.B. (1989). Bronchial biopsies in asthma: an ultrastructural, quantitative study and correlation with hyperreactivity. *Am. Rev. Respir. Dis.* **140**, 1745–1753.

Jeffery, P.K., Godfrey, R.W., Adelroth, E., Nelson, F., Rogers, A. and Johansson, S.-A. (1993). Effects of treatment on airway inflammation and thickening of reticular collagen in asthma: a quantitative light and electron microscopic study. *Am. Rev. Respir. Dis.* **145**, 890–899.

Juniper, E.F., Frith, P.A. and Hargreave, F.E. (1981). Airway responsiveness to histamine and methacholine: relationship to minimum treatment to control symptoms of asthma. *Thorax* **36**, 575–579.

Kay, A.B., Ying, S., Varney, V., Gaga, M., Durham, S.R., Moqbel, R.,

Wardlaw, A.J. and Hamid, Q. (1991). Messenger RNA expression of the cytokine gene cluster IL-3, IL-4, IL-5 and GM-CSF in allergen-induced late phase cutaneous reactions in atopic subjects. *J. Exp. Med.* **173**, 775–778.

Kirby, J.G., Hargreave, F.E., Gleich, G.J. and O'Byrne, P.M. (1987). Bronchoalveolar cell profiles of asthmatic and non-asthmatic subjects. *Am. Rev. Respir. Dis.* **136**, 379–383.

Laitinen, L.A., Heino, M., Laitinen, A., Kava, T. and Haahtela, T. (1985). Damage of airway epithelium and bronchial reactivity in patients with asthma. *Am. Rev. Respir. Dis.* **131**, 599–606.

Lee, T.H., Nagakura, T., Papageorgiou, N., Iikura, Y. and Kay, A.B. (1983). Exercise-induced late asthmatic reactions with neutrophil chemotactic activity. *New Engl. J. Med.* **308**, 1502–1505.

Lopez, A.F., Williamson, D.J., Gamble, J.R., Begley, C.G., Harian, J.M., Klebanoff, S.J., Waltersdorph, A., Wong, G., Clark, S.C. and Vadas, M.A. (1986). Recombinant human granulocyte-macrophage colony stimulating factor stimulates *in vitro* mature human eosinophil and neutrophil function, surface receptor expression and survival. *J. Clin. Invest.* **78**, 1220–1228.

Lopez, A.F., Sanderson, C.J., Gamble, J.R., Campbell, H.D., Young, I.G. and Vadas, M.A. (1988). Recombinant human interleukin-5 is a selective activator of eosinophil function. *J. Exp. Med.* **167**, 219–224.

Maggi, E., Del Prete, G.F., Macchia, D., Parronchi, P., Tiri, A., Chretien, I., Ricci, M. and Romagnani, S. (1988). Profile of lymphokine activities and helper function for IgE in human T-cell clones. *Eur. J. Immunol.* **18**, 1045–1050.

Mattoli, S., Mattoso, V.L., Soloperto, M., Allegra, L. and Fasoli, A. (1991). Cellular and biochemical characteristics of bronchoalveolar lavage fluid in symptomatic nonallergic asthma. *J. Allergy Clin. Immunol.* **87**, 794–802.

Metzger, W.J., Zavala, D., Richerson, H.B., Moseley, P., Iwamota, P., Monick, M., Sjoerdsma, K. and Hunninghake, G.W. (1987). Local allergen challenge and bronchoalveolar lavage of allergic asthmatic lungs: description of the model and local airway inflammation. *Am. Rev. Respir. Dis.* **135**, 433–440.

Mosmann, T.R. and Coffman, R.L. (1989). TH_1 and TH_2 cells: different patterns of lymphokine secretion lead to different functional properties. *Annu. Rev. Immunol.* **7**, 145–173.

Paliard, X., de Waal Malefijt, R., Yssel, H., Blanchard, D., Chretien, I., Abrams, J., de Vries, J. and Spits, H. (1988). Simultaneous production of IL-2, IL-4 and IFN-γ by activated human $CD4^+$ and $CD8^+$ T-cell clones. *J. Immunol.* **141**, 849–855.

Parronchi, P., Tiri, A., Macchia, D., De Carli, M., Biswas, P., Simonelli, C., Maggi, E., Del Prete, G.F., Ricci, M. and Romagnani, S. (1990). Noncognate contact-dependent B-cell activation can promote IL-4 dependent *in vitro* human IgE synthesis. *J. Immunol.* **144**, 2102–2108.

Platts-Mills, T.A.E. and Chapman, M.D. (1987). Dust mites: immunology, allergic disease and environmental control. *J. Allergy Clin. Immunol.* **80**, 755–775.

Platts-Mills, T.A.E., Tovey, E.R., Mitchell, E.B., Moszoro, H., Nock, P. and Wilkins, S.R. (1982). Reduction of bronchial hyperreactivity during prolonged allergen evidence. *Lancet* **ii**, 675–677.

Quint, D.J., Bolton, E.J., MacNamee, L.A., Solan, R., Hissey, P.H., Champion, B.R., Mackenzie, A.R. and Zanders, E.D. (1989). Functional and phenotypical analysis of human T-cell clones which stimulate IgE production *in vitro*. *Immunology* **67**, 68–74.

Raghavachar, A., Fleischer, S., Frickhofen, N., Heimpel, H. and Fleischer, B. (1987). T-lymphocyte control of human eosinophilic granulopoiesis. *J. Immunol.* **139**, 3753–3758.

Reynolds, D.S., Boom, W.H. and Abbas, A.K. (1987). Inhibition of B-lymphocyte activation by interferon-γ. *J. Immunol.* **139**, 767–773.

Romagnani, S., Maggi, E., Del Prete, G.F. and Ricci, M. (1987). Activation through CD3 molecule leads a number of human T-cell clones from allergic and non-allergic individuals to promote IgE synthesis. *J. Immunol.* **138**, 1744–1749.

Romagnani, S., Del Prete, G., Maggi, E., Parronchi, P., Tiri, A., Macchia, D., Giudizi, M.G., Almengogna, F. and Ricci, M. (1989). Role of interleukins in induction and regulation of human IgE synthesis. *Clin. Immunol. Immunopathol.* **50**, 513–518.

Rothenberg, M.E., Owen, W.F., Silberstein, D.S., Soberman, R.J., Austen, K.F. and Stevens, R.L. (1987). Eosinophils cocultured with endothelial cells have increased survival and functional properties. *Science* **237**, 645–647.

Rothenberg, M.E., Owen, W.F., Silberstein, D.S., Woods, J., Soberman, R.J., Austen, K.F. and Stevens, R.L. (1988). Human eosinophils have prolonged survival, enhanced functional properties and become hypodense when exposed to human interleukin-3. *J. Clin. Invest.* **81**, 1986–1992.

Rothenberg, M.E., Petersen, J., Stevens, R.L., Silberstein, D.S., McKenzie, D.T., Austen, K.F. and Owen, W.F. (1989). IL-5 dependent conversion of normodense human eosinophils to the hypodende phenotype uses 3T3 fibroblasts for enhanced viability, accelerated hypodensity and sustained antibody-dependent cytotoxicity. *J. Immunol.* **143**, 2311–2316.

Salvato, G. (1968). Some histological changes in chronic bronchitis and asthma. *Thorax* **23**, 168–172.

Sanderson, C.J., Warren, D.J. and Strath, M. (1985). Identification of a lymphokine that stimulates eosinophil differentiation *in vitro*: its relationship to interleukin-3 and functional properties of eosinophils produced in cultures. *J. Exp. Med.* **162**, 60–74.

Silberstein, D.S., Owen, W.F., Gasson, J.C., Di Persio, J.F., Golde, D.W., Bina, J.C., Soberman, R., Austen, K.F. and David, R. (1986). Enhancement of human eosinophil cytotoxicity and leukotriene synthesis by biosynthetic (recombinant) granulocyte-macrophage colony stimulating factor. *J. Immunol.* **137**, 3290–3294.

Solley, G.O., Gleich, G.J., Jordan, R.E. and Schroeter, A.L. (1976). The late phase of the immediate wheal and flare skin reaction. Its dependence upon IgE antibodies. *J. Clin. Invest.* **58**, 408–420.

Stevens, R.L. and Austen, K.F. (1989). Recent advances in the cellular and molecular biology of mast cells. *Immunol. Today* **10**, 381–386.

Stevens, T.L., Bossie, A., Sanders, V.M., Fernandez-Botran, R., Coffman, R.L., Mosmann, T.R. and Vitetta, E.S. (1988). Subsets of antigen-specific helper T-cells regulate isotype secretion by antigen-specific B-cells. *Nature* **334**, 255–258.

Valerius, T., Repp, R., Kalden, J.R. and Platzer, E. (1990). Effects of IFN on human eosinophils in comparison with other cytokines. *J. Immunol.* **145**, 2950–2958.

Walker, C., Virchow, J.-C., Bruijnzeel, P.L.B. and Blaser, K. (1991). T cell subsets and their soluble products regulate eosinophilia in allergic and nonallergic asthma. *J. Immunol.* **146**, 1829–1835.

Walsh, G.M., Hartnell, A., Wardlaw, A.J., Kurihara, K., Sanderson, C.J. and Kay, A.B. (1990). IL-5 enhances the *in vitro* adhesion of human eosinophils, but not neutrophils, in a leukocyte integrin (CD11/18) dependent manner. *Immunology* **71**, 258–265.

Walsh, G.M., Hartnell, A., Mermod, J.-J., Kay, A.B. and Wardlaw, A.J. (1991). Human eosinophil, but not neutrophil adherence to IL-1 stimulated HUVEC is $\alpha 4\beta 1$ (VLA-4) dependent. *J. Immunol.* **146**, 3419–3423.

Wang, J.M., Rambaldi, A., Biondi, A., Chen, Z.G., Sanderson, C.J. and Mantovani, A. (1989). Recombinant human interleukin-5 is a selective eosinophil chemoattractant. *Eur. J. Immunol.* **19**, 701–705.

Wardlaw, A.J., Dunnette, S., Gleich, G.J., Collins, J.V. and Kay, A.B. (1988). Eosinophils and mast cells in bronchoalveolar lavage in mild asthma: relationship to bronchial hyperreactivity. *Am. Rev. Respir. Dis.* **137**, 62–69.

Warner, J.O. (1976). Significance of late reactions after bronchial challenge with house dust mite. *Arch. Dis. Child.* **51**, 905–910.

Warner, J.O., Price, J.F., Soothill, J.F. and Hey, E.N. (1978). Controlled trial of hypersensitisation to *Dermatophagoides pteronyssinus* in children with asthma. *Lancet* **ii**, 912–915.

Wierenga, E.A., Snoek, M., de Groot, C., Chretien, L., Bos, J.D., Jansen, H.M. and Kapsenberg, M.I. (1990). Evidence for compartmentalisation of functional subsets of $CD4^+$ T-lymphocytes in atopic patients. *J. Immunol.* **144**, 4651–4656.

Discussion

J.M. Drazen

Do you now know which of these cytokines are transcriptionally regulated? The finding of the messenger RNA suggests that the message is being made but, once the protein comes off and is excreted into the microenvironment, does the cell have to continue to make RNA, or is it a transient phenomenon that occurs at one point during a cell life?

A.B. Kay

It is one of many interesting questions that need to be asked now that the initial observation has been made. We have not got much further than this initial observation and I cannot answer the question precisely in any way – except just to remind you that these are resting asthmatics, people who have the day-to-day disease, mild asthmatics who are well controlled. I will soon be able to say what the situation will be after antigen challenge.

T.R. Mosmann

I was struck again by the very beautiful *in situ* hybridizations – there are spectacular amounts of hybridization. The frequency of the responding cell appears to be quite high. The numbers for T cells in general are that one T cell can make enough cytokine to satisfy perhaps of the order of 10^4 target cells for cytokines such as interleukin-4 (IL-4). It appears that very high numbers of T cells are responding. Can you give some idea of the ratio between the responding T cells and the target cells – in other words, the ratio of IL-5-producing T cells versus eosinophils in the actual tissue?

A.B. Kay

That is an interesting point. About 10% of that cell population are T cells, of which about half are producing the IL-4 or IL-5 message. The number of eosinophils will range, on a percentage basis, from about 3% up to 20%.

T.R. Mosmann

If about 5% of the T cells are perhaps responding, this is more than enough to saturate any cells in the immediate vicinity, so perhaps it is not surprising that this is a very powerful response.

B.B. Vargaftig

Can the T-lymphocytes isolated from the bronchoalveolar lavage (BAL), as compared to the lymphocytes from the blood, produce enough cytokines to influence the eosinophils present in the BAL and thus account for the hyperresponsiveness?

A.B. Kay

I cannot do any more than speculate and enlarge on what I have already said. However, I think there is another factor in this equation that should be borne in mind: that is, terminal differentiation of the eosinophil which might be taking place locally. The relationship between the T cell and the eosinophil may thus not be simply calling cells in from the vasculature, but perhaps also terminal differentiation in the tissue.

T.H. Lee

These questions on T cell–eosinophil interactions are very difficult to answer because there are so many different cell types in the airway producing all sorts of cytokines. There is tremendous redundancy in the system. To try to understand a ratio of one cell against another must be virtually impossible to answer *in vivo*. The question that needs to be asked is *why* is there so much redundancy in the system and what is it doing there?

A.R. Leff

One of the other issues, and one reason why this all appears so redundant, is that the data that we have seen, and with which I think everyone here agrees, are taken retrospectively. They are snapshots of what goes on during the process. Has anyone done it the other way round and used activated T cells or activated eosinophils to induce hyperresponsiveness? Otherwise, it becomes very difficult, and the number of possibilities enlarges greatly, as we look at all the correlates of asthmatic hyperresponsiveness without actually demonstrating causality.

A.B. Kay

Perhaps it is possible in the experimental animal situation, but of course that question cannot be answered in these clinical studies.

All the queries and comments are very interesting, but I should perhaps emphasize that we are at very early days. We have put forward the hypothesis that the T cell may be involved in these reactions. We must now convince ourselves that its presence goes together with disease severity. The extra information required is to show that these cells, at least theoretically, are capable of producing mediators which can explain the well-known local eosinophilia.

J.-A. Karlsson

There is now plenty of data showing TH_2 cell type and IL-5 message in human airways. It is interesting too that we find IL-5 message and IL-5, measured either directly by enzyme-linked immunoadsorbent assay (ELISA) techniques or in the eosinophil viability assays in serum or BAL not only from asthmatics but also (presented by Gleich's group) in people with the hypereosinophilic syndrome and with parasite infections. Is it possible that the IL-5 is acting like a maturation factor and a chemotactic agent rather more than as an activator of the cell in man since symptoms are very different in these patients?

A.B. Kay

IL-5 is a very weak chemoattractant by itself, but it primes eosinophils so that they respond more vigorously to agents such as platelet activating factor. IL-5 transgenic mice, which have now been described by two groups, have lots of eosinophils but not a lot of tissue damage. This is interesting, and suggests that several cytokines may be involved.

2

Immune Regulation by T Cells Secreting Different Cytokines

T. MOSMANN

Department of Immunology, University of Alberta, Edmonton, Alberta, Canada

Introduction

The discovery of two T cell types, originally defined according to their patterns of cytokine secretion, has provided some information on the regulation of different effector functions in the immune response to different infectious agents. In particular, the allergic response appears to be induced mainly by one of these two types of T helper cell (TH), while the other type can suppress several aspects of allergic responses. In the sections below, the current state of knowledge of mouse T cell diversity is summarized, together with a description of some of the cytokines involved in the cross-regulation of allergic responses.

TH Subtypes Defined by Cytokine Secretion Patterns

As originally defined by mouse T cell clones, the TH_1 pattern of cytokines includes interleukin-2 (IL-2), Interferon-γ (IFN-γ) and lymphotoxin (LT). TH_2 cells produce IL-4, IL-5, IL-6, IL-10 and P600, and both types produce several other cytokines including granulocyte–macrophage colony-stimulating factor (GM-CSF) and IL-3 (Mosmann *et al.*, 1986; Cherwinski

T-Lymphocyte and Inflammatory Cell Research in Asthma
ISBN 0-12-388170-6

et al., 1987; Mosmann and Moore, 1991). As would be expected from the differential synthesis of several potent cytokines, TH_1 and TH_2 cells have markedly different functions. In general, TH_2 cells induce high levels of antibody production by B cells, whereas TH_1 cells induce delayed-type hypersensitivity (DTH).

Although the TH_1 and TH_2 phenotypes have been well characterized in both mouse and human T cell clones and normal cells (Del Prete *et al.*, 1991; Kay *et al.*, 1991; Mosmann and Moore, 1991), these may represent the extremes of a spectrum of TH cell phenotypes. Among effector T cells induced during an immune response, there appear to be several other phenotypes, notably the TH_0 pattern (Firestein *et al.*, 1989; Street *et al.*, 1990), which includes most or all of the cytokines of the TH_1 and TH_2 patterns. All of the phenotypes identified as *in vitro* clones probably represent activated effector T cells, whereas resting T cells probably secrete only IL-2 the first time they are stimulated by antigen (Mosmann and Moore, 1991). Since the TH_1 and TH_2 phenotypes are the most thoroughly characterized, and because they appear to control a major dichotomy in immune responses, these two types will be emphasized in this article.

Appropriate and Inappropriate Immune Responses

In response to different pathogens, different types of effector mechanisms need to be induced. In general, antibody responses are more effective against extracellular infectious agents and toxins, whereas intracellular organisms are more effectively dealt with by various cytotoxic mechanisms, including DTH. Thus the TH_1 and TH_2 responses are most appropriate for intracellular and extracellular pathogens, respectively (Mosmann and Coffman, 1989). During an extreme TH_2 response, immunoglobulin E (IgE) is produced at high levels, since IL-4 induces B cells to switch to IgE production. This effect is only seen in the relative absence of a TH_1 response, since IFN-γ inhibits this effect of IL-4 (Coffman *et al.*, 1988).

Cytokine Cross-Regulation of TH_1 and TH_2 Response

Strong antibody and DTH responses are often mutually exclusive. At least part of the regulation of this choice is due to cytokine regulation of the differentiation and activation of TH_1 and TH_2 cells. IFN-γ inhibits the proliferation of TH_2 cells, and IL-4 enhances the differentiation of TH_2-like cells, while inhibiting the differentiation of cells that secrete

IFN-γ (Mosmann and Moore, 1991). Since TH_2-like responses often included suppression of TH_1 responses, we searched for a TH_2-derived inhibitor of TH_1 function, and discovered IL-10 (Fiorentino *et al.*, 1989), which inhibits cytokine synthesis by TH_1 cells. This effect occurs at the level of the antigen-presenting cell, since IL-10 inhibits the ability of macrophages to activate TH_1 but not TH_2 cells (Fiorentino *et al.*, 1991). After isolation of the cDNA clone (Moore *et al.*, 1990), IL-10 was found to have several other functions, many in common with IL-4, such as induction of major histocompatibility complex (MHC) class II antigens on B cells, enhancement of mast cell proliferation, and inhibition of cytokine synthesis by macrophages (Mosmann and Moore, 1991).

Role of TH_1 and TH_2 Cells in Allergic Responses

TH_2 cells enhance allergic responses in several ways, as seen during several parasite responses. IL-4 induces IgE secretion, IL-3, IL-4 and IL-10 cause mast cell proliferation, and IL-5 induces eosinophil growth and differentiation. IL-4 enhances the production of more TH_2-like cells, and IL-10 inhibits the production of IFN-γ. In contrast, TH_1 cells inhibit allergic reactions, mainly by production of IFN-γ, which inhibits mast cell activation, switching to IgE, and proliferation of TH_2 cells. Thus if a TH_2 response becomes dominant, several aspects of allergy are amplified, whereas a TH_1 response can prevent many of these functions.

Conclusion

TH_1 and TH_2 cells are, respectively, inducers and suppressors of allergic responses. Since each of these types of cell can establish dominance over the other type, it is possible that allergic response can be diminished by preferentially inducing a TH_1-like response, or at least a mixed response in which many of the allergy-stimulating functions of TH_2 cells can be inhibited.

References

Cherwinski, H.M., Schumacher, J.H., Brown, K.D. and Mosmann, T.R. (1987). Two types of mouse helper T cell clone. III. Further differences in lymphokine synthesis between Th_1 and Th_2 clones revealed by RNA hybridization, functionally monospecific bioassays, and monoclonal antibodies. *J. Exp. Med.* **166**, 1229–1244.

Coffman, R.L., Seymour, B.W., Lebman, D.A., Hiraki, D.D., Christiansen, J.A., Shrader, B., Cherwinski, H.M., Savelkoul, H.F., Finkelman, F.D., Bond, M.W. and Mosmann, T.R. (1988). The role of helper T cell products in mouse B cell differentiation and isotype regulation. *Immunol. Rev.* **102**, 5–28.

Del Prete, G.F., De Carli, M., Mastromauro, C., Biagiotti, R., Macchia, D., Falagiani, P., Ricci, M. and Romagnani, S. (1991). Purified Protein Derivative (PPD) of Mycobacterium tuberculosis and Excretory-Secretory Antigen(s) (TES) of Toxocara canis expand *in vitro* human T cells with stable and opposite (type 1 T helper or type 2 T helper) profiles of cytokine production. *J. Clin. Invest.* **88**, 346–350.

Fiorentino, D.F., Bond, M.W. and Mosmann, T.R. (1989). Two types of mouse T helper cell. IV. TH_2 clones secrete a factor that inhibits cytokine production by TH_1 clones. *J. Exp. Med.* **170**, 2081–2095.

Fiorentino, D.F., Zlotnik, A., Vieira, P., Mosmann, T.R., Howard, M., Moore, K.W. and O'Garra, A. (1991). IL-10 acts on the antigen-presenting cell to inhibit cytokine production by Th_1 cells. *J. Immunol.* **146**, 3444–3451.

Firestein, G.S., Roeder, W.D., Laxer, J.A., Townsend, K.S., Weaver, C.T., Hom, J.T., Linton, T., Torbett, B.E. and Glasebrook, A.L. (1989). A new murine $CD4^+$ T cell subset with an unrestricted cytokine profile. *J. Immunol.* **143**, 518–525.

Kay, A.B., Ying, S., Varney, V., Gaga, M., Durham, S.R., Moqbel, R., Wardlaw, A.J. and Hamid, Q. (1991). Messenger RNA expression of the cytokine gene cluster, Interleukin-3 (IL-3), IL-4, IL-5, and granulocyte/macrophage colony-stimulating factor, in allergen-induced late-phase cutaneous reactions in atopic subjects. *J. Exp. Med.* **173**, 775–778.

Moore, K.W., Vieira, P., Fiorentino, D.F., Trounstine, M.L., Khan, T.A. and Mosmann, T.R. (1990). Homology of cytokine synthesis inhibitory factor (IL-10) to the Epstein-Barr virus gene BCRFI. *Science* **248**, 1230–1234.

Mosmann, T.R. and Coffman, R.L. (1989). TH_1 and TH_2 cells: Different patterns of lymphokine secretion lead to different functional properties. *Annu. Rev. Immunol.* **7**, 145–173.

Mosmann, T.R. and Moore, K.W. (1991). The role of IL-10 in cross-regulation of TH_1 and TH_2 responses. *Immunol. Today* **12**, 49–53.

Mosmann, T.R., Cherwinski, H., Bond, M.W., Giedlin, M.A. and Coffman, R.L. (1986). Two types of murine helper T cell clone. I. Definition according to profiles of lymphokine activities and secreted proteins. *J. Immunol.* **136**, 2348–2357.

Street, N.E., Schumacher, J.H., Fong, T.A.T., Bass, H., Fiorentino, D.F., Leverah, J.A. and Mosmann, T.R. (1990). Heterogeneity of mouse helper T cells: Evidence from bulk cultures and limiting dilution cloning for precursors of Th_1 and Th_2 cells. *J. Immunol.* **144**, 1629–1639.

Discussion

A.B. Kay

In human skin biopsies from the allergen-induced late phase reaction in atopics we found a lot of major histocompatibility complex (MHC) class

2 upregulation with an anti-HLA-DR-antibody. Those of course are interferon-γ negative. Would you agree with our speculation that this was probably GM-CSF?

T.R. Mosmann
Could they have been B cells, because both IL-4 and IL-10 will induce MHC class 2?

A.B. Kay
This is MHC class 2 upregulation largely on endothelial cells. I raise the point because it does not quite fit in with some of your data.

T.R. Mosmann
In terms of the endothelial cells, I am not sure which agents induce MHC class 2.

A.B. Kay
Secondly, and slightly more difficult to understand, I think I have said previously that we have shown that the tuberculin reaction in non-atopic human subjects is essentially a T helper (TH) 1 pattern, as would be expected, with significantly more messenger RNA-positive cells for interferon-γ and IL-2 in both the injected and the control sites. For IL-3 and GM-CSF it was very low – which I suppose was a surprise. One or two sites expressed IL-4 and IL-5: interestingly, though, they also had a little eosinophilia. The story is becoming rather complex.

T.R. Mosmann
Perhaps we should make it much more complex. I short-circuited quite a few points. One is that delayed-type hypersensitivity (DTH) is probably not a single phenomenon. If DTH is separated into tuberculin-type reactions or Jones-Mote (?) type reactions, the mouse TH_1-induced DTH appears to be the latter type. There is a granulocytic infiltration in the mouse and not much in the way of monocytes. It has relatively short kinetics, and it appears to have a lot of oedema – the swelling is more oedema than cellular infiltration. By those criteria, it is more of a Jones-Mote (?) type reaction.

At some point we have to come to grips with the functions of all the other types of T cells, such as the TH_0, the cell that makes IL-2, IL-4 and IL-5, and so on. It may be, for example, that the TH_0 cell has some strong functions in a tuberculin-type DTH.

We are still just scratching at the surface of all the possible functions. This is one reason why we tend to focus on the parasite infections. I am glad to see that the allergic reactions are now going the same way – but they are probably more extreme reactions, whereas many of our immune responses may involve a mixture of these cell types and be much more complex.

M.K. Church

Unfortunately, the majority of the cytokine work on the stimulation of mast cell growth has been done in mouse and rat cell lines and perhaps the extrapolation to human may be a little difficult at the moment.

Secondly, I thoroughly enjoyed the explanation that the mast cell may possibly kick-start the TH_2 engine, if you like. Professor Holgate and I have just put forward exactly the same hypothesis in a paper now being prepared for publication. This hypothesis is based on two lines of evidence. First, that human mast cells from the nose, lung and skin, using immunocytochemical staining for the products, have been shown to contain IL-4, and also IL-5 and IL-6.

With IL-4, certainly in biopsies, more than 80% of the cells staining for IL-4 appear to be mast cells. This means that they store it. It does not mean that lymphocytes do not make it. They may do, and probably transport it – therefore, it is not picked up by the same techniques. From the studies we have done with immunoglobulin E (IgE)-dependent systems using purified mast cells, on immunological stimulation the mast cells will release that IL-4 – preliminary experiments suggest between 10 and 25 fm/cell (fm = fentomol), which I think is enough to invade the local environment and start the T-cell reaction which I think keeps the whole system going. I think that, taken together, the studies that Professor Holgate and I have done provide evidence for Dr Mosmann's thesis in man.

T.R. Mosmann

In relation to the cytokine effects on mast cells, I have not heard yet whether the IL-3, IL-4 and IL-10 combination has been tried. I know that the IL-3 and IL-4 combination was very frustrating.

S.T. Holgate

It has been extremely frustrating and disappointing so far. All three have been tried in various combinations. There is mast cell growth, but nothing like the sort of replication seen in the bone marrow-derived mast cells with these stimuli being put in.

IL-9 is probably the most promising, C-kit ligand the next, and then there is a hierarchy. None of them, even together, look as if they are yet in the same ballpark as with the mouse mast cell.

R. Moqbel
We have to be very careful with some of the parasitic infection systems that you described, in the sense that some of them are TH_1-dependent and some are not. *Schistosoma mansoni* in the mouse, for instance, appears to be interferon-γ-dependent rather than IL-5-dependent. The interpretation has to be based on that understanding. It has been shown in the past that, unlike the rat which is IL-5 eosinophil and IgE-dependent, the mouse system behaves in a different fashion with schistosoma, and responds to treatment with anti-interferon-γ.

T.R. Mosmann
By "dependent" you mean that resolution of the infection is dependent? I was using the schistosoma system as an example of an extremely powerful TH_2 response, which the worms do not induce but the eggs do. If the egg antigen alone is injected it gives an extremely powerful TH_2 response. One of the speculations in this area has been that some of these parasites induce a TH_2 response for the express purpose of interfering with the immune response and preventing it from making the more effective TH_1 response. Certainly, in the case of *leishmania* this would be one explanation why some people make the TH_2 response which then leads to death rather than making the TH_1 which cures very effectively. It is an important distinction between what is useful and what is the major response.

R. Moqbel
Is there any information about the effect of IL-10 directly on the eosinophil?

Secondly, could you explain a little more the ability of the same cell to produce interferon-γ and IL-10?

T.R. Mosmann
The TH_0 cells seem able to produce both. Since the action is indirect, we would really need to look at the presenting cells for the TH_0 as opposed to the TH_1 and TH_2, which we have not done yet. Clearly, the ability of B cells to present antigen to either TH_1 or TH_2 is not inhibited by IL-10. This appears to be selective for macrophage-like cells, so perhaps, in a sense, it does not really matter whether the TH_0 is inhibited in the same way as TH_1, because there would still be other presenting cells that could stimulate it. To my knowledge, though, this has not yet been tested.

N.C. Barnes
Patients who first develop asthma as adults or adults who have worsening of their asthma will often attribute it to a viral infection – and there is some reasonable evidence that in at least a proportion this is correct. What is the pattern of lymphocyte response following a viral infection?

T.R. Mosmann
In the mouse, I think, there tends to be a rather TH_1-biased response against viruses as compared to other antigens. In a sense, that seems appropriate because the TH_1 response is much more effective at killing intracellular parasites, whereas the TH_2 responses would be more effective for extracellular forms. That is not as extreme a form as is found in some of the parasites, but is much more mixed.

N.C. Barnes
Is there any evidence for differences between different mouse strains? It is people with a family history of asthma, hay fever and atopy who, when they are adults, get a viral infection and develop asthma.

T.R. Mosmann
I think there is a slight tendency to think of a balb/C mouse as being a more TH_2 mouse and a C57Bl as more of a TH_1 mouse – but there is not a very strong effect yet.

3

T Cell Subtypes in Allergy

S. ROMAGNANI, E. MAGGI, G.F. DEL PRETE, P. PARRONCHI, M. DE CARLI, M.P. PICCINI and R. MANETTI

Division of Clinical Immunology and Allergology, Istituto di Clinica Medica 3, University of Florence, Italy

$CD4^+$ T Helper (TH) Cells and TH Cell-Derived Cytokines are Involved in the Regulation of Human IgE Synthesis

In the last few years, a pathway of human immunoglobulin E (IgE) regulation, essentially based on the reciprocal activity of interleukin-4 (IL-4) and interferon-γ (IFN-γ), has been discovered (reviewed by Romagnani, 1990). The first demonstration that IL-4- or IFN-γ-producing $CD4^+$ T helper TH cell subsets play a reciprocal role in the regulation of human IgE synthesis was provided by assaying the activity of large numbers of phytohaemagglutinin (PHA)-induced T cell clones derived from different lymphoid organs. When T cell clones or their supernatants were assayed for their ability to induce the synthesis of IgE and to produce IL-2, IL-4 and IFN-γ, a significant positive correlation between helper function for IgE and production of IL-4 was found. In contrast, there was a significant inverse correlation between the IgE helper activity of T cell clones (or supernatants derived from them) and their ability to produce IFN-γ (Del Prete *et al.*, 1988). The opposite regulatory role of IL-4 and IFN-γ on the synthesis of human IgE was confirmed by two additional observations. First, human recombinant IL-4 can induce the synthesis of IgE in peripheral blood mononuclear cells (PBMNC). Second, this effect is inhibited by addition of recombinant IFN-γ (Del Prete *et al.*, 1988; Pene *et al.*, 1988). However, both recombinant IL-4 and IL-4-

T-Lymphocyte and Inflammatory Cell Research in Asthma
ISBN 0-12-388170-6

containing supernatants are consistently ineffective in inducing IgE synthesis by highly purified B cells (Del Prete *et al.*, 1988; Pene *et al.*, 1988). IL-4 alone is able to induce germ-line Cϵ but not mature Cϵ transcripts in human B cells (Gauchat *et al.*, 1990). IgE synthesis requires the presence of both IL-4 and appropriate concentrations of CD4$^+$ T cells. Both cognate- and noncognate-type interactions between CD4$^+$ T cells and B cells may support the IL-4-dependent human IgE synthesis (Parronchi *et al.*, 1990).

CD4$^+$ (TH$_2$-like) Cells May Play a Pathogenic Role in Helminthic Infections and Allergic Disorders

Patients with helminthic infections or atopic disorders usually exhibit both elevated IgE serum levels and eosinophilia. Based on the findings mentioned above, as well as on the knowledge that IL-5 (another T cell-derived cytokine) acts as a selective differentiation factor for eosinophils (Sanderson *et al.*, 1985), it was reasonable to suggest that both atopic patients and patients with helminth infections may harbour TH cells resembling the TH$_2$ subset described in mice (Mosmann *et al.*, 1986) for their ability to produce IL-4 and IL-5, but not IFN-γ. To test this possibility, we first investigated the profile of cytokine production of PHA-induced T cell clones obtained from the blood of patients with helminthic infections or severe atopic diseases. Significantly higher proportions of IL-4-producing and significantly lower proportions of IFN-γ-producing T cell clones were recovered from the blood of both groups of patients in comparison with healthy controls (Romagnani, 1990). Furthermore, PHA-induced T cell clones derived from the conjunctival infiltrates of three patients suffering from vernal conjunctivitis (VC) were examined. The great majority of T cell clones obtained from VC infiltrates were CD4$^+$ T cells inducible to the production of high concentrations of IL-4 and able to provide helper function for IgE synthesis by B cells. In contrast, even after maximal stimulation, such as that delivered by phorbol myristate acetate (PMA) plus anti-CD3 monoclonal antibody, a few T cell clones expressed IFN-γ mRNA and could produce IFN-γ (Maggi *et al.*, 1991). By using a different experimental approach, strong IL-5, but poor IL-2 and no IFN-γ, message has recently been found in T cells from biopsies of both allergen-induced late phase cutaneous reactions (Kay *et al.*, 1991) and bronchi of patients with allergic asthma (Hamid *et al.*, 1991). More recently, high frequency of IL-4-producing CD4$^+$ allergen-specific T lymphocytes in atopic dermatitis lesional skin has also been reported (van Reijsen *et al.*, 1992). Taken together, these data suggest that in patients with helminthic infections or atopic disorders both production of IgE and eosinophilia probably result from the activation of TH_2-like cells and from their accumulation in target organs.

$CD8^+$ T Cells May Play a Pathogenic Role in Toluen-diisocyanate (TDI)-Induced Asthma

$CD4^+$ TH_2-like cells are probably not the only subtype of T cells involved in the pathogenesis of bronchial asthma. We have examined recently the phenotype and the functional attitude of T cell lines and T cell clones derived from the bronchial biopsies of three patients with toluen-diisocyanate (TDI)-induced asthma. Biopsies were taken 48 h after the challenge with TDI and cultured in medium supplemented with IL-2 alone. T cell lines derived from all three patients mainly consisted of $CD8^+$ T cells and developed into T cell clones, the majority of which showed the $CD8^+$ phenotype. As expected, all $CD8^+$ T cell clones displayed cytolytic activity and produced elevated concentrations of IFN-γ and IL-2, but not IL-4. Interestingly, however, many $CD8^+$ T cell clones showed the ability to produce IL-5. Thus, the involvement of such a type of cells might explain the eosinophilia which occurs in the absence of an increased IgE production as in the majority of patients with TDI-induced and even in those with intrinsic asthma.

Helminth Antigens and Allergens Preferentially Expand $CD4^+$ TH_2-like T Cell Clones, whereas Protein Purified Derivative Expands TH_1

In order to investigate the nature of TH_2-like cells present in the blood and/or target organs of patients with helminthic infections or allergic disorders, as well as on the mechanisms responsible for their development, our strategy has been to establish T cell clones specific for allergens (*Dermatophagoides pteronyssinus* group I (Der p I) and *Lolium perenne* Group I (Lol p I), helminthic components (excretory/secretory antigen of *Toxocara canis* (TES)) or bacterial components (protein purified derivative (PPD) of *Mycobacterium tuberculosis* and tetanus toxoid (TT)).

When large series of PPD- or TES-specific T cell clones derived from two healthy individuals were compared, a clear-cut dichotomy in the profile of cytokine secretion was observed. Virtually all PPD-specific clones produced IL-2 and IFN-γ, but not IL-4 and IL-5, whereas the great majority of TES-specific clones produced IL-4 and IL-5, but not

IL-2 and IFN-γ. PPD-specific T cell clones that failed to secrete IL-4 and IL-5, and TES-specific T cell clones that failed to secrete IL-2 and IFN-γ, were found to lack transcripts for IL-4 and IL-5 or for IL-2 and IFN-γ, respectively (Del Prete *et al.*, 1991a). As expected, TH_2-like TES-specific T cell clones consistently supported the synthesis of IgE by autologous B cells under MHC-restricted conditions, whereas TH_1-like PPD-specific T cell clones did not. These results demonstrate that PPD and TES antigens expand helper T cells with opposite (TH_1 or TH_2) phenotype of cytokine secretion.

High numbers of Der p I- or Lol p I-specific T cell clones could be obtained from mite- or grass-sensitive atopic individuals and compared for their phenotype of cytokine secretion with PPD- or TT-specific T cell clones derived from the same donors. Virtually all the allergen-specific T cell clones produced IL-4 (and IL-5) and variable amounts of IL-2 in response to stimulation with PMA plus anti-CD3 antibody, and a small proportion of them failed to produce IFN-γ. When assessed with the specific antigen under MHC-restricted conditions, the great majority of allergen-specific T cell clones behave as TH_2-like helper T cells. While most T cell clones specific for TT produced both IL-4 and IFN-γ (particularly in response to PMA plus anti-CD3 antibody), all T cell clones specific for PPD produced high amounts of IFN-γ, but most of them did not produce IL-4 and IL-5 (Parronchi *et al.*, 1991). These data are partially at variance with those recently reported by Wierenga *et al.* (1990), who showed clear-cut TH_1 and TH_2 dichotomy between TT- and allergen-specific T cell clones derived from atopic donors. However, they support the view that the immune response to environmental allergens results in the preferential activation of TH_2-like clones. These cells are responsible for both the induction of IgE antibody production and increase in eosinophils via the release of IL-4 and IL-5, respectively.

PPD-Specific T Cell Clones Derived from Atopics Show Enhanced Ability to Produce IL-4

Additional elements of complexity emerged when the phenotype of cytokine secretion of a total number of 158 PPD- and 202 TT-specific T cell clones obtained from three atopic and three non-atopic donors was compared. The proportions of TT-specific T cell clones with TH_2-like profile of cytokine production were significantly higher in atopics than in non-atopics. More importantly, even if all PPD-specific clones from both atopic and non-atopic donors were able to produce elevated concentrations of IFN-γ, a clear difference emerged with regard to their ability to produce IL-4. Indeed, 37% of PPD-specific T cell clones derived from atopic patients, but only 4% of those obtained from non-atopic individuals, produced IL-4 in response to stimulation with the specific antigen (Parronchi *et al.*, 1992). These data suggest that atopic patients have enhanced ability to produce IL-4 even in response to antigens other than common environmental allergens or helminthic components. The molecular alteration(s) responsible for the enhanced ability of TH cells from atopic patients to produce IL-4 are at present unknown.

Human TH_1 and TH_2 T Cell CLones also Differ for Cytolytic Potential and Mode of B-Cell Help for Immunoglobulin Synthesis

With a large series of human T cell clones exhibiting clear-cut TH_1 or TH_2 phenotypes, we then determined other functional properties of the two subsets. The majority of TH_1 (77%), but only a minority of TH_2 (18%), clones exhibit cytolytic activity in a 4 h PHA-dependent assay (Del Prete *et al.*, 1991b). All TH_2 (non-cytolytic) clones induced IgM, IgG, IgA, and IgE synthesis by autologous B cells in the presence of the specific antigen and the degree of response was proportional to the number of TH_2 cells added to B cells. Under the same experimental conditions, TH_1 (cytolytic) clones provided B cell help for IgM, IgG and IgA, but not IgE, synthesis with a peak response at a T cell:B cell ratio of 1:1. At higher T cell:B cell ratios, a decline in B cell help was observed (Del Prete *et al.* 1991b). Interestingly, all these TH_1 clones lysed Epstein–Barr virus (EBV)-transformed autologous B cells pulsed with the specific antigen and the decrease of Ig production correlated with the lytic activity of TH_1 clones against autologous antigen presenting B cell targets (Del Prete *et al.*, 1991b). This may represent an important mechanism for the downregulation of antibody responses *in vivo* (Romagnani, 1991a,b).

Interestingly, none of the 13 allergen (Der p I or Lol p I)-specific TH_2-like T cell clones tested exhibited cytolytic activity against EBV-transformed autologous B cells, whereas 6 out of 7 PPD-specific T cell clones established from the same donor did (Romagnani *et al.*, 1992). Thus, the ability of TH_2-like cells to produce IL-4 (but no or limited amounts of IFN-γ) together with their inability to kill the antigen presenting cell may explain, at least in part, the chronicity of IgE antibody responses to common environmental allergens. Taken together, these data clear up all doubt about the existence of human $CD4^+$ T cell subsets secreting different patterns of cytokines similar to those described in mice and support the view that these T cell subsets are of major importance in determining the class of immune effector function.

Cytokines Can Regulate the *In Vitro* Development of TH Cells into TH_1- or TH_2-like T Cell Clones

More recently, the effects exerted on the *in vitro* development of PPD-specific or Der p I-specific T cell lines and T cell clones by IL-4 or IFN-γ addition or neutralization in human PBMNC cultures were examined. As expected, PBMNC from normal individuals, which were stimulated with PPD and then cultured in IL-2 alone, developed into PPD-specific T cell lines and T cell clones able to produce IFN-γ and IL-2, but not IL-4 and IL-5 (TH_1-like). IFN-γ or anti-IL-4 antibody addition in bulk cultures before cloning did not influence the PPD-specific T cell line profile of cytokine production. In contrast, the addition of IL-4 resulted in the development of PPD-specific T cell lines and T cell clones able to produce not only IFN-γ and IL-2, but also IL-4 and IL-5.

PBMNC from one atopic *Dermatophagoides pteronyssinus* group I (Der p I)-sensitive patient, which were stimulated with Der p I and then cultured in IL-2 alone, developed into Der p I-specific T cell lines and T cell clones able to produce IL-5 and high amounts of IL-4 but no, or limited amounts of, IFN-γ (TH_2-like). The development of Der p I-specific T cells into IL-4 (and IL-5)-producing T cell lines and into TH_2-like T cell clones was markedly inhibited by the addition in bulk cultures before cloning of either IFN-γ or anti-IL-4 antibody (Maggi *et al.*, 1992). These data suggest that the presence or absence of IL-4 and IFN-γ in bulk cultures of PBMNC before cloning may have strong regulatory effects on the *in vitro* development of human $CD4^+$ T cells into TH_1 or TH_2 T cell clones.

Possible Role of Cytokines in the Development of TH_1 and TH_2 Cells *In Vivo*

The most important question to be solved, however, is why circulating PPD-specific memory T cells are apparently conditioned to produce IFN-γ, but no IL-4, whereas Der p I-specific memory T cells usually produce IL-4 and IL-5, but no IFN-γ upon *in vitro* re-stimulation with the specific antigen. This question involves both the origin of TH_1 and TH_2 cells and the factors influencing their development *in vivo*. So far, the most clear-cut requirements for the generation of murine TH_1 or TH_2 effector cells *in vivo* also include lymphokines. IL-2 promotes effector cell development in general regardless of other lymphokines (Swain, 1991). Studies with the murine leishmaniasis model have provided significant evidence that IFN-γ can strongly influence TH cell precursors to differentiate into cells that produce the TH_1 set of cytokines and that IL-4 may be the counterpart that promotes TH_2 differentiation of the same precursors (Coffman *et al.*, 1991). These findings suggest that the endogenous levels of IFN-γ and/or IL-4 may regulate the differentiation process of naive TH cells *in vivo*. If IL-4 is responsible for *in vivo* generation of human TH_2 cells, we can wonder what kind of cells can produce IL-4. One likely possibility is that IL-4 is provided by cells other than T-lymphocytes. It is known that mouse mast cell lines, as well as splenic and bone marrow non-B, non-T cells can secrete IL-4 (Plaut *et al.*, 1989; Ben Sasson *et al.*, 1990). The IL-4-producing capacity of non-B, non-T cells expands dramatically in *Nippostrongylus brasiliensis* infection and in association with anti-IgD injection (Conrad *et al.*, 1990), suggesting that these cells play an important role in lymphokine production in helminthic infections and other situations marked by striking elevations of serum IgE levels. More recently, we have demonstrated the existence of human bone marrow non-B, non-T cells, probably belonging to mast cell/basophil lineage, capable of producing IL-4 in response to Fcϵ receptor cross-linkage (Piccinni *et al.*, 1991). Thus, IL-4 production by cells of the mast cell/basophil lineage might very well reflect a means through which TH_2 cells could be strikingly amplified *in vivo* during allergic reactions and parasitic infestations.

The results of our studies indicate that a better knowledge of factors that modulate the activation of TH_2 cells may provide a means for therapeutic interventions in IgE-mediated disorders through successful transformation of a TH_2-like into a TH_1-like response. For instance, a bias toward TH_1 activation could be achieved *in vitro* either by addition of IFN-γ or neutralization of IL-4 in the microenvironment where the TH cell–allergen interaction occurs. A further characterization of the events required for selective activation of TH_1 or TH_2 cells might offer potential sites for pharmacological manipulation of TH_1 and TH_2 activation, leading to the development of drugs that selectively activate or inhibit specific TH subsets *in vivo*.

References

Ben Sasson, S.Z., Le Gros, G., Conrad, D.H., Finkelman, F. and Paul, W.E.

(1990). Cross-linking Fc receptors stimulate splenic non-B, non-T cells to secrete interleukin 4 and other lymphokines. *Proc. Natl. Acad. Sci. U.S.A.* **87**, 1421–1425.

Coffman, R.L., Chatelain, R., Leal, L.M.C.C. and Varkila, K. (1991). Leishmania major infection in mice: a model system for the study of $CD4^+$ T-cell subset differentiation. *Res. Immunol.* **142**, 36–39.

Conrad, D.H., Ben Sasson, S.Z., Le Gros, G., Finkelman, F.D. and Paul, W.E. (1990). Infection with *Nippostrongylus brasiliensis* or injection of anti-IgD antibodies markedly enhances Fc-receptor-mediated interleukin 4 production by non-B, non-T cells. *J. Exp. Med.* **171**, 1497–1507.

Del Prete, G.F., Maggi, E., Parronchi, P., Chretien, I., Tiri, A., Macchia, D., Ricci, M., Banchereau, J., de Vries, J.E. and Romagnani, S. (1988). IL-4 is an essential factor for the IgE synthesis induced in vitro by human T cell clones and their supernatants. *J. Immunol.* **140**, 4193–4198.

Del Prete, G.F., De Carli, M., Mastromauro, C., Biagiotti, R., Macchia, D., Falagiani, P., Ricci, M. and Romagnani, S. (1991a). Purified protein derivative (PPD) of *Mycobacterium tuberculosis* and excretory/secretory antigen(s) (TES) of Toxocara canis expand in vitro human T cells with stable and opposite (Th_1 or Th_2) profile of cytokine production. *J. Clin. Invest.* **88**, 346–350.

Del Prete, G.F., De Carli, M., Ricci, M. and Romagnani, S. (1991b). Helper activity for immunoglobulin synthesis of T helper type 1 (Th_1) and Th_2 human T cell clones: the help of Th_1 clones is limited by their cytolytic capacity. *J. Exp. Med.* **174**, 809–814.

Gauchat, J.-F., Lebman, D., Coffman, R.L., Gascan, H. and de Vries, J.E. (1990). Structure and expression of germline ϵ transcripts in human B cells induced by interleukin 4 to switch to IgE production. *J. Exp. Med.* **172**, 463–472.

Hamid, Q., Azzawi, M., King, S., Moqbel, R., Wardlaw, A.J., Corrigan, C.J., Bradley, B., Durham, S.R., Collins, J.V., Jeffery, P.K., Quint, D.J. and Kay, A.B. (1991). Expression of mRNA for interleukin-5 in mucosal bronchial biopsies from asthma. *J. Clin. Invest.* **87**, 1541–1545.

Kay, A.B., Ying, S., Varney, V., Gaga, M., Durham, S.R., Moqbel, R., Wardlaw, A.J. and Hamid, Q. (1991). Messenger RNA expression of the cytokine gene cluster, Interleukin 3 (IL-3), IL-4, IL-5, and Granulocyte/Macrophage Colony-stimulating factor, in allergen-induced late phase cutaneous reactions in atopic subjects. *J. Exp. Med.* **173**, 775–778.

Maggi, E., Biswas, P., Del Prete, G.F., Parronchi, P., Macchia, D., Simonelli, C., Emmi, L., De Carli, M., Tiri, A., Ricci, M. and Romagnani, S. (1991). Accumulation of Th_2-like helper T cells in the conjunctiva of patients with vernal conjunctivitis. *J. Immunol.* **146**, 1169–1174.

Maggi, E., Parronchi, P., Manetti, R., Simonelli, C., Piccinni, M.-P., Santoni Rugiu, F., De Carli, M., Ricci, M. and Romagnani, S. (1992). Reciprocal regulatory effects of IFNγ and IL-4 on the in vitro development of human Th1 or Th2 clones. *J. Immunol.* **148**: 2142–2147.

Mosmann, T.R., Cherwinski, H., Bond, M.W., Giedlin, M.A. and Coffman, R.L. (1986). Two types of murine helper T cell clone. Definition according to profiles of lymphokine activities and secreted proteins. *J. Immunol.* **136**, 2348–2357.

Parronchi, P., Tiri, A., Macchia, D., Biswas, P., Simonelli, C., Maggi, E., Del Prete, G.F., Ricci, M. and Romagnani, S. (1990). Noncognate contact-dependent B cell activation can promote IL-4-dependent in vitro human IgE synthesis. *J. Immunol.* **144**, 2102–2108.

Parronchi, P., Macchia, D., Piccinni, M.-P., Biswas, P., Simonelli, C., Maggi, E., Ricci, M., Ansari, A.A. and Romagnani, S. (1991). Allergen- and bacterial antigen-specific T cell clones established from atopic donors show a different profile of cytokine production. *Proc. Natl. Acad. Sci. U.S.A.* **88**, 4538–4542.

Parronchi, P., De Carli, M., Manetti, R., Simonelli, C., Piccinni, M.-P., Macchia, D., Maggi, E., Del Prete, G.F., Ricci, M. and Romagnani, S. (1992) Aberrant interleukin (IL)-4 and IL-5 production in vitro by CD4 helper T cells from atopic subjects. *Eur. J. Immunol.* **22**: 1615–1620.

Pene, J., Rousset, F., Briere, F., Chretien, I., Bonnefoy, J.-Y., Spits, H., Yokota, T., Arai, N., Arai, K.-I., Banchereau, J. and de Vries, J. (1988). IgE production by normal human lymphocytes is induced by interleukin 4 and suppressed by interferons γ and α and prostaglandin E_2. *Proc. Natl. Acad. Sci. U.S.A.* **85**, 6880–6884.

Piccinni, M.-P., Macchia, D., Parronchi, P., Giudizi, M.G., Bani, D., Bellesi, G., Grossi, A., Ricci, M., Maggi, E. and Romagnani, S. (1991). Human bone marrow non-B, non-T cells produce IL-4 in response to cross-linkage of Fcϵ and Fcγ receptors. *Proc. Natl. Acad. Sci. U.S.A.* **88**, 8656–8661.

Plaut, M., Pierce, J.H., Watson, C.J., Hanley-Hyde, J., Nordan, R.P. and Paul, W.E. (1989). Mast cell lines produce lymphokines in response to cross-linkage of FcϵRI or to calcium ionophores. *Nature* **339**, 64–67.

Romagnani, S. (1990). Regulation and deregulation of human IgE synthesis. *Immunol. Today* **1**, 316–321.

Romagnani, S. (1991a). Human Th_1 and Th_2: doubt no more. *Immunol. Today* **12**, 256–257.

Romagnani, S. (1991b). Type 1 T helper and type 2 T helper cells: functions, regulation and role in protection and disease. *Int. J. Clin. Lab. Res.* **21**, 152–158.

Romagnani, S., Del Prete, G.F., Maggi, E., Parronchi, P., De Carli, M., Macchia, D., Piccinni, M.-P., Simonelli, C., Manetti, R., Santoni Ruju, F., Giudizi, M.-G., Biagiotti, R., Almerigogna, F. and Ricci, M. (1992). Cellular and molecular regulatory mechanisms of human IgE synthesis. *In Progress in Allergy and Clinical Immunology* (T. Miyamoto and M. Okuda eds), pp. 519–524. Hogzefe & Huber, Gottingen.

Sanderson, C.J., Warren, D.J. and Strath, M. (1985). Identification of a lymphokine that stimulates eosinophil differentiation *in vitro*. Its relationship to interleukin 3, and functional properties of eosinophils produced in culture. *J. Exp. Med.* **162**, 60–68.

Swain, S.L. (1991). Regulation of the development of distinct subsets of $CD4^+$ T cells. *Res. Immunol.* **142**, 14–18.

van Reijsen, F.C., Bruijnzeel-Koomen, C.A., Kalthoff, F.S., Maggi, E., Romagnani, S., Westland, J.K.T. and Mudde, G.C. (1992). Skin-derived aeroallergen specific T cell clones of Th2 phenotype in patients with atopic dermatitis. *J. Allergy Clin. Immunol.* **90**: 184–193.

Wierenga, E.A., Snoek, M., de Groot, C., Chretien, I., Bos, J.D., Jansen, H.M. and Kapsenberg, M. (1990). Evidence for compartmentalization of functional subsets of CD4 T lymphocytes in atopic patients. *J. Immunol.* **144**, 4651–4656.

Discussion

J.M. Drazen

Are any of your clones steroid-responsive? If steroids are included in the cultures, is the ability to isotype switch from T helper (TH) 1 to TH_2 changed?

S. Romagnani

If steroids are put on well-established T cell clones, there are no qualitative variations in their ability to produce cytokines. Recently we have used steroids and cyclosporin A in the system I described at the end of my presentation. Cyclosporin A strongly influences and enhances the development of T cells into TH_2 clones. The only steroid so far tried is hydrocortisone, with which we found only one, not so strong type of variation – a decrease in the interferon-γ production.

J.M. Drazen

The steroid does not make a difference in interleukin (IL)-4?

S. Romagnani

At least at the T cell line level it does not. We are now developing clones, and do not know yet if there is such a change in the subsequent phases of the development, but at least after 15 days of culture there is no significant change in IL-4 or IL-5 production by hydrocortisone.

M.K. Church

I know your experiments cannot answer definitively, but what is your view on the commitment of the progenitors or the ability of a TH_1 to switch to a TH_2 and back?

T.R. Mosmann

I think it is still open. If I had to guess, it would be that the precursor is not committed in a particular direction, but I do not know of any information yet that allows us to give any proof for that.

4

Hyposensitization of Allergic Immune Responses and T Cell Anergy

R.E. O'HEHIR, J.A. HIGGINS, E.R. JARMAN and J.R. LAMB

Department of Immunology, St. Mary's Hospital Medical School, Imperial College of Science, Technology and Medicine, Norfolk Place, London W2 1PG, UK

Introduction

In many individuals exposure to environmental allergens triggers a cascade of physiopathological mechanisms that results in a broad spectrum of clinical symptoms ranging from extrinsic asthma and allergic rhinitis to atopic dermatitis. Although immunocompetent $CD4^+$ T-lymphocytes represent only one of the heterogeneous cellular components mobilized in atopic disease, they are central to the induction of the specific (IgE) and non-specific (polymorphonuclear granulocytes) effector arcs involved in allergic inflammation (Kay, 1988; O'Hehir *et al.*, 1991b). The potential to treat allergic disease through the downregulation of these aberrant or unwanted immune responses has long been realized and forms the theoretical basis of hyposensitization.

Despite widespread clinical use of hyposensitization regimens a systematic approach to the development of immunotherapy has been hampered, in part due to a lack of knowledge of the immunological principles that determine the downregulation of established immune responses. Different mechanisms, including increased membrane stability

T-Lymphocyte and Inflammatory Cell Research in Asthma
ISBN 0-12-388170-6

of mediator-releasing cells, decreased IgE antibody levels, increased IgG antibodies, altered lymphocyte reactivity, the generation of suppressor T cells and the induction of anti-idiotypic networks, have all been offered to account for the clinical effectiveness of desensitization (Rocklin, 1983). Furthermore, effective immunotherapy may be achieved at a practical level by mimicking the natural mechanisms of T cell non-responsiveness that occur *in vivo* to prevent self-reactivity in the periphery. These mechanisms of tolerance may result in either physical elimination (clonal deletion) or functional inactivation (clonal anergy) of specific cells from the T cell repertoire (Blackman *et al.*, 1990; Ramsdell and Fowlkes, 1990). Clonal deletion is attributed to the neonatal thymus and involves the physical removal of self-reactive thymocytes during the maturation of the T cell repertoire. Anergy differs from deletion in two fundamental aspects. First, the autoreactive T cells are functionally, but not physically, removed from the repertoire and, secondly, anergy may be induced in mature T cells which have already survived thymic deletion and been released into the periphery. Therefore, the ability to render selected subsets of peripheral T cells of atopic individuals anergic to rechallenge with specific allergen may prevent the development of disease. The focus of this chapter will be directed towards the potential contribution of T cell anergy in hyposensitization of allergic immune responses.

In Vivo Models of Allergen Hyposensitization

Animal Studies

Analysis of the effects of physicochemical modification of allergen structure on immunoresponsiveness has been the primary aim of several animal studies (Sehon and Lee, 1979). Both chemical modification of intact molecules, such as carboxymethylation (Allen and Unanue, 1984) and glutaraldehyde polymerization (HayGlass and Stefura, 1991), and enzymatic degradation of proteins (Ferguson *et al.*, 1983; Litwin *et al.*, 1991) may alter their immunogenicity. The results of a recent study have demonstrated that immunization with glutaraldehyde-polymerized ovalbumin (OVA-POL), but not the native protein, leads to the induction of specific tolerance affecting both *de novo* and ongoing IgE responses, that is accompanied by enhanced production of anti-OVA IgG antibodies (HayGlass and Stefura, 1991). Two distinct functional subsets of $CD4^+$ T cells, designated TH_1 and TH_2 have been identified in the peripheral T cell compartment in mice (Mossman and Coffman, 1987) and to a lesser degree in humans (O'Hehir *et al.*, 1989; Wierenga *et al.*, 1990;

Romagnani, 1990). Each subset is characterized by the profile of lymphokines released; TH_1 cells secrete interleukin-2 (IL-2), interferon-γ (IFN-γ), tumour necrosis factor-α (TNF-α), TNF-β and granulocyte-macrophage colony-stimulating factor (GM-CSF), whilst TH_2 cells secrete IL-3, IL-4, IL-5, IL-6 and IL-10. In addition to the pleomorphic effects of TH_2-derived lymphokines on the non-specific effector cells of the allergic immune response, IL-4 is primarily responsible for regulating the IgG to IgE isotype switch (Esser and Radbruch, 1990). Lymphokines derived from TH_1 cells also influence eosinophils and indirectly modulate B cell function, but of major importance is the ability of IFN-γ to antagonize IL-4, and so prevent IgE production (Finkleman *et al.*, 1990). The effects of chemically modified OVA were inhibited by the *in vivo* administration of anti-IFN-γ antibodies, suggesting that the mode of action of OVA-POL may be mediated through the preferential induction of IFN-γ-secreting (TH_1) T cells, and operate by diverting the nature of the immune response towards IgG production. Therefore, the selective stimulation of distinct profiles of lymphokine production may be dictated, in part, by the physical characteristics of antigen encountered and influence the nature of the immune response generated.

In a series of experimental models using bovine serum albumin (BSA), phospholipase A_2 (PLA_2) and ragweed pollen (*Amb a* I) peptic fragment derivatives of these allergens were investigated for their ability to modulate the immune response to the native molecule (Ferguson *et al.*, 1983; Michael *et al.*, 1985; Litwin *et al.*, 1991). In each of these systems immunization with fragments downregulated specific IgE production to the intact protein. Different fragments of BSA of 40–300 amino acids in length, and each containing a single serological determinant, inhibited the response to the native protein. The adoptive transfer of T cells from non-responsive donors prevented the induction of immune responses in naive recipients to subsequent specific antigen challenge and the authors interpreted these findings as indicating that inhibition was due to suppressor T cells (Ferguson *et al.*, 1983). The pepsin-derived cleavage fragment P-1 of honey bee venom PLA_2, although able to bind to anti-PLA_2 antibodies, failed to elicit an immediate hypersensitivity reaction in the form of a passive cutaneous anaphylaxis reaction. Furthermore, the intravenous administration of P-1 inhibited an ongoing murine anti-PLA_2-specific IgE response (Michael *et al.*, 1985; Litwin *et al.*, 1988). In similar studies on the modulation of the immune response to *Amb a* I, the injection of peptic fragments suppressed specific IgE production (Litwin *et al.*, 1991). The cellular and molecular basis of the inhibitory effects mediated by these allergen-derived fragments remains ill-defined.

As many environmental allergens are inhaled they encounter initially immunocompetent cells residing locally in the lung and respiratory tract. Consequently, the immune defence systems of the lung and their response to inhaled allergens have become a focus of attention (Holt and McMenamin, 1989). The repeated administration of allergens, such as OVA, ragweed and house dust mite (HDM), in the form of aerosols induced transient IgE responses in rodents which were spontaneously downregulated despite continued aerosol exposure. Rechallenge of these animals up to 6 months after their final exposure elicited normal allergen-specific IgG antibody levels, whereas the specific IgE response was suppressed (Sedgwick and Holt, 1985). The adoptive transfer of phenotypically defined cell populations indicated that the $CD8^+$ T cells mediated the suppression of the IgE response. The failure to induce this regulatory cell pathway would facilitate allergen-specific IgE production and contribute to the development of allergic disease. In recent studies, making use of the selective homing of activated T cells to the lung, Holt and his colleagues (Nelson *et al.*, 1990; and personal communication) have adoptively transferred allergen-specific T cell clones into naive recipients and observed that the T cells are anergic to rechallenge, and that this phenomenon is characterized by phenotypic modulation. Additionally, the tight network of dendritic cells present within the lung epithelium (Holt *et al.*, 1989), expressing major histocompatibility complex (MHC) class II gene products, and the presence of tissue macrophages, may play vital roles in regulating the second signals that differentiate T cell clonal expansion from anergy.

In summary, animal models suggest that a wide variety of effector mechanisms, which include induction of regulatory T cells and anergy, may be operational in allergen-mediated hyposensitization.

Clinical Studies

Although there is a wealth of literature describing clinical studies of allergen hyposensitization, the interpretations offered to account for the physiological basis of this are varied and inconsistent. The list of variables that may explain these differences ranges from patient selection and allergen preparation to laboratory assay systems. Therefore, to embark upon a detailed discussion of these studies would be beyond the scope of this chapter. However, the selected recent reports discussed here will provide an indication of variation in the potential regulatory mechanisms that are activated in hyposensitization.

Immunotherapy with honey bee venom (PLA_2) has been demonstrated to provide significant protection against further stings (Hunt *et al.*, 1978). Analysis of specific cellular and antibody responses after rush therapy suggested that both proliferative and suppressor T cell activity was initially increased, as were specific IgG_1 and IgG_4 (Lesourd *et al.*, 1989a). Suppressor T cell activity was determined by the inhibition of proliferative responses in coculture systems in the absence of exogenous lymphokines. When reassessed one year later while IgG_4 levels remained high, specific IgE antibody was decreased. The authors suggest that there is an interrelationship between the modulation of the specific T and B cell responses to venom in immunotherapy, even though they are temporally dissociated. In the absence of further information on the T cell subsets activated and their lymphokine profiles it is difficult to identify the immunoregulatory mechanisms involved. These studies were extended and the immunological parameters of T cell proliferation, suppression and antibody synthesis assessed at two years after rush immunotherapy (Lesourd *et al.*, 1989b). The investigators noted that both the T cell proliferative and suppressive activities remained elevated. The transient rises in both specific IgG_1 and IgE, occurring immediately after immunotherapy, were decreased, in contrast to IgG_4 which was elevated. These findings were again interpreted to suggest that the activation of suppressor networks in the hyposensitized individuals was responsible for the reduction in specific IgE. A related study on the immune status of patients at one year after immunotherapy with cat extract (*Fel d* I) reported a decrease in skin sensitivity but both IgG and IgE antibodies reactive with extract were increased (van Metre *et al.*, 1989). In a continuation of their evaluation of the P-1 peptic fragment of PLA_2 in desensitization to honey bee venom, Litwin *et al.* (1988) reported that there was no initial rise in IgE following cutaneous injection of P-1, and the decrease in both PLA_2-reactive IgE and IgG was rapid. This was accompanied by a reduction in skin sensitivity to PLA_2. However, although the immunological status of the hyposensitized individuals appeared to parallel that of non-atopics, the clinical benefits of the treatment were not assessed. The authors postulated that the effect of pepsin hydrolysis on PLA_2 may be to alter the balance between helper and suppressor epitopes in the protein. Nevertheless, details of the immunological mechanisms underlying P-1-mediated hyposensitization still remained to be determined, since the capacity of P-1 to induce T cell anergy would also be compatible with their observations. Alternative immunoregulatory mechanisms have been identified to account for effective desensitization to Hymenoptera venom. These include release of a $CD8^+$ T cell-derived suppressor supernatant of 25 kDa molecular weight that inhibits platelet cytotoxic function (Tsicopoulos *et al.*, 1990). From the same laboratory, it was also reported in longitudinal studies, that the lymphocyte cell surface molecules CD23 and CD25, associated with activation, were decreased in patients undergoing rush hyposensitization (Tilmant *et al.*, 1989). Although little variation in the overall $CD4^+$ T cell population was observed in the treated patients, the percentage increase in $CD45R^+$ cells was accompanied by a reduction in $CDw29^-$ T cells. It has been suggested that $CD2w29^+$, $CD45R^-$ are equivalent to murine TH_2 cells (Umetsu *et al.*, 1988), therefore, one interpretation of these findings is that in hyposensitization the allergen reactive T cell repertoire is diverted from a predominance of TH_2 to TH_1 cells. The phenotype of T cells infiltrating the dermis after local allergen provocation of patients who had received immunotherapy with grass pollen extract was characterized by increased CD25 and MHC class II expression with downregulation of CD3 and CD4 as compared with the placebo control group (Durham *et al.*, 1991; Varney *et al.*, 1991). In approximately 50% of the patient group that received immunotherapy IFN-γ transcripts were increased as compared with the placebo controls (Durham, personal communication). The authors suggested that this might represent selective recruitment of TH_1 cells in the hyposensitized patients, in contrast to the untreated atopics where TH_2 cells migrate to the site of allergen challenge. However, these changes observed in both the T cell surface proteins and lymphokine profiles are compatible with the induction of peripheral T cell non-responsiveness (O'Hehir and Lamb, 1990; O'Hehir *et al.*, 1991a,c). In contrast, in immunotherapy mediated with peptic fragments of ragweed pollen, Litwin *et al.* (1991) attributed the effectiveness to the activation of suppressor activity. Therefore, although the immunological mechanisms that have been proposed to account for successful immunotherapy are varied, several of the experimental findings could equally support a role for peripheral T cell anergy. Standardization of desensitizing agents, perhaps based on defined non-IgE binding peptides, may resolve some of the conflicts arising from the assessment of these clinical studies.

In Vitro Models of T Cell Non-responsiveness

Many of the clinical protocols of hyposensitization mimic the features of T cell-dependent low zone tolerance and, as discussed above, may modulate allergen-specific IgE levels, T cell proliferative responses and the pattern of recruitment of T cell subsets. Recently, *in vitro* models using human T cell clones have been established for the analysis of antigen-specific anergy (Lamb *et al.*, 1983; Lamb and O'Hehir, 1989; O'Hehir and Lamb, 1990). It was observed that after repeated exposure to escalating concentrations of *Dermatophagoides farinae* extract house dust mite (HDM)-reactive T cells, capable of supporting specific IgE synthesis *in vitro*, failed to proliferate in response to an immunogenic challenge with specific allergen (Lamb and O'Hehir, 1989). Enhanced responsiveness to exogenous IL-2 indicated that the loss of antigen-dependent proliferation was not the result of cytolysis. The exposure of *Der p* I allergen-reactive cloned T cells to a single pulse of specific peptide (residues 89–117) at a supraimmunogenic concentration in the presence of antigen presenting cells delivered a negative signal to the T cells, the result of which was to inhibit proliferation (O'Hehir *et al.*, 1991c). The induction of anergy was associated with phenotypic modulation; CD3 and, in some instances, CD4 were downregulated, in contrast to CD2, CD25 and CD45RO cell surface expression which was enhanced (O'Hehir *et al.*, 1991a; Faith, Higgins, O'Hehir and Lamb, unpublished results). During the induction phase of anergy, IL-2, IL-4 and IFN-γ were synthesized and the levels were equal to that of activated T cells. However, restimulation of anergic allergen-reactive T cell clones with peptide or whole extract of HDM failed to induce IL-4 production, whereas IFN-γ release remained intact (O'Hehir *et al.*, 1991c). The ability to regulate selectively the synthesis of these lymphokines by HDM-reactive T cell clones such that IL-4 production is inhibited and IFN-γ is maintained would be advantageous in downregulating aberrant responses in allergic disease. These changes in both the phenotype and lymphokine profiles of the anergic T cells parallel the findings reported by Durham and his colleagues (1991) in studies on immunotherapy with pollen and indicate that T cell tolerance may be operational in hyposensitization. T cell anergy appears to be induced more efficiently with peptides than either complex mixtures of multideterminant antigens or intact proteins. This may contribute to the inability of certain studies to identify this as a primary immunological mechanism underlying immunotherapy. If a limited set of "major determinants" can be identified within an allergenic protein, the administration of synthetic peptides, derived from these determinants, under defined conditions, may modulate T cell antigen recognition and induce anergy. Furthermore, structural modification of the peptides may allow their tolerogenic activity to be enhanced and their ability to bind IgE diminished. The specific allergic response in atopic individuals undoubtedly will involve the recognition of multiple epitopes. Nevertheless, T cell receptor (TcR) usage may be restricted, as appears to occur in certain infectious (Choi *et al.*, 1990) and autoimmune (Paliard *et al.*, 1991) diseases. Therefore, an alternative approach would be to tolerize antigen-specific T cells using antigens that bind to shared sequences on the specific receptors of T cell families, such as the variable (V) regions of TcR β-chains. A family of antigens has been termed "superantigens" based on their ability to stimulate proliferative responses of T cells that express particular TcR-Vβ gene products (Marrack and Kappler, 1990). The staphylococcal enterotoxins, which are included in the family of superantigens, are able both to activate T cells and induce anergy (O'Hehir and Lamb, 1990). After exposure to the appropriate bacterial toxin, HDM-reactive T cells fail to respond when restimulated with their natural ligand but retain responsiveness to exogenous IL-2 (O'Hehir *et al.*, 1991a). It must be emphasized that chemical modification and genetic manipulation may remove the toxicity of these bacterial superantigens without affecting their tolerogenicity. The mechanism of toxin-mediated T cell anergy parallels those underlying non-responsiveness induced by nominal peptide (O'Hehir *et al.*, 1991c). These studies indicate that families of allergen-reactive T cells may be functionally inactivated by the interaction with non-allergen-derived ligands, which offers an alternative approach to hyposensitization.

Concluding Comments

The evidence supporting a central role for $CD4^+$ T cells in the initiation and regulation of allergic immune responses is now firmly established. Therefore, the induction of non-responsiveness in selective populations and clones of specific $CD4^+$ T cells may potentially prevent the development of allergic immune responses. Non-responsiveness to self peptides is maintained in the peripheral T cell repertoire by clonal anergy. The presentation of allergen in a non-immunogenic form may result in the delivery of negative signals to T cells of distinct specificities and, thus, induce clonal anergy. The interpretation of the results of recent clinical trials of immunotherapy in the context of *in vitro* models of T cell anergy indicate that tolerance may be an operational modality in allergen hyposensitization. As the molecular mechanisms of T cell anergy unfold and defined peptide components of allergens are applied in hyposensitization studies it will be possible to determine further the relationship between tolerance and immunotherapy.

Acknowledgements

We thank Dr S.R. Durham for his helpful discussions and the contribution of results prior to publication. This work was supported by grants from the Medical Research Council and the Wellcome Trust. R.E. O'Hehir is the recipient of a Wellcome Senior Fellowship in Clinical Science and E.R. Jarman is a Rodney Porter Scholar.

References

Allen, P.M. and Unanue, E.R. (1984). Differential requirements for antigen processing by macrophages for lysozyme-specific T cell hybridomas. *J. Immunol.* **133**, 1077–1082.

Blackman, M., Kappler, J. and Marrack, P. (1990). The role of the T cell receptor in positive and negative selection of developing T cells. *Science* **248**, 1335–1341.

Choi, Y., Lafferty, J.A., Clements, J.R., Todd, J.K., Gelfand, E.W., Kappler, J., Marrack, P. and Kotzin, B.L. (1990). Selective expansion of T cells expressing V beta 2 in toxic shock syndrome. *J. Exp. Med.* **172**, 981–984.

Durham, S.R., Varney, V.A., Gaga, M., Jacobson, M.R., Frew, A.J. and Kay, A.B. (1991). Immunotherapy suppresses T lymphocyte infiltration in the cutaneous late-phase reaction. *J. Allergy Clin. Immunol.* **87**, 299 (abst.).

Esser, C. and Radbruch, A. (1990). Immunoglobulin class switching: molecular and cellular analysis. *Annu. Rev. Immunol.* **8**, 717–735.

Ferguson, T.A., Peters, T.A., Reed, R., Pesce, J.A. and Michael, J.G. (1983). Immunoregulatory properties of antigenic fragments from bovine serum albumin. *Cell Immunol.* **78**, 1–12.

Finkleman, F.D., Holmes, J., Katona, I.M., Urban, J.F., Beckman, M.P., Park, L.S., Schooley, K.A., Coffman, R.L., Mossman, T.R. and Paul, W.E. (1990). Lymphokine control of *in vivo* immunoglobulin isotype selection. *Annu. Rev. Immunol.* **8**, 303–333.

HayGlass, K.T. and Stefura, W.P. (1991). Anti-interferon gamma treatment blocks the ability of glutaraldehyde-polymerised allergens to inhibit specific IgE responses. *J. Exp. Med.* **173**, 279–285.

Holt, P.G. and McMenamin, C. (1989). Defence against allergic sensitization in the healthy lung: the role of inhalation tolerance. *Clin. Exp. Allergy* **19**, 255–262.

Holt, P.G., Schon-Hegrad, M.A., Phillips, M.J. and McMenamin, C. (1989). Ia-positive dendritic cells form a tightly meshed network within the human airway epithelium. *Immunology* **19**, 597–601.

Hunt, K.J., Valentine, M.D., Sobotka, A.K., Amodio, F.J. and Lichenstein, L.M. (1978). A controlled trial of immunotherapy in insect hypersensitivity. *New Engl. J. Med.* **299**, 157–159.

Kay, A.B. (1988). Mechanisms in allergic and chronic asthma which involve eosinophils, neutrophils, lymphocytes and other inflammatory cells. *In* "The Allergic Basis of Asthma". Baillière Tindall, London, 1–14.

Lamb, J.R. and O'Hehir, R.E. (1989). Cellular and molecular mechanisms of T lymphocyte unresponsiveness induced *in vitro*. *Thymus Update* **3**, 71–95.

Lamb, J.R., Skidmore, B.J., Green, N., Chiller, J. and Feldmann, M. (1983). Induction of tolerance in influenza-virus stimulated immune T lymphocyte clones with synthetic peptides of influenza haemagglutinin. *J. Exp. Med.* **157**, 1434–1447.

Lesourd, B., Paupe, J., Thiollet, M., Moulias, R., Sainte-Laudy, J. and

Scheinmann, P. (1989a). Hymenoptera venom immunotherapy. I. Induction of T cell-mediated immunity by honeybee venom immunotherapy: Relationships with specific antibody responses. *J. Allergy Clin. Immunol.* **83**, 563–571.

Lesourd, B., Paupe, J., Melani, M., Sainte-Laudy, J., Moulias, R. and Scheinmann, P. (1989b). Hymenoptera venom immunotherapy. II. T proliferative and T suppressive activities induced by *Vespula* immunotherapy: Effects on long-term antibody responses. *J. Allergy Clin. Immunol.* **83**, 572–580.

Litwin, A., Pesce, A.J. and Michael, J.G. (1988). Regulation of the immune response to allergens by immunosuppressive allergenic fragments. *Int. Arch. Allergy Appl. Immunol.* **87**, 361–366.

Litwin, A., Pesce, A.J., Fischer, T., Michael, M. and Michael, J.G. (1991). Regulation of human immune responses to ragweed pollen by immunotherapy. A controlled trial comparing the effect of immunosuppressive peptic fragments of short ragweed with standard treatment. *Clin. Exp. Allergy* **21**, 457–465.

Marrack, P. and Kappler, J. (1990). The staphylococcal enterotoxins and their relatives. *Science* **248**, 705–711.

Michael, J.G., Pesce, A.J., Litwin, A. and Freisheim, J. (1985). Immunosuppressive properties of a phospholipase A2 antigen fragment. *J. Allergy Clin. Immunol.* **75**, 200 (abstract).

Mossman, T.R. and Coffman, R.L. (1987). Two types of mouse helper T-cell clone. *Immunol. Today* **8**, 223–227.

Nelson, D., Strickland, D. and Holt, P.G. (1990). Selective attrition of non-circulating T cells during normal passage through the lung vascular bed. *Immunology* **69**, 476–481.

O'Hehir, R.E. and Lamb, J.R. (1990). Induction of specific clonal anergy in human T lymphocytes by *Staphylococcus aureus* enterotoxins. *Proc. Natl. Acad. Sci. U.S.A.* **87**, 8884–8888.

O'Hehir, R.E., Bal, V., Quint, D., Moqbel, R., Kay, A.B., Zanders, E.D. and Lamb, J.R. (1989). An *in vitro* model of allergen dependent IgE synthesis by human B cells: comparison of the response of an atopic and non-atopic individuals. *Immunology* **66**, 499–504.

O'Hehir, R.E., Aguilar, B.A., Schmidt, T.J., Gollnick, S.O. and Lamb, J.R. (1991a). Functional inactivation of *Dermatophagoides* spp. (house dust mite) reactive T cell clones. *Clin. Exp. Allergy* **21**, 209–215.

O'Hehir, R.E., Garman, R.D., Greenstein, J.L. and Lamb, J.R. (1991b). The specificity and regulation of T-cell responsiveness to allergens. *Annu. Rev. Immunol.* **9**, 76–95.

O'Hehir, R.E., Yssel, H., Verma, S., de Vries, J.E., Spits, H. and Lamb, J.R. (1991c). Clonal analysis of differential lymphokine production in peptide and superantigen induced T cell anergy. *Int. Immunol.* **3**, 819–826.

Paliard, X., West, S.G., Lafferty, J.A., Clements, J.R., Kappler, J.W., Marrack, P. and Kotzin, B.L. (1991). Evidence for the effects of a superantigen in rheumatoid arthritis. *Science* **253**, 325–329.

Ramsdell, F. and Fowlkes, B.J. (1990). Clonal deletion versus clonal anergy: the role of the thymus in inducing self tolerance. *Science* **248**, 1342–1348.

Rocklin, R.E. (1983). Clinical and immunologic aspects of allergen-specific immunotherapy in patients with seasonal allergic rhinitis and/or allergic asthma. *J. Allergy Clin. Immunol.* **72**, 323–328.

Romagnani, S. (1990). Regulation and deregulation of human IgE synthesis. *Immunol. Today* **11**, 316–321.

Sedgwick, J.D. and Holt, P.G. (1985). Induction of IgE-secreting cells and IgE isotype specific suppressor T cells in the respiratory lymph nodes of rats in response to antigen inhalation. *Cell Immunol.* **56**, 182–194.

Sehon, A.H. and Lee, W.Y. (1979). Suppression of immunoglobulin E antibodies with modified allergens. *J. Allergy Clin. Immunol.* **64**, 242–250.

Tilmant, L., Dessaint, J.P., Tsicopoulos, A., Tonnel, A.B. and Capron, A. (1989). Concomitant augmentation of $CD4^+$ $CD45R^+$ suppressor/inducer subset and diminution of $CD4^+CDw29^+$ helper/inducer subset during rush hyposensitization in hymenoptera venom allergy. *Clin. Exp. Immunol.* **76**, 13–18.

Tsicopoulos, A., Tonnel, A.B., Vorng, H., Wallaert, B., Kusnierz, J.P., Pestel, J. and Capron, A. (1990). Lymphocyte-mediated inhibition of platelet cytotoxic functions during Hymenoptera venom desensitization: characterisation of a suppressive lymphokine. *Eur. J. Immunol.* **20**, 1201–1207.

Umetsu, D.T., Jabara, H.H., Dekruyff, R.H., Abbas, A.K., Abrams, J.S. and Geha, R.S. (1988). Functional heterogeneity among human inducer T cell clones. *J. Immunol.* **140**, 4211–4216.

van Metre, T.E., Marsh, D.G., Adkinson, N.F., Kagey-Sobotka, A., Khattignavong, A., Norman, P.S. and Rosenberg, G.L. (1989). Immunotherapy decreases skin sensitivity to cat extract. *J. Allergy Clin. Immunol.* **83**, 888–899.

Varney, V.A., Gaga, M., Frew, A.J., Aber, V.R., Kay, A.B. and Durham, S.R. (1991). Usefulness of immunotherapy in patients with severe summer hay fever uncontrolled by antiallergic drugs. *Brit. Med. J.* **302**, 265–269.

Wierenga, E.A., Snoek, M., de Groot, C., Chretien, I., Bos, J.D., Jansen, H.M. and Kapsenberg, M.L. (1990). Evidence for compartmentalisation of functional subsets of $CD4^+$ lymphocytes in atopic patients. *J. Immunol.* **144**, 4651–4656.

Discussion

S. Romagnani

Can you comment on the CD28 signal stabilizing the message for cytokines?

J. Lamb

The original experiments were done by Carl June and Craig Thompson. They showed that if T cells are activated with anti-CD28 antibodies, IL-2 production was resistant to modulation with cyclosporin, whereas with normal activation through the T cell receptor IL-2 production could be blocked with cyclosporin. They suggested that it was a different pathway for cytokine regulation, and have shown in a recent paper that the breakdown of the message is much more delayed if there is stimulation with anti-CD2, so they believe that it stabilizes the IL-2, IL-4 and, I think, other cytokine messages.

A.B. Kay

In some, as yet unpublished, work we have shown that after successful immunotherapy there is a change in the phenotype profile in the cells which have infiltrated the site of reaction by antigen. This is similar to what you are describing, which is a downregulation of CD3 and CD4 and an upregulation of CD25. It would fit in very nicely with what you have said.

However, all the patients we studied who had immunotherapy got better. There was not a range of clinical improvement: they all got markedly better, although there was quite a range of upregulation of CD25. Another explanation for our findings is that immunotherapy causes more antigen-specific T cells to infiltrate the site of the reaction. This would seem to be a much simpler explanation for the finding, which might in fact have nothing to do with the mechanism of immunotherapy.

J. Lamb

That is true. I would be very surprised if we find it is a single mechanism. I think we will find a very complex set of reactions occurring, a very broad spectrum, which will vary from patient to patient. In some patients I think it will be much more an anergic type of therapy, if you like, in others, a different subset migrating in and replacing the one that is there.

F.P. Nijkamp

With induction of bronchial hyperresponsiveness with Gram-negative bacteria like *Bordetella pertussis* or endotoxins from Gram-negative bacteria is something similar observed to what was described for the enterotoxins – that is, after increasing doses the response is lost, and sometimes even reversed? How specific is the kind of phenomenon that you described for the enterotoxins?

J. Lamb

I think we will find that a wide range of pathogens have evolved to produce these, if you like, superantigens (if that is what we should call them), these very potent stimulators of the immune response. The enterotoxins can go both ways. Depending upon concentration, how you present it, either an enormous activation of the T cell repertoire can be induced or it can just be pushed slightly one way and there is a complete shutting down. I think a number of pathogens have evolved this way of trying to regulate the response of the host.

5

New Prospects for Immunotherapy in Asthma

J. BOUSQUET and F.B. MICHEL

Clinique des Maladies Respiratoires, Hôpital Arnaud de Villeneuve, 555, Route de Ganges, 34059 Montpellier, France

Specific immunotherapy (SIT) was introduced in 1911 and remains in many countries one of the most prescribed treatments in adolescents and young adults. However, the therapeutic index of SIT has been contested for many years. In the 1970s SIT was found to be ineffective for asthma (Lichtenstein, 1978) and recently it has been shown that allergen injections have, using potent extracts, resulted in a number of systemic reactions and possibly of deaths, especially in asthmatics (Committee on Safety of Medicine, 1986; Norman, 1987). Thus, despite significant progress in the past 15 years (Grant, 1986; Dreborg *et al.*, 1988; Bousquet *et al.*, 1990b), the place of SIT in asthma therapy is again contested and threatened with some decline for pneumoallergens.

Before starting any SIT course, it is essential to compare the therapeutic index of SIT and other anti-allergic treatments by examining several factors:

1) Potential severity of the condition to be treated
2) Efficacy of available treatments
3) Cost and duration of each type of treatment
4) Risk incurred by the patient due to the allergic disease and the treatments.

The outdoor and indoor allergenic and non-allergenic environment should always be considered before starting SIT. When possible, environmental control measures should always be applied before starting SIT, even if their efficacy is not complete, as they may improve the patient, reduce

T-Lymphocyte and Inflammatory Cell Research in Asthma
ISBN 0-12-388170-6

the need for further treatment and will always improve the efficacy and safety of SIT.

Mechanisms

The mechanisms of action of SIT in general and in asthma in particular are still unclear and several possibilities have been proposed. For decades it has been postulated that allergen-specific immunoglobulin G (IgG) present in serum and secretions may block allergens before their interaction with cell-bound IgE. This blocking activity may have some relevance in the protective effect of venom immunotherapy (VIT) but is unlikely to be a major mechanism in asthma or rhinoconjunctivitis caused by inhalant allergens. IgG subclasses have also been examined extensively but, to date, there is no definite conclusion since, in some studies, IgG_4 was associated with a poor efficacy of SIT, whereas in others the opposite effect was observed (Van der Zee and Aalberse, 1987). Recent studies on the idiotypic network have highlighted the putative role of specific IgG, possibly explaining the decrease in IgE production after SIT.

The evolution of allergen-specific IgE has also been examined. In the 1970s, it was postulated that SIT might induce a reduction in IgE synthesis, but this only occurs after several months of treatment and cannot explain the early clinical efficacy of this form of treatment. Animal studies have provided evidence that a series of modified extracts elicit a suppressive activity on the IgE response. However, most of these studies were done on primary or secondary responses and rarely on ongoing ones. Many of these extracts have been used in humans, and although they had a protective activity, specific IgE was unaffected (Juniper *et al.*, 1985; Dreborg and Akerblom, 1990).

In the 1930s, some studies showed that skin tests with allergen were decreased during specific SIT but no explanation could be given. These studies were almost forgotten until recent years. Since 1980, many experiments performed with pollens, mites, animal danders or moulds have consistently found that skin tests (Bousquet *et al.*, 1985b, 1988b), conjunctival (Moller *et al.*, 1986), nasal (Bousquet *et al.*, 1988b, 1990c, 1991a; Creticos *et al.*, 1989; Ilioupoulos *et al.*, 1991) and bronchial challenges (Warner *et al.*, 1978; Van Bever *et al.*, 1988; Bousquet *et al.*, 1985a) are decreased after treatment. Both the early and the late phase reactions are inhibited. It was observed that these changes in sensitivity were allergen-specific. They appear very rapidly after the onset of SIT and far before any specific IgG change (Juniper *et al.*, 1986; Hedlin *et al.*, 1989). Studies with nasal challenges showed that the release of inflammatory mediators was decreased after treatment (Bousquet *et al.*, 1991a; Creticos *et al.*, 1989) and these changes were correlated with the efficacy of SIT (Bousquet *et al.*, 1988b, 1990c, 1991a). Moreover, *in vitro* studies using histamine release from blood basophils or platelets have also found a decreased sensitivity of these cells to the allergen after SIT. Finally, it has been elegantly demonstrated that eosinophils were downregulated (Rak *et al.*, 1988) during SIT, possibly because SIT decreases the generation of chemotactic factors.

These changes in cell sensitivity may be due to cytokines since it has been shown recently that after 3 days of VIT, a serum factor decreased the sensitivity of platelets to venom (Tsicopoulous *et al.*, 1990). During pollen SIT mononuclear cells synthesize less histamine-releasing factors (Kuna *et al.*, 1989) and *in situ* hybridization studies have suggested a change in the phenotype of T cells during SIT (Durham *et al.*, 1991). These studies showed that skin tests with allergen elicited a late phase reaction in which interleukin-4 (IL-4) and IL-5 were released whereas in a proportion of subjects after SIT, the late reaction was decreased and this was accompanied by the presence of interferon-γ (IFN-γ), suggesting a switch from TH_2 to TH_1 type cells.

Objectives of Immunotherapy in Asthma

Asthma is a complex disease in which allergic factors and non-allergic triggers (viral infections, irritants, exercise, drugs, aspirin, occupational factors, stress, air pollution) interact and result in bronchial obstruction and inflammation. The role of inhalant allergens in asthma exacerbations has been clearly demonstrated both for perennial allergens like house dust mites or insect dusts (Platts Mills *et al.*, 1989; Platts Mills and De Wek, 1989; Pollart *et al.*, 1989), seasonal allergens such as grass pollens (Reid *et al.*, 1986; Pollart *et al.*, 1989) or moulds (Salvaggio and Aukrust, 1981; Reed, 1985) and animal dander (Van Metre *et al.*, 1986). The inhalation of allergens leads to a complex activation of various cell types and the release of inflammatory and neurogenic mediators (Barnes, 1989).

In allergic asthma, two different situations seem to exist. Although very few pollen grains can reach the lower airways (Michel *et al.*, 1977), these allergens frequently elicit asthma (Reid *et al.*, 1986; Pollart *et al.*, 1989) and an IgE-mediated mechanism is the most likely to explain bronchial symptoms. Allergic reactions prolonged over several days almost always lead to non-specific bronchial hyperreactivity (BHR), but BHR is usually transient in patients only allergic to pollens, lasting from a few weeks to a few months after the cessation of the pollen season (Boulet *et al.*, 1983; Sotomayor *et al.*, 1984). Moreover, pollen-allergic patients do not have severe bronchial alterations. On the other hand, house dust mites and other perennial allergens induce a long-sustained inflammation of the bronchi (Bousquet *et al.*, 1990a; Djuranovic *et al.*, 1990), leading to a variable degree to BHR (Pauwels, 1989) and symptoms are due to allergens, inflammation and BHR. It has been shown that patients with chronic asthma present a pseudo-fibrosis of the bronchi due to collagen deposition beneath the basement membrane (Roche *et al.*, 1989) and alterations of the elastic fibre network of the airways (Bousquet *et al.*, 1993) leading to the concept of airway remodelling in asthma. Inflammation and airway remodelling may be involved in the "accelerated decline" of the pulmonary function characterized by a poorly reversible bronchial obstruction appearing after some decades of chronic asthma (Peat *et al.*, 1987; Bousquet *et al.*, 1987b; O'Connor *et al.*, 1989) as well as permanent bronchial wall alterations as shown by computerized tomography scans (Paganin *et al.*, 1993). After a long course of the disease, inflammation is a major cause of symptoms, suggesting that the immunologic treatment should be replaced by anti-inflammatory drugs (Bousquet *et al.*, 1990b).

These considerations suggest that (1) SIT may be more effective in grass pollen allergic patients than in those sensitized to perennial allergens and (2) grass pollen allergy may be an adequate model to study the effects of specific SIT in patients with normal bronchi, whereas SIT in mite allergy may be used to examined the effects of the treatment in patients with a variable degree of bronchial inflammation and damage.

The objective of immunologic treatment is, in the short term, to reduce the allergic triggers precipitating symptoms and, in the long term, to decrease bronchial inflammation and BHR when it is not too severe and when bronchial damage is not prominent.

Pollen Asthma

Efficacy of Subcutaneous Immunotherapy

Grass pollen allergy

Only a few controlled studies have investigated the efficacy of SIT in grass pollen asthma. Using several types of grass pollen extracts, Frankland and Augustin (1954) were the first to demonstrate that timothy and orchard grass pollen extracts were significantly more effective than the placebo. Recent studies using aqueous (Reid *et al.*, 1986) or standardized extracts (Østerballe, 1980; Bousquet *et al.*, 1985b; Armentia *et al.*, 1989; Varney *et al.*, 1991) or formaldehyde-allergoids (Bousquet *et al.*, 1989b, 1990c) (Fig. 5.1) showed that SIT had a beneficial effect on bronchial symptoms during the pollen season. European studies indicated that bronchial symptoms were better relieved than nasal ones (Bousquet *et al.*, 1985b, 1989b; Østerballe, 1980). However, Hill *et al.* (1982) using rush immunotherapy (RIT) with timothy grass pollen, Bousquet *et al.* (1985b) with a pyridine-extracted orchard grass pollen and alum adjuvant did not find that SIT induced any significant protection. The differences between conclusive and inconclusive studies may be related to the differences in extracts and schedules used or in the doses of allergens administered. Another explanation for discrepancies may be due to differences in pollen counts in various countries, since in Australia

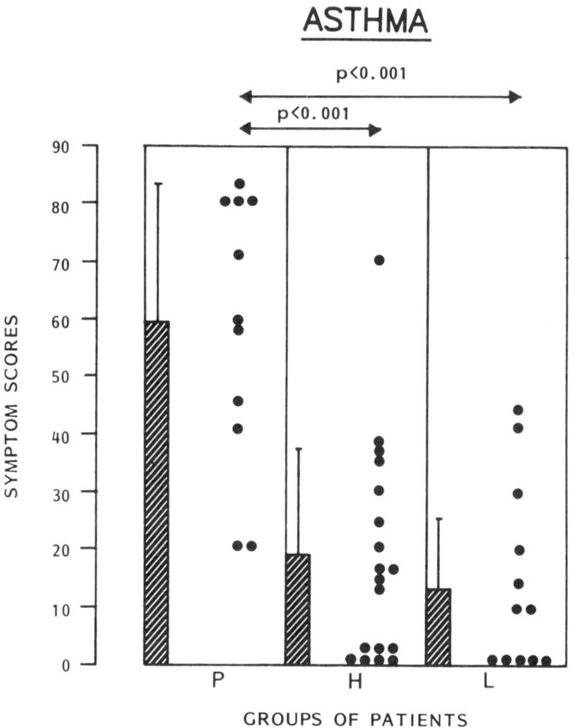

Fig. 5.1 Asthmatic symptoms during the grass pollen season in patients receiving placebo (P) or a high molecular weight allergoid at a high (H) or a lower (L) dose. (From Bousquet *et al.*, 1990c.)

grass pollen counts are extremely high and the study of Hill and colleagues did not find efficacy (Hill *et al.*, 1982).

Using bronchial challenges, McAllen (1961) but not Ortolani *et al.* (1984) observed that the threshold dose eliciting an immediate positive challenge was significantly increased after SIT. In a study examining the efficacy of SIT on bronchial challenge with grass pollen extracts, Van Bever *et al.* (1988) observed no difference in the immediate phase reaction and a significant reduction of the late phase reaction in children who received SIT by comparison with a control group of untreated children.

Other pollen allergens

The observations in grass pollen allergy indicate clearly that grass pollen asthma is improved by SIT, but only when optimal conditions are achieved. These conclusions are, however, at present restricted to grass and birch pollen allergy (Rak *et al.*, 1988) since conflicting results have been produced in ragweed pollen asthma. In 1957, Johnstone and Dutton (see Johnstone and Dutton, 1968) suggested that high doses of ragweed pollen extracts were helpful in treating children with asthma whereas Bruce *et al.* (1977) found that autumnal asthma induced by ragweed pollens was not improved by allergen injections. However, in the latter study, the lack of effectiveness of SIT might be related to the sensitization of some patients to moulds.

The IgE immune response to environmental allergens depends both on genetic and environmental factors and is highly heterogeneous. It was shown that patients only allergic to grass pollens differ clinically and immunologically from those allergic to many pollen species (Bousquet *et al.*, 1991a,b). A double-blind placebo-controlled study compared the efficacy of SIT in these two groups of patients. Grass pollen allergic patients were treated with an optimal maintenance dose of a standardized orchard grass pollen extract whereas those allergic to multiple pollen species received the same biologically equivalent dose of all standardized allergens to which they were sensitized. The results of the study indicated that grass pollen allergic patients but not polysensitized patients were significantly protected (Bousquet *et al.*, 1991a). Using a higher allergen dose, it might be possible to show efficacy in the polysensitized group but the rate of systemic reactions would have been unacceptable.

Studies on bronchial hyperresponsiveness

During the pollen season, patients with asthma often have an increased BHR. The effect of SIT on bronchial reactivity measured by methacholine was investigated in birch pollen asthmatics (Rak *et al.*, 1988). Untreated patients had a decreased threshold to inhaled methacholine (i.e. BHR), whereas those who received SIT did not present a significant change in sensitivity to methacholine.

Safety of Subcutaneous Immunotherapy

Life-threatening reactions are not rare with high-quality extracts and deaths have been reported. The rate of systemic reactions is greater with standardized pollen extracts than with either non-standardized extracts or high molecular weight preparations, but does not differ from SIT performed with standardized extracts of other allergen species. The occurrence of systemic reactions was studied in over 500 individuals allergic to grass pollen who received the same rush SIT protocol with the same standardized extracts (Hejjaoui *et al.*, 1993). It was observed that the rate of systemic reactions was increased in patients who had presented asthma (and rhinoconjunctivitis) during the previous pollen season than in those who had rhinoconjunctivitis alone. The incidence of generalized urticaria and anaphylaxis was similar in both groups, but bronchial symptoms occurred mostly in asthmatic patients. This study indicates that asthmatic patients are at higher risk during SIT. Rush immunotherapy may expose to a high risk of systemic reactions and attempts have been made to reduce the incidence of reactions (Fig. 5.2) (Hejjaoui *et al.*, 1993). With premedication, exclusion of asthmatic patients with FEV_1 (forced expiratory volume in 1 second) under 70% of predicted values at the time of the injection and stopping the rush schedule if large local reactions were noticed, systemic reactions were decreased to an acceptable rate and the severity of these reactions was always mild. Step protocols decrease even further the rate and severity of systemic reactions. Polymerized high molecular weight preparations consistently induced few systemic reactions in grass, ragweed and tree pollen allergy (Østerballe, 1980; Lessof, 1983; Bousquet *et al.*, 1990c; Varney *et al.*, 1991).

Duration

Duration of SIT is another matter of debate. In the case of inhalant allergy in atopic individuals, data are lacking to support any definite conclusion, but it appears that a long-term treatment, at least 3 years, is required. For nasal symptoms, in a retrospective study, Mosbech and Østerballe (1988) observed that the effect of grass pollen SIT lasted several years after its cessation. Grammer and co-workers, using high-

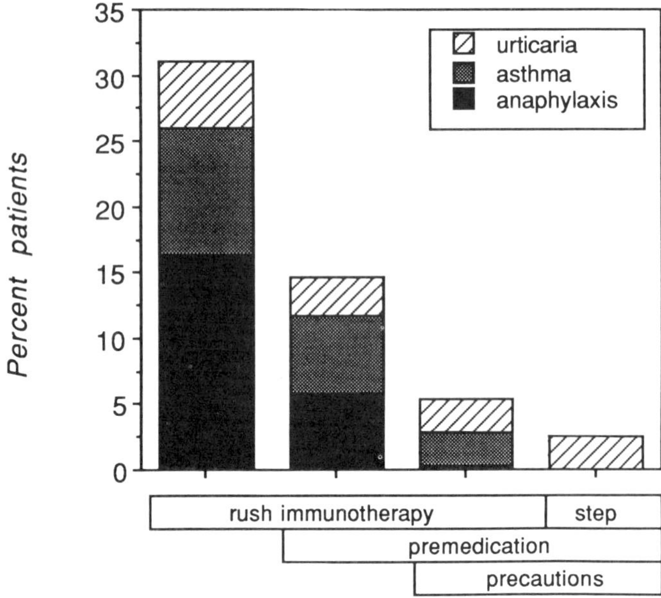

Fig. 5.2 Systemic side reactions observed in patients undergoing immunotherapy with standardized pollen extracts according to the schedule. (From Hejjaoui *et al.*, 1993.)

molecular weight polymerized extracts, reached similar conclusions (Grammer *et al.*, 1984). However, prospective controlled studies are lacking and no definite conclusion can be made.

Indications for Subcutaneous Immunotherapy

Clinical efficacy does not mean clinical indication, especially since pharmacologic treatment is also available for the treatment of allergic diseases. The specific indications of pollen SIT have been studied extensively and the position papers of the European Academy of Allergy and Clinical Immunology (EAACI) (Malling, 1988) and WHO/IUIS (Thompson *et al.*, 1989) have proposed some guidelines. Since rhinoconjunctivitis is present in most if not all patients suffering from pollen allergy, and asthma occurs generally in the most severe patients, it is impossible to propose indications without considering all symptoms. It is commonly accepted and recently confirmed by Varney *et al.* (1991) that SIT is indicated in severe pollinosis. It also appears that SIT is indicated when asthma complicates rhinoconjunctivitis, although this recommendation is not accepted by all investigators. Varney *et al.* (1991) pointed out that patients with perennial asthma should be specifically excluded, but this recommendation appears to be important only if asthma is moderately severe or severe.

Other Routes for Allergen Administration

The usual route of administration of SIT is the subcutaneous one. Recent studies have examined the efficacy of oral SIT in asthma. In grass and birch pollen asthma, oral SIT is ineffective even when administered at a high dose (Cooper *et al.*, 1984; Rebien *et al.*, 1987), whereas a recent Chinese study showed efficacy in mugwort asthma (Leng *et al.*, 1990). There are no data on nasal SIT in asthma. Sublingual SIT is currently under investigation but definite results are not available yet.

House Dust Mite Asthma

House dust mites of the species *Dermatophagoides* are among the most prevalent perennial allergens throughout the world and have been shown to cause asthma, especially during childhood (Platts Mills and De Weck, 1989; Platts Mills *et al.*, 1989).

Efficacy

Symptom-medication scores

Review of the literature (Table 5.1) indicates that SIT with mites is more effective than with house dust (McAllen, 1961; British Tuberculosis Association, 1968; Aas, 1971; Maunsell *et al.*, 1971; Smith, 1971; D'Souza *et al.*, 1973; Tuchinda and Chai, 1973; Taylor *et al.*, 1974; Bessot *et al.*, 1975; Gaddie *et al.*, 1976; Gabriel *et al.*, 1977; Marques and Avila, 1978; Newton *et al.*, 1978; Warner *et al.*, 1978; British Thoracic Association, 1979; Smith and Pizzaro, 1982; Formgren *et al.*, 1984; Pauli *et al.*, 1984; Price *et al.*, 1984; Bousquet *et al.*, 1985a, 1988a, 1990b; Mosbech *et al.*, 1988, 1989a,b, 1990a,b; Wahn *et al.*, 1988; Van Bever and Stevens, 1989; Mosbech, 1990; Machiels *et al.*, 1990). Although some studies are conclusive (Aas, 1971), SIT with house dust extracts should not be used any more, owing to the great heterogeneity of house dust and the impossibility of appropriately standardizing house dust extracts (Malling *et al.*, 1986; Thompson *et al.*, 1989). Both asthma and rhinitis have been

Table 5.1
Controlled studies of the effect of immunotherapy with house dust mite extracts

Author	Age (years)	N	Allergen	Extraction protocol	Duration of treatment	Study design	Symptoms	Bronchial challenge	Non-specific hyperreactivity
Bessot	–	44	Der p/HD	Aluminium-adjuved	> 6 months	dbc	Improved	Improved ipr	
Bousquet	14–36	27	Der p	Standardized, rush	7 weeks	dbpc		Improved ipr, lpr	
Bousquet	5–72	150	Der p	Standardized, rush	1 year	c:u	Improved		
Crimi	13–57	22	Der p + f	Standarized, bronchial	9 weeks	dbpc		Improved: ipr ns: lpr	
D'Souza	10–50	96	Der p	Aqueous, classical	1 year	dbpc	Improved		
Formgren		35	Der f	Standardized, rush	1 year	dbpc	Improved	Improved lpr	ns
Gabriel	8–ad	66	Der p	Aqueous, classical	1 year	dbpc	Improved		
Gaddie	13–68	55	Der p	Tyrosine-adsorbed	1 year	dbpc	ns		
Machiels	16–57	39	Der p	Der p-ab complexes	1 year	dbpc	Improved	Improved, epr	Improved
Marques	12–55	28	Der p	Tyrosine-adsorbed	1 year	dbpc	Improved		
Maunsell	16–56	34	Der f/HD	Aqueous, classical	6–9 months	dbc	Improved		

Mosbech	18–56	46	Der p	Standardized	18 months	c:u	Improved 1 year ns: 18 months	ns	ns
				PEG-adjuved	18 months	c:u	ns	ns	ns
Newton	18–44	14	Der p	Alum-pyridine	1 year	dbpc	ns	Improved ipr	
Pauli	19–40	18	Der p	Tyrosine-adsorbed	1 year	dbpc	ns		
Price	5–15	51	Der p	Tyrosine-adsorbed	2 years	dbpc	Improved		
A.P. Smith	11–48	22	Der p/SS	Aqueous, classical	1 year	dbc	Improved		
J.M. Smith	7–21	30	Der p/HD	Aqueous, classical		dbc	ns		
Van Bever	7–15	24	Der p	Standardized, semi-rush	1 year	c:u		Improved ipr, lpr	
Wahn	8–15	24	Der p	Standardized, classical	2 years			Improved ipr	
Warner	5–14	85	Der p	Tyrosine-adsorbed	1 year	dbpc	Improved	Improved lpr	
BTS		46	Der p	Aluminium-adjuved	4–18 months	dbpc	ns		

Der p: *Dermatophagoides pteronyssinus*, Der f: *Dermatophagoides farinae*, HD: house dust, SS: human skin scales
PEG: polyethylene glycol-adjuved allergen
dbpc: double-blind placebo-controlled; dbc: double-blind controlled; c:u: untreated control group; ns: non significant results; ipr: immediate phase reaction; lpr: late phase reaction.

Modified from Bousquet *et al.* (1990b).

improved with mite SIT, but there are some inconclusive data, and standardized extracts have been used in a few studies only.

Using aqueous or standardized mite extracts (D'Souza *et al.*, 1973; Gaddie *et al.*, 1976; Lessof, 1983; Formgren *et al.*, 1984; Bousquet *et al.*, 1985a, 1988a), many studies found that patients treated with mite extract were significantly protected in comparison with the placebo or the control groups. However, the results were not always impressive (Mosbech *et al.*, 1989a) especially in adults. Using rush SIT, efficacy was noticeable after a few weeks of treatment. Bousquet and co-workers examined who would be candidates for mite SIT (Bousquet *et al.*, 1988a). Two hundred and fifteen patients were enrolled in a controlled trial. They were followed-up for 1 year by means of symptom-medication scores and pulmonary function tests (Figs 5.3 and 5.4). One hundred and fifty eight received allergen injections and the others were taken as a control group. Patients who had other perennial allergies, or aspirin intolerance and/or chronic sinusitis did not improve. Moreover, among the patients allergic only to *Dermatophagoides pteronyssinus*, children

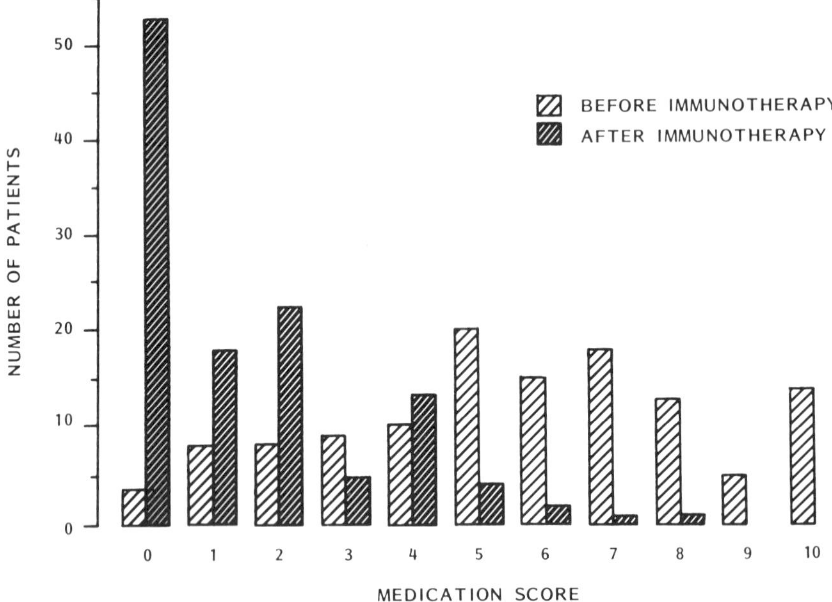

Fig. 5.3 Medication score in 125 asthmatic patients before and after immunotherapy with a standardized *Dermatophagoides pteronyssinus* extract ($P < 0.00001$). Patients used as control group (no immunotherapy) did not present any significant change in medication scores during the survey period. (From Bousquet *et al.*, 1988a.)

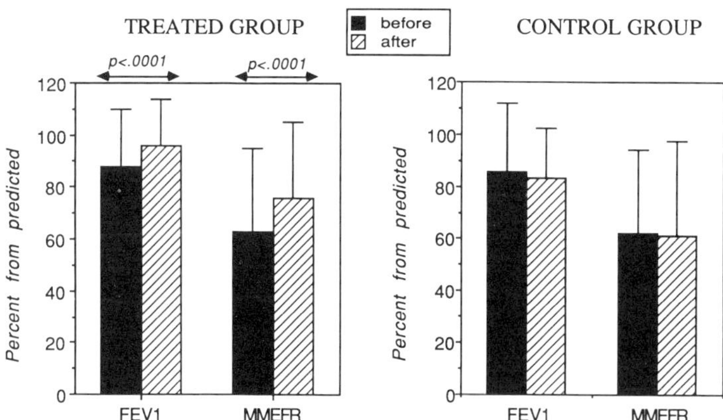

Fig. 5.4 Evolution of the pulmonary function tests in 125 asthmatics treated with a standardized *Dermatophagoides pteronyssinus* extract for 1 year (treated group) and in 25 control patients (control group) who were tested at 1 year intervals. (From Bousquet *et al.*, 1988a.)

presented a significantly greater improvement than adults (Fig. 5.5) and patients with irreversible airflow limitation (FEV_1 under 70% from predicted values after an adequate pharmacologic treatment) did not benefit from SIT (Fig. 5.5).

With other extracts, results are more variable. One study done with a pyridine-extracted *D. pteronyssinus* extract showed with aluminium no major difference between the placebo and the control groups (Newton *et al.*, 1978). With tyrosine-adsorbed *D. pteronyssinus* extracts, it was noticed that asthmatic children were significantly protected in comparison to placebo, whereas results in adults were not always conclusive (Warner *et al.*, 1978; Marques and Avila, 1978; Pauli *et al.*, 1984) and efficacy was only seen after long-term allergen administration. A study with polyethylene glycol (PEG)-modified extracts was inconclusive (Newton *et al.*, 1978; Mosbech *et al.*, 1989a,b; 1990a,b). Machiels *et al.* (1990) used allergen-antibody complexes made from allergens of *D. pteronyssinus* and an excess of purified autologous specific antibodies to treat patients and claimed that the treatment was safe and highly effective, as assessed by symptoms scores and bronchial challenge with allergen. However, the complexes are difficult to prepare and until human monoclonal antibodies become available, it will be difficult to apply this technique to a large scale.

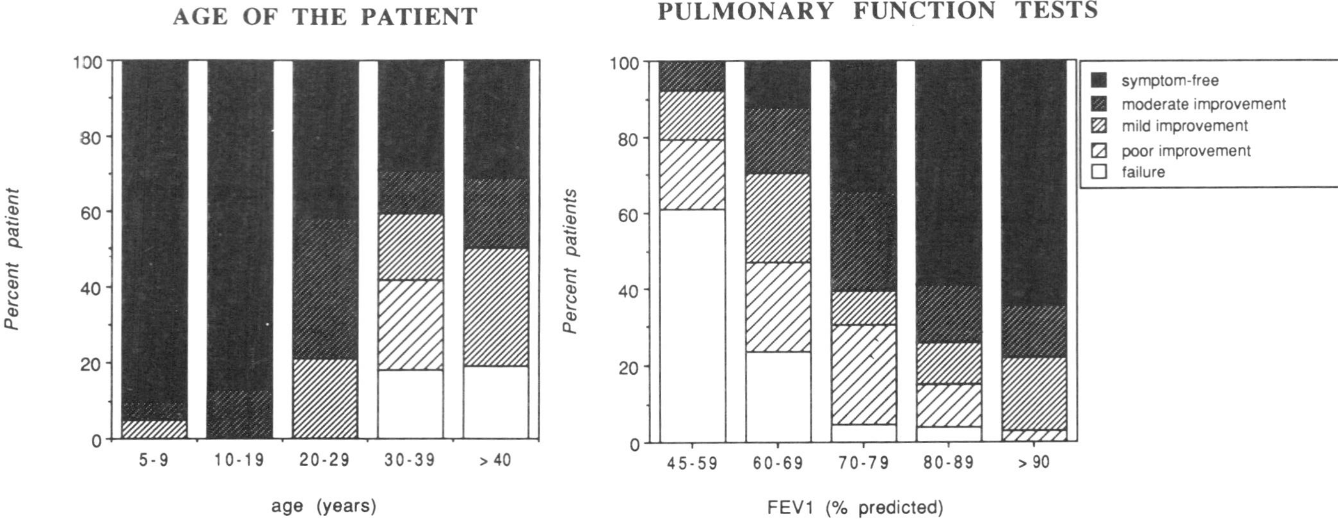

Fig. 5.5 Efficacy of immunotherapy with a standardized *Dermatophagoides pteronyssinus* extract in 125 patients according to their age and pulmonary function test. (From Bousquet *et al.*, 1988a.)

Bronchial challenges

Bronchial challenges with mite extracts confirmed symptom scores, since the threshold dose eliciting an immediate bronchial obstruction was increased (McAllen, 1961; D'Souza *et al.*, 1973; Bousquet *et al.*, 1985a; Wahn *et al.*, 1988) after treatment and even more important, the late phase reaction was inhibited (Warner *et al.*, 1978; Bousquet *et al.*, 1985a; Van Bever *et al.*, 1988). Crimi *et al.* (1991) used the so-called "local immunotherapy" in which allergens are administered by inhalation concomitantly with cromoglycate in order to reduce possible bronchoconstriction due to allergens. In a double-blind placebo-controlled study performed in 22 patients, they showed a reduction of the early but not the late reaction to allergen during bronchial challenge.

Non-specific bronchial hyperreactivity

BHR is a cardinal feature of asthma which can be decreased by allergen avoidance (Platts Mills *et al.*, 1982). Bousquet *et al.* (1987a) found that after 1–4 years of treatment with a standardized *D. pteronyssinus* extract, treated patients had a lower sensitivity to carbachol (i.e. reduced BHR) than untreated patients, but the difference was significant only in patients allergic to *D. pteronyssinus*. Similar results were observed by Machiels *et al.* (1990). On the other hand, Murray *et al.* (1985) observed a slight but insignificant increase in BHR to histamine in 7 children treated with a mite extract for 1 year, whereas 4 subjects treated with placebo had a small reduction. However, with such a low number of patients, no conclusion can be drawn from this study. Mosbech *et al.* (1989b) observed with *D. pteronyssinus* PEG-modified or standardized extracts that BHR was decreased after 1 year of treatment, but returned to normal values during the second year of treatment.

Taken together, these studies suggest that mite SIT is only effective under optimal conditions including an appropriate selection of patients and the use of high-quality extracts administered with an adequate schedule.

Safety

The safety of mite SIT is critical since many, if not most patients who recently died from an allergen injection were asthmatics and, in these patients, death was caused by an irreversible bronchial obstruction. Although some investigators suggest that SIT is indicated in severe patients, Bousquet and co-workers performed a controlled study in over

1000 patients who received the same maintenance dose using a rush or a step procedure (Bousquet *et al.*, 1989a; Hejjaoui *et al.*, 1990). Most patients with FEV_1 under 70% of predicted values developed asthma during SIT, highlighting the importance of avoiding SIT in severe asthmatics (Fig. 5.6). The age of the patient also appears to be of importance. Children under 5 years of age present a significantly greater risk of systemic reaction (Hejjaoui *et al.*, 1990). The symptoms of the systemic reactions were different in pollen and mite allergic individuals. In the latter group, as expected, bronchial symptoms were more prevalent than either urticaria or anaphylaxis (Fig. 5.7), whereas in pollen allergic individuals, asthma was less common (Fig. 5.2). Attempts have been made to reduce systemic reactions and, as in the case of pollen immunotherapy, it was observed that premedication and exclusion of severe asthmatics led to an acceptable rate of mild systemic reactions (Fig. 5.7).

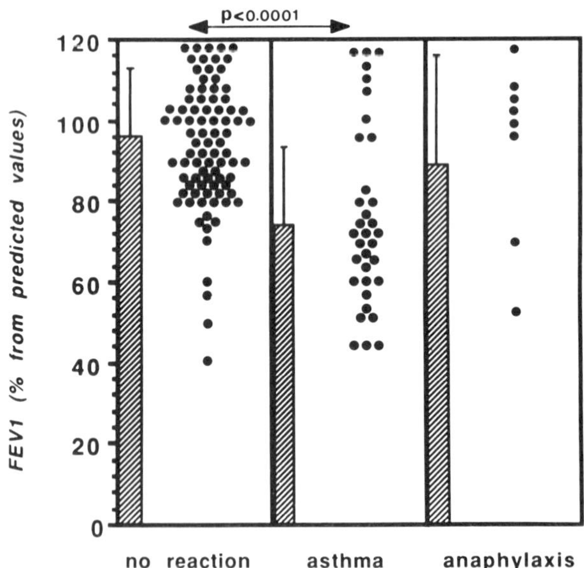

Fig. 5.6 Incidence of systemic reactions observed in asthmatic patients undergoing immunotherapy with standardized *Dermatophagoides pteronyssinus* extract according to their pulmonary function. Patients with $FEV_1 < 70\%$ had a great incidence of asthma. (From Bousquet *et al.*, 1989a.)

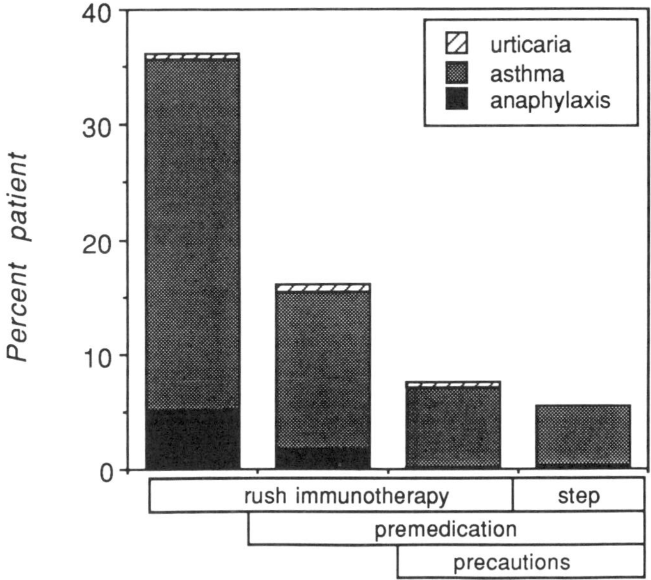

Fig. 5.7 Systemic side reactions observed in asthmatic patients undergoing immunotherapy with a standardized *Dermatophagoides pteronyssinus* extract. (From Hejjaoui *et al.*, 1990.)

Indications

The indication of SIT in mite allergy is not easy to propose and definite indications will not be available until the NIH-sponsored study on mite allergy has been published. From the current studies, the following recommendations may be proposed: (1) Only patients with house dust mites as perennial allergens should be treated. (2) Patients with aspirin intolerance or non-specific triggers of asthma such as chronic sinusitis should not receive SIT. (3) Efficacy and safety studies suggest that patients with irreversible airflow obstruction (FEV_1 under 70% of predicted after an adequate pharmacologic treatment) should not receive SIT. (4) The age of the patient should also be considered. On the one hand, children and young adults usually respond more efficiently to SIT but, on the other hand, children under 5 years of age may not receive SIT because of an increased risk of systemic reactions, an increased severity of the systemic reactions and also because the sensitivity of young patients may vary.

Duration

The duration of SIT with mite extracts is still a subject of debate. Price *et al.* (1984) stopped SIT after 1 year of treatment in half of the children enrolled in a double-blind placebo-controlled study and noticed that most children who stopped SIT presented a relapse within a year after the end of the treatment. Bousquet *et al.* (1990b) observed 10 patients (out of 250 followed over 3 years) who completely lost their sensitivity to *Dermatophagoides pteronyssinus* after 3 years of SIT (negative skin tests, radioallergosorbent test (RAST) and nasal challenge) which led them to stop the treatment. The symptoms and signs of allergy reappeared between 6 and 18 months in six of them. In an unpublished study, Bousquet and co-workers followed 40 asthmatics who received SIT with the same schedule of a standardized *D. pteronyssinus* extract and who, after a duration of SIT ranging from 18 to 96 months, were symptom-free without any pharmacological treatment and presented normal pulmonary function tests. SIT was stopped and patients were followed for up to 3 years every 6 months. The rate of relapse was dependent on the duration of SIT. When SIT was performed for between 18 and 35 months, the rate of relapse was 65% versus 35% in patients with an SIT duration of over 36 months. The estimation of duration of SIT efficacy was carried out using the Kaplan–Meier test. The mean duration of efficacy was 16.0 ± 21.7 months in patients with a SIT duration under 35 months and 32.2 ± 25.2 months ($P < 0.03$) in patients with a duration of SIT of over 36 months.

Asthma to Animal Proteins

Although it has been recommended by the position papers of the European Academy of Allergy and Clinical Immunology (Malling, 1988) and WHO/IUIS (Thompson *et al.*, 1989) that allergen avoidance is preferred to SIT in animal dander allergy, SIT may be envisaged. There are studies showing that SIT is effective in improving the threshold dose inducing positive bronchial challenges with cat or dog dander extract in asthmatic subjects (Taylor *et al.*, 1978; Ohman *et al.*, 1984; Hedlin *et al.*, 1986, 1991; Sundin *et al.*, 1986; Valovirta *et al.*, 1986; Rohatgi *et al.*, 1988; Van Metre *et al.*, 1988; Bertelsen *et al.*, 1989; Bucur *et al.*, 1989; Lilja *et al.*, 1989). One study found that ocular and pulmonary symptoms were significantly delayed on exposure to living cats in the treated group by comparison with either pretreatment and/or the placebo groups (Ohman *et al.*, 1984). However, the clinical efficacy of cat or dog SIT remains to be ascertained since the only two papers examining peak flow rates and symptom-medication scores were inconclusive (Sundin *et al.*, 1986; Lilja *et al.*, 1989). Moreover, BHR was unchanged in all studies with dog extracts and only decreased in one study with cat extracts.

Asthma to Moulds

Moulds are major allergens in asthma but they often induce polysensitizations and the quality of extracts available in the early 1980s was far from being adequate (Yunginger *et al.*, 1976; Aukrust, 1980; Agarwal *et al.*, 1982) so that it was proposed to avoid mould SIT (Salvaggio and Aukrust, 1981). However, efforts have been made to standardize extracts of some moulds such as *Alternaria* and *Cladosporium*, and good-quality allergen extracts are now available (Aukrust, 1980; Yunginger *et al.*, 1980; Helm *et al.*, 1987, 1988). SIT with standardized *Cladosporium* (Dreborg *et al.*, 1986; Karlsson *et al.*, 1986; Malling *et al.*, 1986) and *Alternaria* extracts (Horst *et al.*, 1990) was therefore started and variable results were obtained. In Nordic countries, patients treated with a standardized *Cladosporium* extract were polysensitized and SIT was found to be effective in challenges with the specific allergen but symptom-medication scores were only minimally improved by SIT (Dreborg *et al.*, 1986; Karlsson *et al.*, 1986; Malling *et al.*, 1986). On the other hand, in the double-blind placebo-controlled study of Horst *et al.* (1990) performed over 1 year in 24 highly selected patients allergic only to *Alternaria*, both challenges and symptom-medication scores were improved in the treated group and remained unchanged in the placebo group (Fig. 5.8). Metzger *et al.* (1983) found that *Alternaria* SIT with an uncharacterized extract improved both specific and non-specific bronchial challenges.

SIT with *Cladosporium* induced a high number of systemic reactions (Dreborg *et al.*, 1986; Karlsson *et al.*, 1986; Malling *et al.*, 1986) whereas SIT with *Alternaria* was better tolerated, possibly because Horst *et al.* (1990) attempted to define an "optimal maintenance dose" before starting SIT. Long-term safety of mould SIT has also been questioned and type III allergic reactions have been described (Busse *et al.*, 1976; Kaad and Østergaard, 1982).

These studies indicate that mould SIT may be effective in asthma, but they do not, however, favour SIT with mould species or with extracts of unknown quality (Malling, 1988; Thompson *et al.*, 1989).

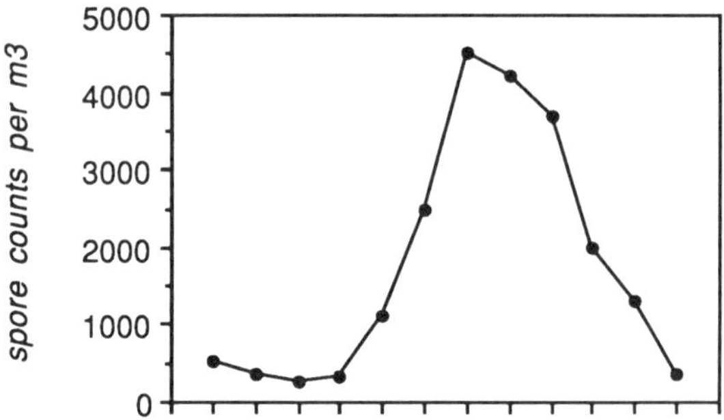

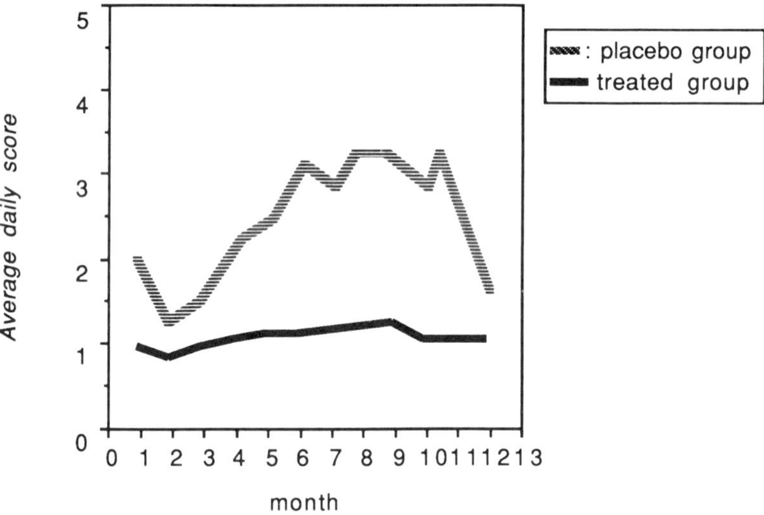

Fig. 5.8 Bronchial symptom-medication scores of patients receiving immunotherapy with a standardized *Alternaria* extract or placebo. (From Horst *et al.*, 1990.)

Immunotherapy with Other Extracts

Although SIT may be administered by oral or sublingual routes, there is no controlled study showing that it is effective in asthma with perennial allergens. SIT with extracts of undefined allergens (bacteria, foods, *Candida albicans*, insect dusts, etc.) should not be used any longer in clinical practice, but controlled trials may be started (Malling, 1988; Thompson *et al.*, 1989).

Conclusions

Specific immunotherapy was introduced in 1911 and for many years remained based on empiricism. Although this form of treatment has been seriously criticized, it still represents an effective treatment of allergic diseases and asthma. Administered with care by specialists, it has gained an increased safety. Using high-quality extracts, SIT may be envisaged in severe pollinosis and mite asthma, though its use may be questioned in asthma due to animal dander and moulds. New forms of SIT have been made available, but oral and sublingual routes deserve further studies. Speculations on the prevention of asthma by administering SIT in patients with rhinitis are currently being tested. New technologies might lead to improved forms of immunologic treatment and immunotherapy may be one of the treatments of the future.

References

Aas, K. (1971). Hyposensitization in house dust allergy asthma. A double-blind controlled study with evaluation of the effect on bronchial sensitivity to house dust. *Acta Paed. Scand.* **60**, 264–268.

Agarwal, M.K., Jones, R.T. and Yunginger, J.W. (1982). Immunochemical and physico-chemical characterization of commercial *Alternaria* extracts: a model for standardization of mold allergen extracts. *J. Allergy Clin. Immunol.* **70**, 432–436.

Armentia, A., Blanco, A. and Martin, J.M. (1989). Rush immunotherapy with a standardized Bermuda grass pollen extract. *Ann. Allergy* **63**, 127–135.

Aukrust, L. (1980). Allergens in *Cladosporium herbarum*. *In* "Advances in Allergology and Applied Immunology" (A. Oehling, I. Glazer, E. Mathov and C. Arbesman, eds), pp. 475–481. Pergamon Press, New York.

Barnes, P.J. (1989). New concepts in the pathogenesis of bronchial hyperresponsiveness and asthma. *J. Allergy Clin. Immunol.* **83**, 1013–1026.

Bertelsen, A., Andersen, J.B., Christensen, J., Ingemann, L., Kristensen, T. and Østergaard, P.A. (1989). Immunotherapy with dog and cat extracts in children. *Allergy* **44**, 330–335.

Bessot, J.C., Moreau, G. and Lenz, D. (1975). Etude comparative d'un essai de désensibilisation "en double-insu" aux extraits de poussière et aux extraits d'acariens. *Rev. Franç. Allergol.* **15**, 73–83.

Boulet, L.P., Cartier, A., Thompson, N.C., Roberts, R.S., Dolovich, J. and Hargreave, F.E. (1983). Asthma and increases in nonallergic bronchial responsiveness from seasonal pollen exposure. *J. Allergy Clin. Immunol.* **71**, 399–406.

Bousquet, J., Calvayrac, P., Guérin, B., Hejjaoui, A., Dhivert, H., Hewitt, B. and Michel, F.B. (1985a). Immunotherapy with a standardized *Dermatophagoides pteronyssinus* extract. I. *In vivo* and *in vitro* parameters after a short course of treatment. *J. Allergy Clin. Immunol.* **76**, 734–744.

Bousquet, J., Guérin, B., Dotte, A., Dhivert, H., Djoukhadar, F. and Michel, F.B. (1985b). Comparison between rush immunotherapy with a standardized allergen and an alum adjuved pyridine extracted material in grass pollen allergy. *Clin. Allergy* **15**, 179–194.

Bousquet, J., Clauzel, A.M. and Hejjaoui, A. (1987a). Non-specific bronchial hyperreactivity in asthmatic subjects after immunotherapy with a standardized mite extract. *Am. Rev. Respir. Dis.* **135**, A 135.

Bousquet, J., Godard, P. and Michel, F.B. (1987b). Asthma in adults. *In* "Highlights in Asthmology" (F.B. Michel, J. Bousquet and P. Godard, eds), pp. 394–398. Springer Verlag, Berlin.

Bousquet, J., Hejjaoui, A. and Clauzel, A.M. (1988a). Specific immunotherapy with a standardized *Dermatophagoides pteronyssinus* extract. II. Prediction of efficacy of immunotherapy. *J. Allergy Clin. Immunol.* **82**, 971–977.

Bousquet, J., Maasch, H.J. and Martinot, B. (1988b). Double-blind placebo controlled immunotherapy with mixed grass pollen allergoids. II. Comparison between parameters assessing the efficacy of immunotherapy. *J. Allergy Clin. Immunol.* **82**, 439–446.

Bousquet, J., Hejjaoui, A., Dhivert, H., Clauzel, A.M. and Michel, F.B. (1989a). Specific immunotherapy with a standardized *Dermatophagoides pteronyssinus* extract. III. Systemic reactions during the rush protocol in patients suffering from asthma. *J. Allergy Clin. Immunol.* **83**, 797–801.

Bousquet, J., Maasch, H. and Hejjaoui, A. (1989b). Double-blind placebo controlled immunotherapy with mixed grass pollen allergoids. III. Comparison of an unfractionated allergoid, a fractionated allergoid and a standardized orchard grass pollen extract in rhinitis, conjunctivitis and asthma. *J. Allergy Clin. Immunol.* **84**, 546–556.

Bousquet, J., Chanez, P. and Lacoste, J.Y. (1990a). Eosinophilic inflammation in asthma. *New Engl. J. Med.* **323**, 1033–1039.

Bousquet, J., Hejjaoui, A. and Michel, F.B. (1990b). Specific immunotherapy in asthma. *J. Allergy Clin. Immunol.* **86**, 292–306.

Bousquet, J., Hejjaoui, A., Soussana, M. and Michel, F.B. (1990c). Double-blind, placebo-controlled immunotherapy with mixed grass-pollen allergoids. IV. Comparison of the safety and efficacy of two dosages of a high-molecular weight allergoid. *J. Allergy Clin. Immunol.* **85**, 490–497.

Bousquet, J., Becker, W.M., Hejjaoui, A., Cour, P., Chanal, I., Lebel, B., Dhivert, H. and Michel, F.B. (1991a). Clinical and immunological reactivity of patients allergic to grass pollens and to multiple pollen species. II. Efficacy of a double-blind, placebo-controlled, specific immunotherapy with standardized extracts. *J. Allergy Clin. Immunol.* **88**, 43–53.

Bousquet, J., Hejjaoui, A., Becker, W.M., Cour, P., Chanal, I., Lebel, B., Dhivert, H. and Michel, F.B. (1991b). Clinical and immunological reactivity of patients allergic to grass pollens and to multiple pollen species. I. Clinical and immunological reactivity. *J. Allergy Clin. Immunol.* **87**, 737–746.

Bousquet, J., Lacoste, J.Y. and Chanez, P. (1993). Alteration of bronchial elastic fibers in normal subjects, asthmatic and chronic bronchitis patients. *J. Allergy Clin. Immunol.* (in press).

British Thoracic Association (1979). A trial of house dust mite extract in bronchial asthma. *Br. J. Dis. Chest* **73**, 260–270.

British Tuberculosis Association (1968). Treatment of house dust allergy. *Br. Med. J.* **3**, 774–777.

Bruce, C.A., Norman, P.S., Rosenthal, R.R. and Lichtenstein, L.M. (1977). The role of ragweed pollen in autumnal asthma. *J. Allergy Clin. Immunol.* **59**, 449–459.

Bucur, J., Dreborg, S. and Einarsson, R. (1989). Immunotherapy with dog and cat allergen preparations in dog-sensitive and cat-sensitive asthmatics. *Ann. Allergy* **62**, 355–359.

Busse, W.W., Storms, W.W., Flaherty, D.K., Crandall, M. and Reed, C.E. (1976). *Alternaria* IgG precipitins and adverse reactions. *J. Allergy Clin. Immunol.* **57**, 367–372.

Committee on Safety of Medicine (1986). Desensitizing vaccines. *Br. Med. J.* **293**, 948.

Cooper, P.J., Darbyshire, J., Nunn, A.J. and Warner, J.O. (1984). A controlled trial of oral hyposensitization in pollen asthma and rhinitis in children. *Clin. Allergy* 14, 541–550.

Creticos, P.S., Marsh, D.G. and Proud, D. (1989). Responses to ragweed-pollen nasal challenge before and after immunotherapy. *J. Allergy Clin. Immunol.* **84**, 197–205.

Crimi, E., Voltolini, S. and Troise, C. (1991). Local immunotherapy with *Dermatophagoides* extract in asthma. *J. Allergy Clin. Immunol.* **87**, 721–728.

Djuranovic, R., Roche, W.R. and Wilson, J.H. (1990). Mucosal inflammation in asthma. *Am. Rev. Respir. Dis.* **142**, 434–457.

Dreborg, S. and Akerblom, E.B. (1990). Immunotherapy with monomethoxypoly-ethylene glycol modified allergens. *Critic. Rev. Ther. Drug Carrier Syst.* **6**, 315–365.

Dreborg, S., Agrell, B., Foucard, T., Kjellman, N.I.M., Koivikko, A. and Nilsson, S. (1986). A double-blind, multicenter immunotherapy trial in children using a purified and standardized *Cladosporium herbarum* preparation. I. Clinical results. *Allergy* **41**, 131–140.

Dreborg, S., Mosbech, H. and Weeke, B. (1988). Immunotherapy (hyposensitization) and bronchial asthma. *In* "Clinical Immunology and Allergy" (A.B. Kay, ed.), vol. 2, pp. 245–258. Baillière Tindall, London.

D'Souza, M.E., Pepys, J., Wells, I.D., Tai, E., Palmer, F., Overell, B.G., McGrath, I.T. and Megson, M. (1973). Hyposensitization with *Dermatophagoides pteronyssinus* in house dust allergy: a controlled study of clinical and immunological effects. *Clin. Allergy* **3**, 177–193.

Durham, S.R., Varney, V., Gaga, M., Frew, A.J., Jacobson, M. and Kay, A.B. (1991). Immunotherapy and allergic inflammation. *Clin. Exp. Allergy* **21**, suppl. 1, 206–210.

Formgren, H., Lanner, A., Linholm, N., Löwhagen, O. and Dreborg, S. (1984). Effects of immunotherapy on specific and non-specific sensitivity of the airways. *J. Allergy Clin. Immunol.* **73**, 140.

Frankland, A.W. and Augustin, R. (1954). Prophylaxis of summer hay fever and asthma. A controlled trial comparing crude grass pollen extracts with the isolated main protein component. *Lancet* **i**, 1055–1057.

Gabriel, M., Ng, H.K., Allan, W.G.L., Hill, L.E. and Nunn, A.J. (1977). Study of prolonged hyposensitization with *D. pteronyssinus* extract. *Clin. Allergy* **7**, 325–336.

Gaddie, J., Skinner, C. and Palmer, K.N.V. (1976). Hyposensitization with house dust mite vaccine in bronchial asthma. *Br. Med. J.* **2**, 561–562.

Grammer, L.C., Shaughnessy, M.A. and Suszko, I.M. (1984). Persistence of efficacy after a brief course of polymerized ragweed allergens: a controlled study. *J. Allergy Clin. Immunol.* **73**, 484–489.

Grant, I.W.B. (1986). Does immunotherapy have a role in the treatment of asthma. *Clin. Allergy* **16**, 7–16.

Hedlin, G., Graff-Lonnevig, V. and Heilborn, H. (1986). Immunotherapy with cat- and dog-dander extracts. II. *In vivo* and *in vitro* effects observed in 1-year double-blind placebo study. *J. Allergy Clin. Immunol.* **77**, 488–496.

Hedlin, G., Silber, G. and Schieken, L. (1989). Attenuation of allergen sensitivity early in the course of ragweed immunotherapy. *J. Allergy Clin. Immunol.* **84**, 390–399.

Hedlin, G., Graff-Lonnevig, V. and Heilborn, H. (1991). Immunotherapy with cat- and dog-dander extracts. V. Effects of 3 years of treatment. *J. Allergy Clin. Immunol.* **87**, 955–964.

Hejjaoui, A., Dhivert, H., Michel, F.B. and Bousquet, J. (1990). Specific immunotherapy with a standardized *Dermatophagoides pteronyssinus* extract. IV. Systemic reactions according to the immunotherapy schedule. *J. Allergy Clin. Immunol.* **85**, 473–479.

Hejjaoui, A., Ferrando, R., Michel, F.B. and Bousquet, J. (1993). Systemic reactions occurring during immunotherapy with standardized pollen extracts. *J. Allergy Clin. Immunol.* (in press).

Helm, R.M., Squillace, D.L. and Aukrust, L. (1987). Production of an international reference standard *Alternaria* extract. I. Testing of candidate extract. *Int. Arch. Allergy Appl. Immunol.* **82**, 178–189.

Helm, R.M., Squillace, D.L. and Yunginger, J.W. (1988). Production of an international reference standard *Alternaria* extract. II. Results of a collaborative trial. *J. Allergy Clin. Immunol.* **81**, 651–663.

Hill, D.J., Hosking, C.S., Shelton, M.J. and Turner, K.W. (1982). Failure of hyposensitization in treatment of children with grass-pollen asthma. *Br. Med. J.* **284**, 306–309.

Horst, M., Hejjaoui, A., Horst, V., Michel, F.B. and Bousquet, J. (1990). Double-blind placebo-controlled immunotherapy with a standardized *Alternaria* extract. *J. Allergy Clin. Immunol.* **85**, 460–472.

Ilioupoulos, O., Proud, D. and Adkinson, N.F. (1991). Effects of immunotherapy on the early, late and rechallenge nasal reaction to provocation with allergen: changes in inflammatory mediators and cells. *J. Allergy Clin. Immunol.* **87**, 855–856.

Johnstone, D.E. and Dutton, A. (1968). The value of hyposensitization therapy for bronchial asthma in children. *Pediatrics* **42**, 793–802.

Juniper, E.F., Roberts, R.S., Kennedy, L.K., O'Connor, J., Syty-Golda, M., Dolovich, J. and Hargreave, F.E. (1985). Polyethylene glycol-modified ragweed pollen extract in rhinoconjunctivitis. *J. Allergy Clin. Immunol.* **75**, 578–585.

Juniper, E.F., O'Connor, J., Roberts, R.S., Evans, S., Hargreave, F.E. and Dolovich, J. (1986). Polyethylene glycol-modified ragweed extract: comparison of two treatment regimens. *J. Allergy Clin. Immunol.* **78**, 851–856.

Kaad, P.H. and Ostergaard, P.A. (1982). The hazard of mould hyposensitization in children with asthma. *Clin. Allergy* **12**, 317–320.

Karlsson, R., Agrell, B. and Dreborg, S. (1986). A double-blind multicenter immunotherapy trial in children, using a purified and standardized *Cladosporium herbarum* preparation. II. *In vitro* results. *Allergy* **41**, 140–147.

Kuna, P., Alam, R., Kuzminska, B. and Rozniecki, J. (1989). The effect of preseasonal immunotherapy on the production of histamine-releasing factor (HRF) by mononuclear cells from patients with seasonal asthma: results of a double-blind, placebo-controlled, randomized study. *J. Allergy Clin. Immunol.* **83**, 816–824.

Leng, X., Fu, F.X., Ye, S.T. and Duan, S.G. (1990). A double-blind trial of oral immunotherapy for *Artemisia* pollen asthma with evaluation of bronchial response to the pollen allergen and serum-specific IgE antibody. *Ann. Allergy* **64**, 27–31.

Lessof, M. (1983). Experience with Spectralgen(R)/Pharmalgen(R): a new kind of allergen preparation. Proceedings of an International Allergy Workshop, *Excerpta Medica*, Amsterdam, 88 pages.

Lichtenstein, L.M. (1978). An evaluation of the role of immunotherapy in asthma. *Am. Rev. Respir. Dis.* **117**, 191–193.

Lilja, G., Sundin, B. and Graft-Lonnevig, V. (1989). Immunotherapy with cat- and dog-dander extracts. IV. Effects of 2 years of treatment. *J. Allergy Clin. Immunol.* **83**, 37–44.

Machiels, J.J., Somville, M.A., Lebrun, P.M., Lebecque, S.J., Jacquemin, M.G. and Saint-Rémy, J.M.R. (1990). Allergic bronchial asthma due to *Dermatophagoides pteronyssinus* can be efficiently treated by inoculation of allergen-antibody complexes. *J. Clin. Invest.* **85**, 1024–1035.

Malling, H.J. (1988). Position paper of the European Academy of Allergy and Clinical Immunology: Specific Immunotherapy. *Allergy* suppl. 6, 431–463.

Malling, H.J., Dreborg, S. and Weeke, B. (1986). Diagnosis and immunotherapy of mould allergy. V. Clinical efficacy and side effects of immunotherapy with *Cladosporium herbarum*. *Allergy* **41**, 507–519.

Marques, R.A. and Avila, R. (1978). Results of a clinical trial with *Dermatophagoides pteronyssinus* tyrosine absorbed vaccine. *Allergol. Immunopathol.* **6**, 231–235.

Maunsell, K., Wraith, D.G. and Hugues, A.M. (1971). Hyposensitization in mite asthma. *Lancet* **1**, 967–968.

McAllen, M.K. (1961). Bronchial sensitivity testing in asthma. An assessment of the effect of hyposensitization in house-dust and pollen-sensitive asthmatic subjects. *Thorax* **16**, 30–37.

Metzger, W.J., Donnelly, A. and Richerson, H.B. (1983). Modification of late asthmatic responses (LAR) during immunotherapy for *Alternaria*-induced asthma. *J. Allergy Clin. Immunol.* **71**, 119.

Michel, F.B., Marty, J.P., Quet, L. and Cour, P. (1977). Penetration of inhaled pollen into respiratory tract. *Am. Rev. Respir. Dis.* **119**, 609–616.

Moller, C., Dreborg, S., Lanner, A. and Bjorksten, B. (1986). Oral immunotherapy of children with rhinoconjunctivitis due to birch pollen allergy. A double blind study. *Allergy* **41**, 271–279.

Mosbech, H. (1990). Who will benefit from hyposensitization? Predictive parameters in house dust mite allergic asthmatics. *Allergy* **45**, 209–212.

Mosbech, H. and Østerballe, O. (1988). Does the effect of immunotherapy last after termination of treatment? *Allergy* **43**, 523–529.

Mosbech, H., Dreborg, S. and Pählman, I. (1988). Modification of house dust mite allergens by monoethoxypolyethylene glycol. Allergenicity measured by *in vitro* and *in vivo* methods. *Int. Arch. Allergy Appl. Immunol.* **85**, 145–149.

Mosbech, H., Dreborg, S. and Frolund, L. (1989a). Hyposensitization in

asthmatics with mPEG modified and unmodified house dust mtie extract. I. Clinical effect evaluated by diary cards and a retrospective assessment. *Allergy* **44**, 487–498.
Mosbech, H., Dreborg, S. and Frolund, L. (1989b). Hyposensitization in asthmatics with mPEG modified and unmodified house dust mite extract. II. Effect evaluated by challenges with allergen and histamine. *Allergy* **44**, 499–509.
Mosbech, H., Dirksen, A. and Dreborg, S. (1990a). Hyposensitization in asthmatics with mPEG modified and unmodified house dust mite extract. IV. Occurrence and prediction of side effects. *Allergy* **45**, 142–150.
Mosbech, H., Djurup, R. and Dreborg, S. (1990b). Hyposensitization in asthmatics with mPEG modified and unmodified house dust mite extract. III. Effects on mite-specific immunological parameters and correlation to changes in mite-sensitivity and symptoms. *Allergy* **45**, 130–141.
Murray, A.B., Ferguson, A.C. and Morrison, B. (1985). Non-allergic bronchial hyperreactivity in asthmatic children decreases with age and increases with mite immunotherapy. *Ann. Allergy* **54**, 541–544.
Newton, D.A.G., Maberly, D.J. and Wilson, R. (1978). House dust mite hyposensitization. *Brit. J. Dis. Chest* **72**, 21–28.
Norman, P.S. (1987). Fatal misadventures. *J. Allergy Clin. Immunol.* **79**, 572–573.
O'Connor, G.T., Sparrow, D. and Weiss, S.T. (1989). The role of allergy and nonspecific airway hyperresponsiveness in the pathogenesis of chronic obstructive pulmonary disease. *Am. Rev. Respir. Dis.* **140**, 225–252.
Ohman, J.L., Findlay, S.R. and Leitermann, K.M. (1984). Immunotherapy in cat-induced asthma. Double-blind trial with evaluation of *in vivo* and *in vitro* responses. *J. Allergy Clin. Immunol.* **74**, 230–239.
Ortolani, C., Pastorello, E. and Moss, R.B. (1984). Grass pollen immunotherapy: a single year double blind placebo controlled study in patients with grass pollen induced asthma and rhinitis. *J. Allergy Clin. Immunol.* **73**, 283–290.
Østerballe, O. (1980). Immunotherapy in hay fever with two major allergens 19, 25 and partially purified extract of timothy grass pollen. A controlled double blind study. *In vivo* variables, season I. *Allergy* **35**, 473–489.
Paganin, F., Trussard, V. and Seneterre, E. (1993). High resolution computed tomography in asthma. *Am. Rev. Respir. Dis.* (in press).
Pauli, G., Bessot, J.C. and Bigot, H. (1984). Clinical and immunological evaluation of tyrosine adsorbed *Dermatophagoides pteronyssinus* extract: a double-blind placebo controlled trial. *J. Allergy Clin. Immunol.* **74**, 524–535.
Pauwells, R. (1989). The relationship between airway inflammation and bronchial hyperresponsiveness. *Clin. Exp. Allergy* **19**, 395–398.
Peat, J.K., Woolcock, A.J. and Cullen, K. (1987). Rate of decline of lung function in subjects with asthma. *Eur. J. Respir. Dis.* **70**, 171–179.
Platts Mills, T.A.E. and De Weck, A.L. (1989). House dust mites: a world wide problem. *J. Allergy Clin. Immunol.* **83**, 416–427.
Platts Mills, T.A.E., Mitchell, E.B. and Nock, P. (1982). Reduction of bronchial hyperreactivity in patients with asthma. *Lancet* **ii**, 675–678.
Platts Mills, T.A.E., Pollart, S.M., Luczynska, C.M., Chapman, M.D. and Heymann, P.W. (1989). The role of indoor allergens in asthma. *In* "Progress in Allergy and Clinical Immunology" (W.J. Pichler, ed.), pp. 279–286. Hogrefe & Huber, Toronto.
Pollart, S.M., Chapman, M.D., Fiocco, G.P., Rose, G. and Platts Mills, T.A.E.

(1989). Epidemiology of acute asthma: IgE antibodies to common allergens as a risk factor for emergency room visits. *J. Allergy Clin. Immunol.* **83**, 875–882.

Price, J.F., Warner, J.O.P., Hey, E.N., Turner, M.W. and Soothill, J.F. (1984). A controlled trial of hyposensitization with adsorbed tyrosine *Dermatophagoides pteronyssinus* antigen in childhood asthma: *in vivo* aspects. *Clin. Allergy* **14**, 209–220.

Rak, S., Löwhagen, O. and Venge, P. (1988). The effect of immunotherapy on bronchial hyperresponsiveness and eosinophil cationic protein in pollen-allergic patients. *J. Allergy Clin. Immunol.* **82**, 470–480.

Rebien, W., Puttonen, E., Maasch, H.J., Stix, E. and Wahn, U. (1987). Clinical and immunological response to oral and subcutaneous immunotherapy with grass pollen extracts. *Eur. J. Pediatr.* **38**, 341–344.

Reed, C.E. (1985). What we do and do not know about mold allergy and asthma. *J. Allergy Clin. Immunol.* **76**, 773–775.

Reid, M.J., Moss, R.B. and Hsu, Y.P. (1986). Seasonal asthma in Northern California: allergic causes and efficacy of immunotherapy. *J. Allergy Clin. Immunol.* **78**, 590–600.

Roche, W.R., Williams, J.H., Beasley, R. and Holgate, S.T. (1989). Subepithelial fibrosis in the bronchi of asthmatics. *Lancet* **i**, 520–524.

Rohatgi, N., Dunn, K. and Chai, H. (1988). Cat- or dog-induced immediate and late asthmatic responses before and after immunotherapy. *J. Allergy Clin. Immunol.* **82**, 389–397.

Salvaggio, J. and Aukrust, L. (1981). Mold-induced asthma. *J. Allergy Clin. Immunol.* **68**, 327–346.

Smith, A.P. (1971). Hyposensitization with *Dermatophagoides pteronyssinus* antigen: trial in asthma induced by house dust. *Brit. Med. J.* **4**, 204–206.

Smith, J.M. and Pizzaro, Y. (1982). Hyposensitization with extracts of *Dermatophagoides pteronyssinus* and house dust. *Clin. Allergy* **2**, 281–283.

Sotomayor, H., Badier, M. and Vervloet, D. (1984). Seasonal increase in carbachol airway responsiveness in patients allergic to grass pollen, *Am. Rev. Respir. Dis.* **130**, 56–65.

Sundin, B., Lilja, G. and Graft-Lonnevig, V. (1986). Immunotherapy with partially purified and standardized animal dander extracts. I. Clinical results from a double-blind study on patients with animal dander asthma. *J. Allergy Clin. Immunol.* **77**, 478–487.

Taylor, B., Sanders, S.S. and Norman, A.P. (1974). A double-blind controlled trial of house dust mite fortified vaccine in childhood asthma. *Clin. Allergy* **4**, 35–40.

Taylor, B., Ohman, J.L. and Lowell, F.C. (1978). Immunotherapy in cat-induced asthma. Double-blind trial of bronchial responses to cat allergen and histamine. *J. Allergy Clin. Immunol.* **61**, 283–287.

Thompson, R., Bousquet, J., Cohen, S., Frei, P.C., Jager, L., Lambert, P.H., Lessof, M.H., Loblay, R.H., Malling, H.J., Norman, P.S., De Weck, A.L. and Weeke, B. (1989). The current status of allergen immunotherapy (hyposensitization). Report of WHO/IUIS Working Group. *Lancet* **i**, 259–261.

Tsicopoulos, A., Tonnel, A.B. and Vorng, H. (1990). Lymphocyte-mediated inhibition of platelet cytotoxic functions during Hymenoptera venom desensitization: characterization of a suppressive lymphokine. *Eur. J. Immunol.* **20**, 1201–1207.

Tuchinda, M. and Chai, H. (1973). Effect of immunotherapy in chronic asthmatic children. *J. Allergy Clin. Immunol.* **51**, 131–138.
Valovirta, E., Viander, M., Koivikko, A., Vanto, T. and Ingemann, L. (1986). Immunotherapy in allergy to dog. Immunologic and clinical findings of a double blind study. *Ann. Allergy* **57**, 173–179.
Van Bever, H.P. and Stevens, W.J. (1989). Suppression of the late asthmatic reaction by hyposensitization in asthmatic children allergic to house dust mite (*Dermatophagoides pteronyssinus*). *Clin. Exp. Allergy* **19**, 399–404.
Van Bever, H.P., Bosmans, J., De Clerck, L.S. and Stevens, W.J. (1988). Modification of the late asthmatic reaction by hyposensitization in asthmatic children allergic to house dust mite (*Dermatophagoides pteronyssinus*) or grass pollen. *Allergy* **43**, 378–386.
Van der Zee, J.S. and Aalberse, R.C. (1987). The role of IgG. *In* "Allergy, an International Textbook" (H.M. Lessof, T.H. Lee and D.M. Kenedy, eds), pp. 49–68. John Wiley & Sons, Bath, UK.
Van Metre, T.E. Jr., Marsh, D.G. and Adkinson, N.F. Jr. (1986). Dose of cat (*Felix domesticus*) allergen (*Fel d 1*) that induces asthma. *J. Allergy Clin. Immunol.* **78**, 62–75.
Van Metre, T.E., Marsh, D.G. and Adkinson, N.F. Jr. (1988). Immunotherapy for cat asthma. *J. Allergy Clin. Immunol.* **82**, 1055–1068.
Varney, V.A., Gaga M., Aber, V.R., Kay, A.B. and Durham, S.R. (1991). Usefulness of immunotherapy in patients with severe summer hay fever uncontrolled by antiallergic drugs. *Brit. Med. J.* **302**, 265–269.
Wahn, U., Schweter, C., Lind, P. and Lowenstein, H. (1988). Prospective study on immunologic changes induced by two different *Dermatophagoides pteronyssinus* extracts prepared from whole mite culture and mite bodies. *J. Allergy Clin. Immunol.* **82**, 360–370.
Warner, J.O., Price, J.F. and Soothill, J.F. (1978). Controlled trial of hyposensitization to *Dermatophagoides pteronyssinus* in children with asthma. *Lancet* **ii**, 912–916.
Yunginger, J.W., Jones, R.T. and Gleich, G.J. (1976). Studies on *Alternaria* allergens. II. Measurement of the relative potency of commercial *Alternaria* extracts by the direct RAST and by RAST inhibition. *J. Allergy Clin. Immunol.* **58**, 405–413.
Yunginger, J.W., Jones, R.T., Nesheim, M.E. and Geller, M. (1980). Studies on *Alternaria* allergens. III. Isolation of a major allergenic fraction (*Alternaria* I.). *J. Allergy Clin. Immunol.* **66**, 138–147.

Discussion

A.R. Leff

Is it Dr Bousquet's conclusion that in adults over the age of 41 we should probably not think of immunotherapy as it now exists?

J. Bousquet

In mite allergic patients absolutely – I am not saying this in pollen because we did not test it.

A.R. Leff

From your approach, is there a way of thinking about starting first with the available drugs like inhaled bronchodilators and then going to immunotherapy, or do you think everyone who has allergy should have some form of immunotherapy?

J. Bousquet

Everyone who has allergy does not need immunotherapy. In fact, the international consensus on asthma suggests that with grass pollen immunotherapy should be given in the patients with a severe pollen allergy and in whom asthma is not controlled by conventional β_2-agonists. There is usually very severe hayfever in these patients and the patients who require inhaled steroids for their asthma have such a bad rhinitis that topical steroids are not sufficient. This means that we have very few patients switching – usually these patients have to be started on oral corticosteroids.

J.-A. Karlsson

I am interested in the long-term treatment. How does it compare with inhaled steroids, with which long-term treatment abolishes the inflammation, but 10 years later there is still almost the same degree of hyperreactivity? In your patients who you said had no symptoms after 3 years, has the inflammation gone and is there no evidence of bronchial hyperreactivity?

J. Bousquet

When it is used for mites and pollen allergies, the rate of success is 60% and all pharmacological treatment can be stopped. Immunotherapy is continued for 5 years, and then stopped. We have now followed several patients in this way, and there are usually no symptoms for many years. We are now following bronchial hyperreactivity in an ongoing study, to see if it comes back – but we do not have the data yet.

Part II

Eosinophils in Asthma

6

Possible Role of IL-5 Ligand-Receptor System in Eosinophilia

A. TOMINAGA,* Y. HITOSHI*‡ and K. TAKATSU*‡

*Department of Biology, Institute for Medical Immunology, Kumamoto University Medical School, 2-2-1 Honjo, Kumamoto 860, Japan

‡Department of Immunology, The Institute of Medical Science, The University of Tokyo, 4-6-1 Shiroganedai, Minato-Ku, Tokyo, 108, Japan

Introduction

Interleukin-5 (IL-5) has two histories. One is as a T cell-replacing factor which replaces the function of helper T cells in the differentiation process of antigen-stimulated B cell into immunoglobulin-secreting cells. This concept was proposed in the early 1970s (Schimpl and Wecker, 1972). We started to study this soluble mediator as one of the T cell-replacing factors (Takatsu *et al.*, 1988). At first, we used this activity to replace immune helper T cells in the IgG plaque-forming cell assay of antigen activated B cells as a functional assay for T cell-replacing factor (Takatsu *et al.*, 1970). The other history of IL-5 is as an eosinophil growth and differentiation factor. In 1970, Basten and Beeson (1970) reported the presence of a soluble factor which stimulates eosinophil proliferation from parasite-infected rat T-lymphocytes. It is now known that both B cell and eosinophil growth and differentiation activities are mediated by

T-Lymphocyte and Inflammatory Cell Research in Asthma
ISBN 0-12-388170-6

a single molecule. This was proved by establishing monoclonal antibodies against this molecule and by molecular cloning of the gene for it (Kinashi *et al.*, 1986, Harada *et al.*, 1987). We proposed it to be called interleukin-5 (IL-5) (Kinashi *et al.*, 1986).

Structure of IL-5

Both murine IL-5 (mIL-5) and human IL-5 (hIL-5) have been characterized by cloning, sequencing and expression (Kinashi *et al.*, 1986; Azuma *et al.*, 1986; Yokota *et al.*, 1987). The mIL-5 cDNA encodes a mature polypeptide of 113 amino acids, while the hIL-5 cDNA codes for a mature polypeptide of 115 amino acids. Both have a molecular weight of approximately 13 kDa. Comparison of the cDNA sequence of mIL-5 with that of hIL-5 shows sequence homology of 77% at the DNA level and 70% at the protein level. Recombinant IL-5 produced in mammalian cells has a molecular mass of 45–60 kDa, which is formed by dimerization of a glycoprotein with a molecular mass of 22–30 kDa (glycosylated form of 13 kDa polypeptides). Thus IL-5 is a disulphide-linked dimer that is unusual among the T cell-derived cytokines. This dimerization is essential for the biological activity of the IL-5 molecule (Takahashi *et al.*, 1990). Recent investigations have identified two conserved cysteine residues which cross-link the dimer in an anti-parallel arrangement (Minamitake *et al.*, 1990). The heterogeneity of IL-5 in molecular weight is predominantly due to the addition of *N*-glycosides, which can be removed to leave a fully active molecule (Tominaga *et al.*, 1990). The *N*-glycoside moieties of IL-5 are probably responsible for the stability of this molecule.

While mIL-5 and hIL-5 are equally active in human eosinophil assays, hIL-5 is 100-fold less active than mIL-5 in a murine early B cell line (Mita *et al.*, 1989a). McKenzie *et al.* (1991) clearly identified that the C-terminal region, consisting of 36 amino acids, is responsible for the full activity of IL-5 in the mouse cell assays by constructing mouse/human IL-5 hybrids. A small area of similarity near the C-terminal was originally identified among IL-3, IL-5 and granulocyte–macrophage colony-stimulating factor (GM-CSF) by cDNA sequence comparison (Kinashi *et al.*, 1986) and later this similarity was expanded to include IL-4 and IL-6 using the mutation data matrix based on frequencies of observed substitutions in real proteins over evolutionary time (Sanderson *et al.*, 1988).

IL-5 Transgenic Mouse

As a Tool to Confirm a Physiological Role of IL-5

We established an IL-5 transgenic mouse to confirm *in vitro* activities of IL-5 (Tominaga *et al.*, 1991). Mouse IL-5 cDNA was inserted in the exon of β globin gene and ligated to mouse metallothionein promoter. Expression of IL-5 was observed mainly in spleen, liver and bone marrow cells. Injection of $CdS0_4$ solution (20 μg/0.1 ml/mouse) intraperitoneally enhanced the activity of this promoter and a several-fold increase in the serum level of IL-5 was observed. As shown in Table 6.1, IL-5 is not detectable in the serum of normal mice (under 10 pg/ml). In IL-5 transgenic mice, we could detect 5–20 ng/ml in the sera. This level of IL-5 can also be observed in patients with eosinophilia. The predominant effect of IL-5 was an increased level of eosinophils in peripheral blood. The number of other cells such as lymphocytes, monocytes and neutrophils was doubled. There is no difference in the ratio of $CD4^+$ over $CD8^+$ or

Table 6.1
Characterization of IL-5 transgenic mice

	Control mice (C3H/HeN, 25 week)	IL-5 transgenic mice (Homozygotes, 25 week)
Serum IL-5 (ng/ml)	< 0.01	16.6 ± 13
Serum Ig (μg/ml)		
IgM	293 ± 9.0	1545 ± 261
IgG_1	736 ± 42	876 ± 26
IgG_{2a}	536 ± 24	512 ± 11
IgE	0.24 ± 0.045	2.30 ± 0.36
White blood cells (per mm^3)[a]		
Total	8737 ± 578	29 800 ± 1682
Eosinophils	186 ± 62	13 719 ± 1024
Lymphocytes	5757 ± 574	10 365 ± 845
Monocytes	337 ± 119	653 ± 60
Neutrophils	2460 ± 766	5 063 ± 189

Results are expressed as the mean ± S.E. of five female mice in each group at 25 weeks of age.

[a] Female mice at the age of 25 weeks were examined for their peripheral blood cell populations. Smears of peripheral blood were stained with May–Grünewald and Giemsa solution, and their cell types were examined by microscope. The mean values and S.E. of five mice are shown as number of cells per cubic millimetre.

of α/β^+ over γ/δ^+ among T-lymphocytes, and we could not find any increase in allo-killer or mixed lymphocyte reaction activity in IL-5 transgenic mice. Antibodies raised in this IL-5 transgenic mouse are immunoglobulin M (IgM), IgA and IgE as shown in Table 6.1. IgM antibodies have polyreactivity including binding activity to DNA. These polyreactive IgM antibodies may be related to the increase in $CD5^+$ B cells. In mouse, IL-5 seems to be engaged in the development of $CD5^+$ B cells (Tominaga *et al.*, 1989).

As Experimental Disease Models

Asthma

Eosinophils are implicated in asthma and IL-5 is an important eosinophil maturation and activation factor. Activated eosinophils have a tendency to lodge in areas where connective tissue is rich, such as Glisson's capsule in the liver, muscle, outer membrane of spleen and liver (Takatsu and Tominaga, 1991). From the point of view of the role of IL-5 in asthma, we examined the eosinophils in IL-5 transgenic mice. Although there are not many eosinophils in lymph nodes in other tissues, eosinophils accumulated in the lymph nodes of the lung. In our view, there are two kinds of lymph nodes in the lung: one is full of eosinophils, the other has less eosinophils. Murine eosinophils, as defined, have ring or U-shaped nuclei and red granules which are not as clear as those in human eosinophils. IL-5 is totally responsible for the increase in eosinophils in the lung, because the lymph nodes which are full of eosinophils disappear after serial injections of anti-IL-5R α-chain antibodies (H7). (Fig. 6.1a, b). There is, however, no obvious tissue damage caused by eosinophils (Tominaga *et al.*, 1991). On the other hand, IL-5 is known to induce eosinophils to have antibody-dependent cell-mediated cytotoxicity activity, to have ability to produce superoxide anions and to have an increased adherence. In order to activate eosinophils, there must be an antigen-driven immunobiological response such as antibody production and antigen-specific helper T cells that are induced by airway sensitization. We think that IL-5 is one of the elements involved in asthma and that it is possible to make an asthma model by using this transgenic mouse. Despite the considerable difference between mouse and human – for example, murine tracheal smooth muscle does not respond to histamine, while the human muscle contracts in response to histamine – we can probably examine the possible role of eosinophils induced by IL-5 in asthma by using this transgenic mouse. In particular, it may be usetul for studying the possible mechanism for eosinophil activation.

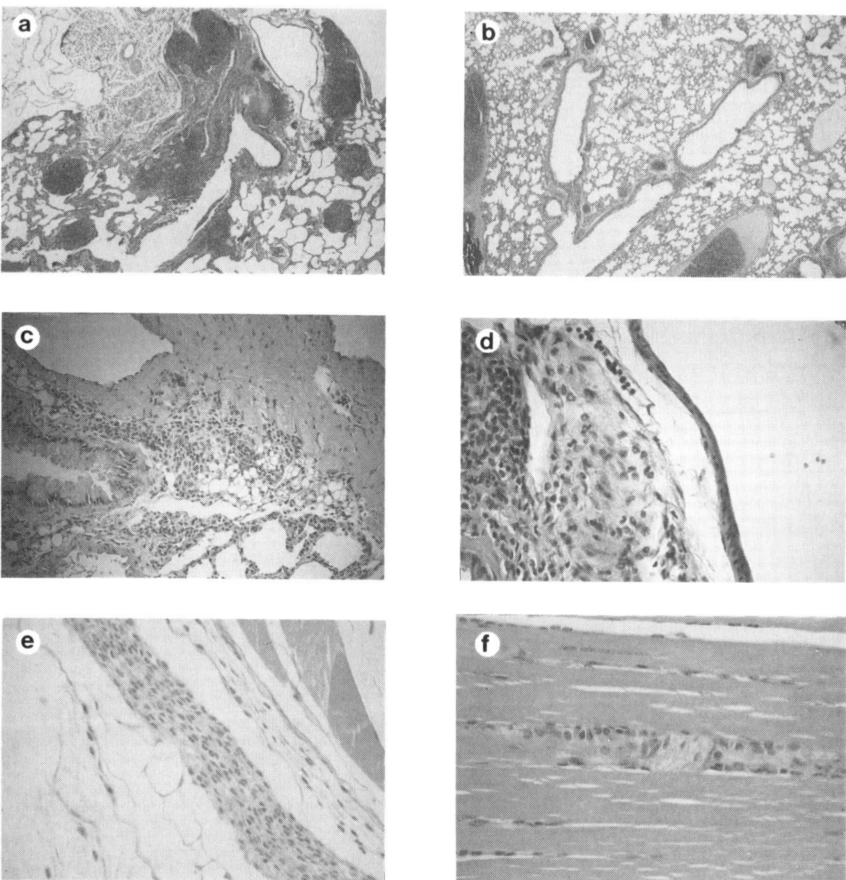

Fig. 6.1 Histology of IL-5 trangenic mice. All tissue was fixed in 10% phosphate-buffered formalin (pH 7.2) and sections were stained with haematoxylin and eosin. (a) In lung, lymph nodes with eosinophils can be recognized as densely stained cell mass. (b) IL-5 transgenic mice received six serial injections of an anti-IL-5R antibody (H7) every 3 days (1 mg/mouse/day, i.p.) and the lung was fixed and stained as described 30 days after the last injection of H7. (c) Eosinophils infiltrated around artery and bronchus in the lung. (d) Eosinophils infiltrated around lung vein. (e) A bundle of eosinophils surrounding femur muscle. (f) Eosinophils infiltrated into the femur muscle and the disappearance of striation and a sign of fibrosis of muscle cells were observed. Photographs were taken at × 100 for (a) and (b), × 500 for (c), × 1000 for (d), × 800 for (e) and × 1200 for (f).

Myocytis (myocarditis) or fascitis

Although IL-5 may not work on human B cells, it may be possible to make this mouse a model of myocytis (Spry, 1988) in which IgE antibodies are often increased as in this transgenic mouse. This mouse can also be used as an experimental system for fascitis. There are infiltrated eosinophils in the muscle and a slight sign of myocytis such as disappearance of striation or fibrosis of muscle cells (Fig. 6.1f). Although this figure shows a femur muscle, we can observe a similar sign in heart muscle. This transgenic mouse may also be the model mouse for myocarditis. Surprisingly, there are bundles of eosinophils surrounding the femur muscle, especially between the muscle and the fat tissue as shown in Fig. 6.1e and there are eosinophils infiltrated between the muscle of blood vessels and the fat tissue in lung as shown in Fig. 6.1c, d. Homing of eosinophils to the fat tissue may be related to the fact that eosinophils release lipid mediators such as prostaglandin E_2, platelet-activating factor, leukotriene C_4, lipoxin A and 15-monohydroxyeicosatetraenoic acid. We think that it is quite possible that cell–cell interactions and/or certain cell surface receptors, including homing receptors, may be responsible for the final activation of eosinophils to release such mediators (Bruijnzeel and Verhagen, 1989).

Difference Between IL-5 Ligand-Receptor Systems of Human and Mouse

Constitution of IL-5R

The murine IL-5R consists of an α-chain (60 kDa) and a β-chain (130 kDa) (Mita *et al.*, 1988, 1989b; Takaki *et al.*, 1990, 1991). The IL-5R α-chain itself binds to IL-5 with an affinity (K_d) of 2–10 nM. Although the IL-5R β-chain does not bind IL-5 by itself, it stabilizes the IL-5 α-chain complex and gives high-affinity IL-5R with a K_d of 30–150 pM.

The human IL-5R is expressed only on human eosinophils, as studied in a ligand-binding assay. Human IL-5R binds IL-5 with a K_d of 170–330 pM (Migita *et al.*, 1991). We have characterized both human and murine IL-5R α-chains by molecular cloning and protein purification using antibodies against the IL-5R (Takaki *et al.*, 1990; Yamaguchi *et al.*, 1991; Murata *et al.*, 1992). The deduced amino acid sequences are compared with other members of the cytokine receptor superfamily in (Fig. 6.2). Their extracellular portions consisted of three domains with fibronectin type III motif. Each of the domains consists of approximately 100 amino acids. The second domains contain two pairs of cysteine residues and the third domains contain a WSxWS motif which is characteristic of the cytokine receptor superfamily. Cytoplasmic domains are relatively short and do not have any known consensus sequences for the protein kinase catalytic domains. However, they have a proline-rich area that may be involved in the association with the β-chain or with other signalling apparatus. Furthermore, we found that most of the intracytoplasmic domain of the IL-5R is homologous to a part of the actin-binding domain of human β-spectrin, suggesting that intracytoplasmic domain of the IL-5R may interact with actin (Yamaguchi *et al.*, 1991).

In spite of their homology (about 70% in terms of amino acid sequence), there is a significant difference in the affinity of the α-chain for IL-5 binding between human and murine IL-5Rs. In contrast to the murine α-chain, the human α-chain of the hIL-5R expressed on COS cells has a much higher affinity (K_d = 250–590 pM). Therefore, it is suggested that the contribution of the β-chain to the increase in affinity for IL-5 binding is much less in the case of the human IL-5R than in the case of the murine IL-5R. We think, however, that the human IL-5R does use the second chain.

In fact, we and others have accumulated evidence for IL-5, GM-CSF and IL-3 sharing the β-chain of their receptors in human and in the mouse (Fig. 6.3) (Rolink *et al.*, 1989; Yonehara *et al.*, 1990; Mita *et al.*, 1991; Takaki *et al.*, 1991; Devos *et al.*, 1991; Kitamura *et al.*, 1991a,b; Tavernier *et al.*, 1991). This shared β-chain does not have any binding ability to any cytokines. The only difference between human and mouse receptors is that there is an extra β-chain for the murine IL-3R called AIC2A (Itoh *et al.*, 1989; Gorman *et al.*, 1990) which has weak affinity for murine IL-3. We do not know the physiological meaning of sharing the β-chain among the receptors for IL-3, IL-5 and GM-CSF. They certainly have redundant function in the development and activation of granulocytes, especially in the case of the eosinophils. In support of this, a similar pattern of phosphorylations of cytoplasmic proteins in early B cells was observed in response to either IL-3 or IL-5 (Murata *et al.*, 1990). It is also reported that both IL-3 and GM-CSF induce tyrosine phosphorylation of an identical set of cellular proteins (Kanakura *et al.*, 1990).

Soluble Form of IL-5R

In the process of the molecular cloning of both murine and human IL-5Rs, we could obtain cDNAs which do not encode transmembrane and cytoplasmic domains. We observed the secreted IL-5Rs from COS cells transfected with those cDNAs (Takaki *et al.*, 1990; Yamaguchi *et*

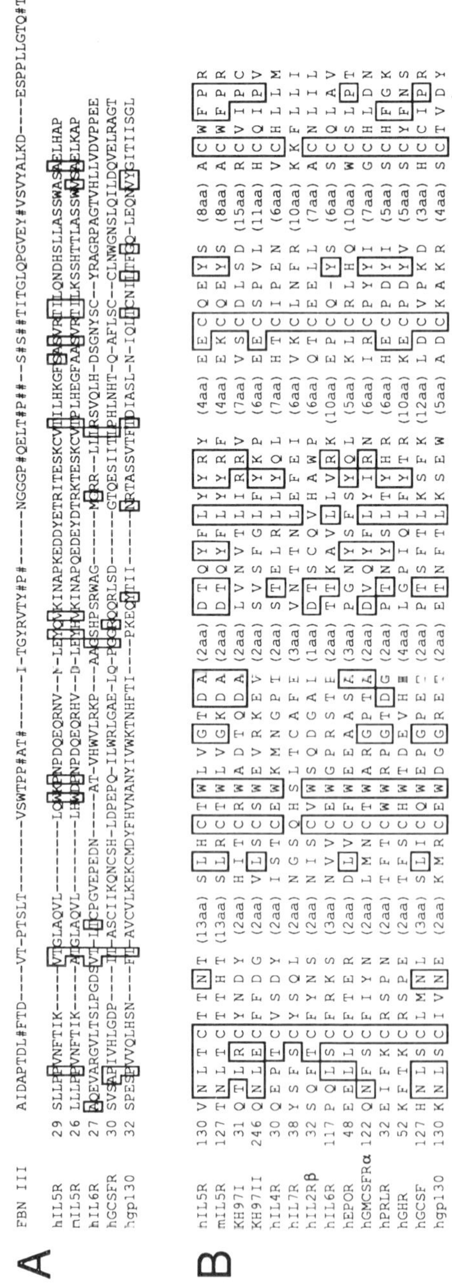
A
FBN III
hIL5R
mIL5R
hIL6R
hGCSFR
hgp130
B
hIL5R
mIL5R
KH97I
KH97II
hIL4R
hIL7R
hIL2Rβ
hIL6R
hEPOR
hGMCSFRα
hPRLR
hGHR
hGCSF
hgp130

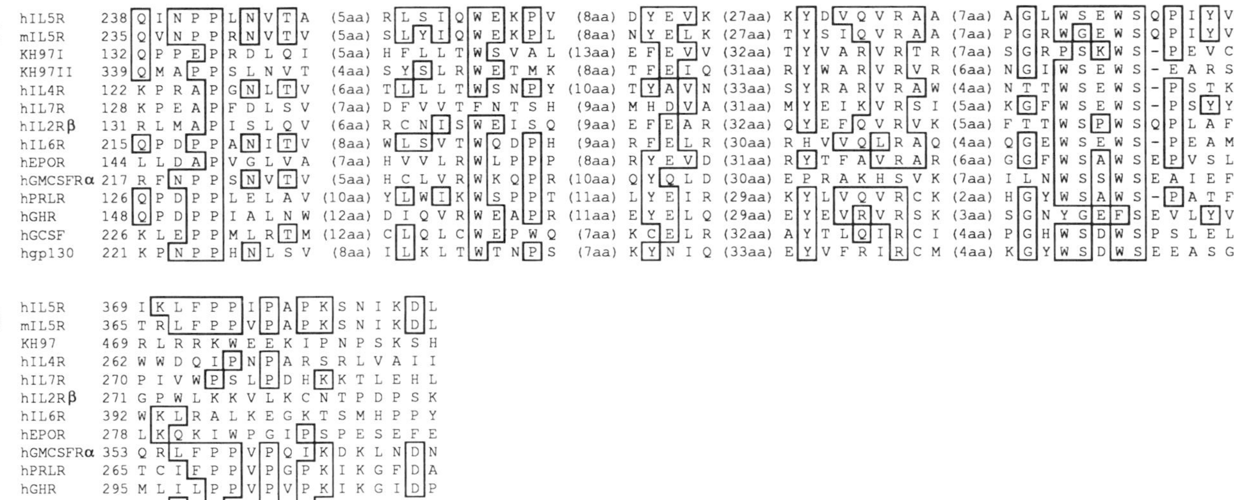

Fig. 6.2 Alignment of human and murine IL-5 receptor amino acid sequences with sequences from hIL-3R β-chain (hIL-3Rβ, KH97) (Itoh *et al.*, 1989), hIL-4R (Idzerda *et al.*, 1990), hIL-7R (Goodwin *et al.*, 1990), hIL-2Rβ (Hatakeyama *et al.*, 1989), hIL-6R (Yamasaki *et al.*, 1988), human erythropoietin receptor (hEPOR) (Jones *et al.*, 1990), hGM-CSFRα (Gearing *et al.*, 1989), human prolactin receptor (hPRLR) (Boutin *et al.*, 1989), human growth hormone receptor (hGHR) (Leung *et al.*, 1987), hG-CSFR (Larsen *et al.*, 1990), and human IL-6R β-chain (hgp 130) (Hibi *et al.*, 1990). Identical amino acids are boxed. Numbers at the left indicate the amino acid number starting from the first methionine. (A) The first domain of IL-5Rs are compared with those of hIL-6R, hG-CSFR and hgp 130 which have fibronectin type III (FBN III) motifs. (B), (C) the second and the third domains of IL-5Rs are compared with other members in cytokine receptor superfamily. Although they also have FBN III motifs, they are aligned to make the best match to other members in the cytokine receptor superfamily, but not to FBN III sequence. (D) Cytoplasmic domains of IL-5Rs are compared with other members of the cytokine receptor superfamily around the proline-rich region.

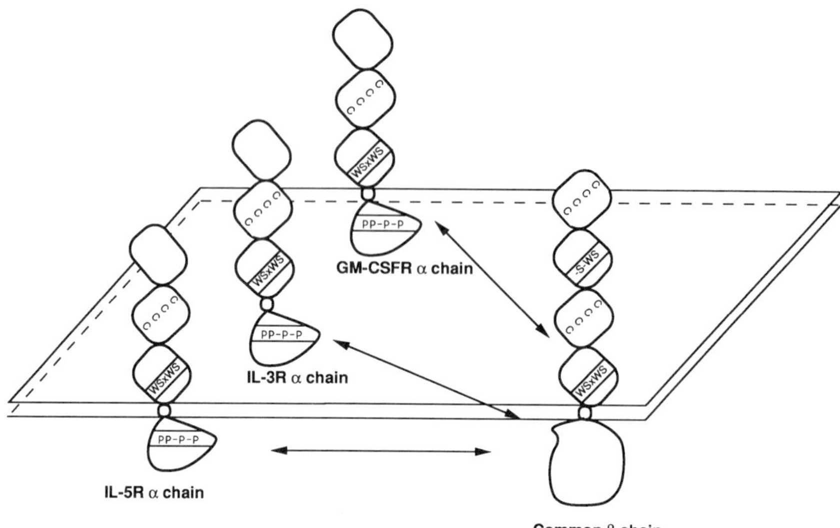

Fig. 6.3 Basic construction of receptors for IL-3, IL-5 and GM-CSF. α-Chains for each cytokine receptor are specialized, although both α- and β-chains belong to the same cytokine receptor superfamily. CCCC indicates the two cysteine pairs. WSxWS motifs are indicated as boxes. PP-P-P is the conserved area in the cytoplasmic region of the cytokine receptor superfamily including growth factor receptor and prolactin receptor.

al., 1991; Murata *et al.*, 1992). It is reported that the human soluble IL-5R inhibited the hIL-5-driven differentiation of eosinophils from human cord blood (Tavernier *et al.*, 1991), while the murine soluble IL-5R is less effective (Yamaguchi *et al.*, 1991). This is probably due to the higher affinity of hIL-5R α-chain for IL-5 binding than that of the murine α-chain.

Effect of IL-5 on B Cells

The major difference in IL-5 function between human and mouse is its role on B cells. Although there is a discrepancy among reports on the role of IL-5 on human B cells (Azuma *et al.*, 1986; Yokota *et al.*, 1987; Clutterbuck *et al.*, 1987), it is true that the antibody-forming cell-inducing ability of IL-5 in human B cells is marginal. We could not detect IL-5Rs on human B cells in a radiolabelled ligand-binding assay (Migita *et al.*, 1991) though this does not exclude the possibility that there is a small number of functional IL-5Rs on human B cells. In particular, we have to examine the effect of IL-5 on human $CD5^+$ B cells, because we know that IL-5 is deeply involved in the development of murine $CD5^+$ B cells as described above.

IL-5 may work indirectly on human B cells through other cells that have IL-5 receptors, such as T cells, eosinophils and basophils. In this sense, the existence of IL-5R on T cells is also a very interesting issue. The effects of IL-5 on human T-lymphocytes still remain obscure, although we reported the killer helper factor activity of IL-5 in the cytotoxic T-lymphocytes generation system from immature thymocytes against hapten-modified self in mouse. It only works in the presence of IL-2. We also have to think of the synergism among cytokines.

We certainly think that antigens, specific antibodies and antigen-specific helper T cells are necessary for causing asthma symptoms, even if IL-5 is not involved in antibody formation in man.

We also think that homing receptors or adherence receptors for eosinophils are necessary to trigger the eosinophils to become active and to work as a causative factor in asthma.

Acknowledgements

We appreciate all the collaborators for their individual work. We especially appreciate Drs Ryoji Matsumoto and Eiichiro Sonoda for the measurement of serum levels of immunoglobulins in IL-5 transgenic mice. We are also grateful to Drs Satoshi Takaki, Yoshiyuki Murata, Masahiro Migita, Seiji Mita and Naoto Yamaguchi in our Medical School and Drs Toshio Kitamura and Atsushi Miyajima of the DNAX Institute in Palo Alto, California, for the molecular characterization of the IL-5R.

References

Azuma, C., Tanabe, T., Konishi, M., Kinashi, T., Noma, T., Matsuda, F., Yaoita, Y., Takatsu, K., Hammerstrom, L., Smith, C.I.E., Severinson, E. and Honjo, T. (1986). Cloning of cDNA for human T-cell replacing factor (interleukin-5) and comparison with the murine homologue. *Nucleic Acids Res.* **14**, 9149–9158.

Basten, A., and Beeson, P.B. (1970) Mechanisms of eosinophilia. II. Role of the lymphocyte. *J. Exp. Med.* **131**, 1288–1305.

Boutin, J.-M., Edery, M., Shirota, M., Jolicoeur, C., Lesueur, L., Ali, S., Gould, D., Djiane, J. and Kelly, P.A. (1989) Identification of a cDNA encoding a long form of prolactin receptor in human hepatoma and breast cancer cells. *Molec. Endocrinol.* **3**, 1455–61.

Bruijnzeel, P.L.B. and Verhagen, J. (1989). Lipid metabolism by eosinophils.

In "Eosinophils in Asthma" (J. Morley and I. Colditz, eds), pp. 69–92. Academic Press, London.

Clutterbuck, E., Shields, J.G., Gordon, J., Smith, S.H., Boyd, A., Callard, R.E., Campbell, H.D., Young, I.G. and Sanderson, C.J. (1987). Recombinant human interleukin 5 is an eosinophil differentiation factor but has no activity in standard human B cell growth factor assays. *Eur. J. Immunol.* **17**, 1743.

Devos, R., Plaetinck, G., Van der Hayden, J., Cornelis, S., Vandekerkhove, J., Fiers, W. and Tavernier, J. (1991). Molecular basis of a high affinity murine interleukin-5 receptor. *EMBO J.* **10**, 2133–2137.

Gearing, D.P., King, J.A., Gough, N.M. and Nicola, N.A. (1989). Expression cloning of a receptor for human granulocyte-macrophage colony-stimulating factor. *EMBO J.* **8**, 3667–3676.

Goodwin, R.G., Friend, D., Ziegler, S.F., Jerzy, R., Falk, B.A., Gimpel, S., Cosman, D., Dower, S.K., March, C.J., Namen, A.E. and Park, L. S. (1990). Cloning of the human and murine interleukin-7 receptors: demonstration of a soluble form and homology to a new receptor superfamily. *Cell* **60**, 941.

Gorman, D.M., Itoh, N., Kitamura, T., Scheurs, J., Yonehara, S., Yahara, I., Arai, K. and Miyajima, A. (1990). Cloning and expression of a gene encoding an interleukin-3 receptor-like protein: identification of another member of the cytokine receptor gene family. *Proc. Natl. Acad. Sci. U.S.A.* **87**, 5459–5463.

Harada, N., Takahashi, T., Matsumoto, M., Kinashi, T., Ohara, J., Kikuchi, Y., Koyama, N., Severinson, E., Yaoita, Y., Honjo, T., Yamaguchi, N., Tominaga, A. and Takatsu, K. (1987). Production of a monoclonal antibody useful in the molecular characterization of murine T-cell-replacing factor/B-cell growth factor II. *Proc. Natl. Acad. Sci. U.S.A.* **84**, 4581–4585.

Hatakeyama, M., Tsudo, M., Minamoto, S., Kudo, T., Doi, T., Miyata, T., Miyasaka, M. and Taniguchi, T. (1989). Interleukin-2 receptor β chain gene: generation of three receptor forms by cloned human α and β chain cDNA's. *Science* **244**, 551–556.

Hibi, M., Murakami, M., Saito, M., Hirano, T., Taga, T. and Kishimoto, T. (1990) Molecular cloning and expression of an IL-6 signal transducer, gp130. *Cell* **63**, 1149–1157.

Idzerda, R.L., March, C.J., Mosley, B., Lyman, S.D., Vanden-Boss, T., Gimpel, S.D., Din, W.S., Grabstein, K.H., Widmer, M.B., Park, L.S., Cosman, D. and Beckmann, M.P. (1990). Human interleukin-4 receptor confers biological responsiveness and defines a novel receptor superfamily. *J. Exp. Med.* **171**, 861–873.

Itoh, N., Yonehara, S., Scheurs, J., Gorman, D.M., Muramatsu, K., Ishii, A., Yahara, I., Arai, K. and Miyajima, A. (1989). Cloning of an interleukin-3 receptor gene family. *Science* **247**, 324–327.

Jones, S.S. D'Andrea, A., Haines, L.L. and Wong, G.G. (1990). Human erythropoietin receptor: cloning, expression, and biological characterization. *Blood* **76**, 31–35.

Kanakura, Y., Druker, Cannistra, S.A., Furukawa, Y., Torimoto, Y. and Griffin, J.D. (1990). Signal transduction of the human granulocyte-macrophage colony stimulating factor and interleukin-3 receptors involves tyrosine phosphorylation of a common set of cytoplasmic proteins. *Blood* **76**, 706–715.

Kinashi, T., Harada, N., Severinson, E., Tanabe, T., Sideras, P., Konishi, M., Azuma, C., Tominaga, A., Bergstedt-Lindqvist, S., Takahashi, M., Matsuda, F., Yaoita, Y., Takatsu, K. and Honjo, T. (1986). Cloning of complementary

DNA encoding T-cell replacing factor and identity with B-cell growth factor II. *Nature* **324**, 70–73.

Kitamura, T., Hayashida, K., Sakamaki, K., Yokota, T., Arai, K. and Miyajima, A. (1991a). Reconstitution of functional receptors for human granulocyte/macrophage colony-stimulating factor (GM-CSF): Evidence that the protein encoded by the AIC2B cDNA is a subunit of murine GM-CSF receptor. *Proc. Natl. Acad. Sci. U.S.A.* **88**, 5082–5086.

Kitamura, T., Sato, N., Arai, K.-I. and Miyajima, A. (1991b). Expression cloning of the human IL-3 receptor cDNA reveals a shared β subunit for the human IL-3 and GM-CSF receptors. *Cell* **66**, 1165–1174.

Larsen, A., Davis, T., Curtis, B.M., Gimpel, S., Sims, J.E., Cosman, D., Park, L., Sorensen, E., March, C.J. and Smith, C.A. (1990). Expression cloning of a human granulocyte colony-stimulating factor receptor: a structural mosaic of hematopoietin receptor, immunoglobulin, and fibronectin domains. *J. Exp. Med.* **172**, 1559–1570.

Leung, D.W., Spencer, S.A., Cachianes, G., Hammonds, R.G., Collins, C., Henzel, W.J., Barnard, R., Waters, M.J. and Wood, W.I. (1987). Growth hormone receptor and serum binding protein: purification, cloning and expression. *Nature* **330**, 537.

McKenzie, A.N.J., Barry, S.C., Strath, M. and Sanderson, C.J. (1991). Structure-function analysis of interleukin-5 utilizing mouse/human chimeric molecules. *EMBO J.* **10**, 1193–1199.

Migita, M., Yamaguchi, N., Mita, S., Higuchi, S., Hitoshi, Y., Yoshida, Y., Tomonaga, M., Matsuda, I., Tominaga, A. and Takatsu, K. (1991). Characterization of the human IL-5 receptors on eosinophils. *Cell. Immunol.* **133**, 484–497.

Minamitake, Y., Kodama, S., Katayama, T., Adachi, H., Tanaka, S. and Tsujimoto, M. (1990). Structure of recombinant human interleukin-5 produced by chinese hamster ovary cells. *J. Biochem. (Tokyo)* **107**, 292–297.

Mita, S., Harada, N., Naomi, S., Hitoshi, Y., Sakamoto, K., Akagi, M., Tominaga, A. and Takatsu, K. (1988). Receptors for T cell replacing factor TRF/interleukin-5 (IL-5): Specificity, quantitation and its implication. *J. Exp. Med.* **167**, 863–878.

Mita, S., Hosoya, Y., Kubota, I., Honjo, T., Nishihara, T., Takahashi, T. and Takatsu, K. (1989a). Rapid purification of human recombinant IL-5 by using monoclonal antibody against murine IL-5. *J. Immunol. Meth.* **125**, 233–241.

Mita, S., Tominaga, A., Hitoshi, Y., Honjo, T., Sakamoto, K., Akagi, M., Kikuchi, Y. and Takatsu K. (1989b). Characterization of high-affinity receptors for interleukin-5 (IL-5) on IL-5 dependent cell lines. *Proc. Natl. Acad. Sci. U.S.A.* **86**, 2311–2315.

Mita, S., Takaki, S., Hitoshi, Y., Rolink, A.G., Tominaga, A., Yamaguchi, N. and Takatsu, K. (1991). Molecular characterization of the β chain of the murine interleukin-5 receptor. *Int. Immunol.* **3**, 665–672.

Murata, Y., Yamaguchi, N., Hitoshi, Y. Tominaga, A. and Takatsu, K. (1990). Interleukin 5 and interleukin-3 induce serine and tyrosine phosphorylations of several cellular proteins in an interleukin-5-dependent cell line. *Biochem. Biophys. Res. Commun.* **173**, 1102–1107.

Murata, Y., Takaki, S., Migita, M., Kikuchi, Y., Tominaga, A. and Takatsu, K. (1992). Molecular cloning and expression of the human interleukin-5 receptor. *J. Exp. Med.* **175**, 341–351.

Rolink, A.G., Melchers, F. and Palacois, R. (1989). Monoclonal antibodies reactive with the mouse interleukin-5 receptor. *J. Exp. Med.* **169**, 1693–1705.

Sanderson, C.J., Campbell, H.D. and Young, I.G. (1988). Molecular and cellular biology of eosinophil differentiation factor (interleukin-5) and its effects on human and mouse B cells. *Immunol. Rev.* **102**, 29–50.

Schimpl, A. and Wecker, E. (1972). Replacement of T-cell function by a T-cell product. *Nature* **237**, 15–17.

Spry, C.J.F. (1988) Musculo-skeletal diseases. In "Eosinophils", pp. 176–182. Oxford Medical Publications, Oxford.

Takahashi, T., Yamaguchi, N., Mita, S., Yamaguchi, Y., Suda, T., Tominaga, A., Kikuchi, Y., Miura, Y. and Takatsu, K. (1990). Structural comparison of murine T cell (B151K12)-derived T-cell-replacing factor (IL-5) with rIL-5: dimer formation is essential for the expression of biological activity. *Molec. Immunol.* **27**, 911–920.

Takaki, S., Tominaga, A., Hitoshi, Y., Mita, S., Sonoda, E., Yamaguchi, N. and Takatsu, K. (1990). Molecular cloning and expression of the murine interleukin-5 receptor. *EMBO J.* **9**, 4367–4374.

Takaki, S., Mita, S., Kitamura, T., Yonehara, S., Yamaguchi, N., Tominaga, A., Miyajima, A. and Takatsu, K. (1991). Identification of the second subunit of the murine interleukin-5 receptor: interleukin-3 receptor-like protein, AIC2B is a component of the high-affinity interleukin-5 receptor. *EMBO J.* **10**, 2833–2838.

Takatsu, K. and Tominaga, A. (1991). Interleukin-5 and its receptor. *Progr. Growth Factor Res.* **3**, 87–102.

Takatsu, K., Tominaga, A. and Hamaoka, T. (1980). Antigen-induced T cell replacing factor (TRF). I. Functional characterization of a TRF producing helper T cell subset and genetic studies on TRF production. *J. Immunol.* **124**, 2414–2422.

Takatsu, K., Tominaga, A., Harada, N., Mita, S., Matsumoto, M., Takahashi, T., Kikuchi, Y., Takahashi, T. and Yamaguchi, N. (1988). T cell replacing factor (TRF)/interleukin-5 (IL-5): Molecular and functional properties. *Immunol. Rev.* **102**, 107–136.

Tavernier, J., Devos, R., Cornelis, S., Tuypens, T., Van der Heyden, J., Fiers, W. and Plaetinck, G. (1991). A human high affinity interleukin-5 receptor (IL-5R) is composed of an IL-5-specific α chain and a β chain shared with the receptor for GM-CSF. *Cell* **66**, 1175–1184.

Tominaga, A., Mita, S., Kikuchi, Y., Hitoshi, Y., Takatsu, K., Nishikawa, S-I. and Ogawa, M. (1989). Establishment of IL-5 dependent early B cell lines by long-term bone marrow cultures. *Growth Factors* **1**, 135–146.

Tominaga, A., Takahashi, T., Kikuchi, Y., Mita, S., Naomi, S., Harada, N., Yamaguchi, N. and Takatsu, K. (1990). Role of carbohydrates moiety of IL-5 in the expression of biological activity: Effect of tunicamycin on the translation of IL-5 and its activity. *J. Immunol.* **144**, 1345–1352.

Tominaga, A., Takaki, S., Koyama, N., Katoh, S., Matsumoto, R., Migita, M., Hitoshi, Y., Hosoya, Y., Yamauchi, Y., Kanai, Y., Miyazaki, J.-I., Usuku, G., Yamamura, K.-I. and Takatsu, K. (1991). Transgenic mice expressing a B cell growth and differentiation factor (interleukin-5) gene develop eosinophilia and autoantibody production. *J. Exp. Med.* **173**, 429–437.

Yamaguchi, N., Hitoshi, Y., Takaki, S., Murata, Y., Migita, M., Kamiya, T., Minowada, J., Tominaga, A. and Takatsu, K. (1991). Murine interleukin-5 receptor isolated by immunoaffinity chromatography: comparison of determined N-terminal sequence and deduced primary sequence from cDNA and implication of a role of the intracytoplasmic domain. *Int. Immunol.* **3**, 889–898.

Yamasaki, K., Taga, T., Hirata, Y., Yawata, H., Kawanishi, Y., Seed, B., Taniguchi, T., Hirano, T. and Kishimoto, T. (1988). Cloning and expression of the human interleukin-6 (BSF-2/IFNβ2) receptor. *Science* **241**, 825–828.

Yokota, T., Coffman, R.L., Hagiwara, H., Rennick, D.M., Takebe, Y., Yokota, K., Gemmell, L., Shrader, B., Yang, G., Meyerson, P., Luh, J., Hoy, P., Pène, J., Briere, F., Spits, H., Banchereau, J., De Vries, J., Lee, F.D., Arai, N. and Arai, K.I. (1987). Isolation and characterization of lymphokine cDNA clones encoding mouse and human IgA-enhancing factor and eosinophil colony-stimulating factor activities: Relationship to interleukin-5. *Proc Natl. Acad. Sci. U.S.A.* **84**, 7388–7392.

Yonehara, S., Ishii, A., Yonehara, M., Koyasu, S., Miyajima, A., Scheurs, J., Arai, K.I. and Yahara, I. (1990). Identification of a cell surface 105 kD protein (Aic-2 antigen) which binds interleukin-3. *Int. Immunol.* **2**, 143–150.

Discussion

M.N. Palfreyman
Have you looked for any chemical agonists or antagonists to your IL-5 receptor?

A. Tominaga
We have not looked for them yet.

M. Capron
I was interested to see the results on the secretion of the soluble form of IL-5 receptor α-chain. Were your experiments performed in murine or human IL-5 receptor α-chain?

A. Tominaga
Murine.

M. Capron
There are no data on the human soluble form?

A. Tominaga
We have no data at this moment.

A.R. Leff
Is the differentiation from marrow stem cells into eosinophils merely

differentiation or is cell division and differentiation being stimulated by the IL-5 receptor?

A. Tominaga
There are no data to answer the question. We do not have the cloned precursors of those eosinophils, so I cannot draw any conclusions. By observing the bone marrow cells of these transgenic mice, however, I think IL-5 can induce both cell division and differentiation of eosinophil precursors.

A.B. Kay
With regard to the transgenic mice, it is quite surprising that in your system, through a B-cell promoter and Colin Sanderson's T cell transgenic mice, there is this massive eosinophilia, and some increase in immunoglobulins, but apparently no real tissue damage – no damage to epithelial surfaces. At first glance, this might come as a surprise. Alternatively, it may simply be that in the diseases that we have been discussing, bronchial asthma and related diseases, something else is also needed.

A. Tominaga
That is right – that is our way of thinking. I would rather ask you what are the other signals to cause the tissue damage. Probably antigen-stimulated T cells are necessary to be present next to the eosinophils.

A.B. Kay
Are there any plans for developing the transgenic model to study epithelial damage? Perhaps there just needs to be some non-specific injury to the bronchi, for example, and it may be that in the transgenic mice this then would accelerate the type of damage that we recognize in asthma and which would not be seen in the controls.

A.R. Leff
Alternatively, though, perhaps the eosinophilia has nothing to do with asthma and there are many conditions with raised eosinophil numbers.

M. Capron
With regard to the lack of tissue damage in the transgenic mice, I think that IL-5 is not sufficient to activate the eosinophils, which resemble true high potency eosinophils seen in patients. In particular, when IL-5 (or even a combination of IL-3, GM-CSF and IL-5) is used to differentiate the cord blood cells *in vitro*, after 30 days the eosinophils differentiated

in vitro in the presence of IL-5 are very different from eosinophils of patients. I think this is evidence that something is lacking.

J. Souness
Dr Tominaga said that he thinks the β-chain is linked to signal transduction mechanisms. Is anything known about the signal transduction mechanisms of the IL-5 receptor?

A. Tominaga
Nothing is known of an IL-5 specific signal, however, we have just analysed the phosphorylation pattern after the IL-5 and IL-3 responsive cells have received the signal from each cytokine.

J. Souness
Is it possible that there is a tyrosine kinase linked to the β-chain.

A. Tominaga
Tyrosine residue phosphorylation and serine residue phosphorylation have been observed in response to either IL-3 or IL-5.

R. Dahl
The transgenic mice with the IL-5 also produce immunoglobulin M, anti-DNA and IgE. This is also seen in eosinophil-associated disease. Have you looked to see whether IL-5 in other situations might also stimulate mast cells?

A. Tominaga
We have not looked at mast cells, but in the mouse it has been reported that the mast cell itself is a potent secretor of IL-5.

7

The IL-5 Receptor on Human Eosinophils

M. CAPRON, J. CHIHARA, J. PLUMAS, J. TAVERNIER,* P. DESREUMAUX and A. CAPRON

Centre d'Immunologie et de Biologie Parasitaire, Unité Mixte INSERM U 16 - CNRS 624, Institut Pasteur – Lille, France

**Roche Research Ghent, Ghent, Belgium*

Introduction

The effector functions of eosinophils have been studied extensively in parasitic diseases and also suspected in asthma. The demonstration of a large variety of membrane receptors (including Fc and complement receptors) and the identification of cytotoxic molecules (mainly the granule basic proteins) in recent years have allowed eosinophils to be considered as effector cells, able to release pharmacologically active mediators after interaction with specific antibodies and antigens (Tomassini *et al.*, 1991). The detection of granule proteins in the tissues or in the bronchoalveolar lavage fluid of patients with asthma, coupled with the well-known cytotoxic properties of these proteins for epithelial or lung cells *in vitro* strongly suggest the pathological potential of eosinophils in asthma (Gleich and Adolphson, 1986). The number of eosinophils, which is relatively low in normal subjects, increases in certain diseases, such as asthma. Not only increased numbers but also activated eosinophils can be detected in the blood and in the tissues from patients. Activated or "hypodense" eosinophils can be distinguished by several biochemical or

T-Lymphocyte and Inflammatory Cell Research in Asthma
ISBN 0-12-388170-6

functional criteria, as well as by the increased expression of membrane receptors. Among these, the expression of $F_C\epsilon$RII/CD23, CR3, (CD11b/CD18) or more recently CD25, is enhanced in eosinophils from patients (Capron and Plumas, 1993). More importantly, the immunoglobulin E (IgE)-dependent release of eosinophil mediators is dramatically increased in the case of hypodense eosinophils, suggesting that hypodense eosinophils have been activated *in vivo* (Capron *et al.*, 1989).

Regarding the factors responsible for eosinophil differentiation and activation, Interleukin-5 (IL-5) appears to promote specifically the proliferation and terminal differentiation of eosinophil precursors, as well as the prolonged survival of eosinophils *in vitro* (Yamaguchi *et al.*, 1988a, b). It is also a potent activator of eosinophil functions such as cytotoxicity or mediator release. The presence of hypodense eosinophils in hypereosinophilic situations can therefore be related to eosinophils in a state of activation, in addition to increased eosinophilopoiesis. IL-5 might represent the major cytokine involved in the induction of hypodense eosinophils and therefore in eosinophil-mediated pathology (Owen *et al.*, 1989). Similarly to other lymphokines, the biological effects of IL-5 are probably linked to the interaction with specific receptors on susceptible targets. Indeed, the existence of specific receptors for IL-5 has been demonstrated recently on human eosinophils, by binding assays (Chihara *et al.*, 1990). More recently, a molecular approach has led to the cloning of the human high-affinity IL-5 receptor (IL-5R), composed of two chains α and β (Tavernier *et al.*, 1991). The possible functions of IL-5R, specially the soluble form of IL-5Rα, will be discussed, in relation to the recently described expression of IL-5 mRNA by human eosinophils (Desreumaux *et al.*, 1992).

Characterization of a Receptor for IL-5 on Human Eosinophils

Binding experiments using ^{125}I-labelled recombinant human IL-5 were performed, in order to demonstrate the existence and to examine the level of expression of a receptor for IL-5 on human eosinophils (Chihara *et al.*, 1990). Radiolabelled IL-5 specifically bound to eosinophils and reached saturation at an approximate concentration of 1–1.25 nM. Very interestingly, the levels of specific binding were significantly higher on hypodense blood and tissue eosinophils than on normodense cells. Specific IL-5R was not detected on human neutrophils, a finding that correlates with the lack of effect of IL-5 on the neutrophil myeloid series. Scatchard analysis revealed that the association constant was five-fold greater for hypodense eosinophils than for normodense eosinophils, a result that suggests the previous *in vivo* activation of hypodense eosinophils. However, the number of receptors per cell was not different between the two subpopulations. Moreover, these data indicated that the binding of IL-5 was to a single affinity class of receptor, in contrast to results obtained on murine B cells (Mita *et al.*, 1988).

To investigate further the mechanisms involved in the heterogeneous expression of IL-5R, human eosinophils were cultured overnight in the presence or absence of granulocyte–macrophage colony-stimulating factor (GM-CSF), a potent activator of eosinophil functions. Whereas the specific IL-5 binding was greater on hypodense than on normodense eosinophils in the preculture conditions, a specific binding was still detected on hypodense eosinophils but not on normodense cells after overnight incubation in the absence of GM-CSF. This is consistent with the fact that hypodense eosinophils have a prolonged lifespan *in vivo* and *ex vivo*. However, cultivation with GM-CSF induced increased IL-5 binding both on normodense and on hypodense eosinophils. These findings are in agreement with the ability of GM-CSF to stimulate eosinophil colonies *in vitro*.

To determine whether the binding of IL-5 to human eosinophils was specific, competition experiments were performed with other lymphokines showing amino acid sequence homology with IL-5. Only unlabelled IL-5 but not IL-3, GM-CSF or interferon-γ (IFN-γ) inhibited the binding of radiolabelled IL-5, suggesting the specificity of the binding site for IL-5 on blood eosinophils from patients (Chihara *et al.*, 1990).

It should be noted that the existence of such receptors for IL-5 has been further confirmed on human eosinophils in two independent studies. In the first one the binding of murine IL-5 was demonstrated on eosinophils from normal peripheral blood, with a single class of high-affinity receptors (Migita *et al.*, 1991). No apparent increase of IL-5 binding was detected in the case of eosinophils from patients with eosinophilia, which might appear to be in contrast to the previously published study (Chihara *et al.*, 1990). Several factors might explain these discrepancies, including the source of IL-5, the aetiology of eosinophilia of the patients under study, the different techniques of purification, and the lack of data on hypodense and normodense subpopulations in the latter study. The second report revealed that normal human eosinophils showed a single high-affinity binding site with a K_d of 450 pmol/litre and an average receptor number of 1000 per eosinophil (Ingley and Young, 1991). No data concerning eosinophils from patients were given. In parallel, binding experiments performed on HL-60 cells grown under alkaline conditions demonstrated similar characteristics of IL-5 binding (Plaetinck *et al.*, 1990; Ingley and Young, 1991) with 550–1405 receptors/cell, and a K_d value of 400 pmol/litre. In addition, cross-linking studies revealed the existence of a cross-linked complex of 75–85 kDa, giving a molecular mass of 55–60 kD for the human IL-5 receptor itself (Plaetinck *et al.*, 1990; Ingley and Young, 1991). Taken together, these results confirm the existence of a high-affinity binding site for IL-5 on human eosinophils and eosinophilic subclones of HL-60, but not on other cell types, including B-lymphoma cells; these results are in agreement with the specific effect of IL-5 on the human eosinophil lineage.

Molecular Basis of a High-Affinity Human IL-5 Receptor

The mouse IL-5 receptor (mIL-5R) on B cells is composed of at least two molecules, of which the mIL-5R α-chain (60 kDa) can bind mIL-5 independently with low affinity (10^{-9}M). The second subunit (β-chain, 130 kDa) does not bind mIL-5 but associates with the mIL-5R α-chain to form a high-affinity mIL-5R complex (10^{-11}M). Recent studies have shown that this β-chain is identical to the mIL-3R-like protein previously described (Devos *et al.*, 1991). The detection of IL-5 binding with a high affinity on eosinophilic subclones of HL-60, led Tavernier and co-workers to initiate a cloning strategy of the human IL 5 receptor (Tavernier *et al.*, 1991). As a source of mRNA they used butyrate-induced eosinophilic subclones of HL-60. A cDNA library was constructed in λgt11 and screened either with oligonucleotide probes of the murine IL-5R α-chain or with a mouse IL-3R-like cDNA, identical to the mIL-5R β-chain.

First, using degenerated oligonucleotides based on the mIL-5R α-chain, 41 positive clones were isolated and one was selected for further analysis. Some particular features of the sequence were characteristic of the cytokine and cytokine receptor family. The open reading frame defined a polypeptide which is 71% homologous to the murine IL-5R α-chain, indicating that hIL-5Rα belongs to the cytokine receptor gene family. Moreover, the human counterpart is also characterized by the presence of a signal peptide which indicates that the IL-5R α-chain can be secreted. The molecular weight calculated from the sequence is 35.9 kDa which is far less than the 60 kDa estimated from cross-linking studies. This is probably due to the existence of six potential glycosylation sites and therefore to the glycosylation of the molecule. One the other hand, the human IL-5R β-chain was shown to be identical to the IL-3R and GM-CSFR β-chains (Tavernier *et al.*, 1991).

Northern blot analysis using the cDNA of the IL-5R α-chain revealed the presence of a major transcript of 1.4 kb in eosinophilic subclones of HL-60, as well as in human cord blood cells differentiated *in vitro* to eosinophils by culture with IL-5. Other weaker transcripts at 2 and 4.4 kb were also detected, the significance of these being unclear. The major transcript probably corresponds to the secreted hIL-5Rα, whereas the other transcripts might be obtained by alternative splicing and correspond to an anchored form of the molecule. A chimeric protein was constructed by fusion between the secreted hIL-5Rα and the C-terminal domain of the anchored mIL-5Rα. When this IL-5Rα construct was transfected in COS cells, only low-affinity binding was observed. Cotransfection with this IL-5Rα and an IL-5Rβ construct led to a four-fold increase in binding affinity, indicating that both chains are required to form the high-affinity receptor (Tavernier *et al.*, 1991).

The functions of the soluble IL-5R α-chain have been explored, using the supernatants of COS cells transfected with the IL-5R α-chain. The supernatants, containing soluble IL-5R α-chain could inhibit the binding of radiolabelled IL-5 to transfected COS cells. In addition, these supernatants also inhibit, in a dose-dependent manner, the IL-5 driven eosinophil differentiation from cord blood cells, indicating the antagonistic properties of the IL-5R α-chain. The functions of this soluble IL-5R α-chain *in vivo* have still to be explored. In particular, it would be interesting to evaluate its regulatory role on eosinophil recruitment and activation. The expression of IL-5R α-chain during eosinophil maturation/differentiation, as well as by hypodense versus normodense eosinophils during diseases has to be investigated, as well as the tissue specificity of expression.

IL-5 mRNA Expression by Human Eosinophils

IL-5, the major factor involved in eosinophil differentiation, is classically produced by T cells. It has been reported that IL-5 mRNA can be detected by *in situ* hybridization in skin and mucosal bronchial biopsies of patients with eosinophil infiltration (Kay *et al.*, 1991, Hamid *et al.*, 1991) but without a precise identification of the labelled cells. It has also been established that IL-5 mRNA expression can be detected in other cell populations such as mast cells (Plaut *et al.*, 1989) or Reed Sternberg cells (Samoszuck and Nansen, 1990). In a recent study (Desreumaux *et al.*, 1992) we demonstrated the presence of IL-5 mRNA in activated eosinophils. First, eosinophils infiltrating the mucosa of four patients with active coeliac disease strongly expressed IL-5 mRNA, by *in situ* hybridization. In contrast, no positive signal was obtained in the cell infiltrate from patients submitted to gluten restriction or in the normal duodenum tissues. These results, in association with electron microscopy analysis or immunostaining with the EG2 mAb, indicated that activated eosinophils present in coeliac disease can synthesize IL-5. Not only tissue-infiltrating eosinophils but also highly purified eosinophils from the peripheral blood of patients with eosinophilia could express IL-5 mRNA (Desreumaux *et al.*, 1992).

Together, these results suggest that eosinophils have the capacity to synthesize IL-5, which could contribute to paracrine interactions with T and B cells and, in autocrine fashion, could participate locally in eosinophil differentiation and activation through binding to the IL-5 receptor. The secretion by eosinophils of both IL-5 and the antagonistic soluble IL-5R α-chain might constitute the basis of a subtle T cell-independent regulation of eosinophil differentiation and activation and should be explored in diseases such as asthma. In addition to their inflammatory and effector functions, eosinophils may thus serve as a source of growth and regulatory factors with a broad range of biological effects.

References

Capron, M. and Plumas, J. (1993) Eosinophil membrane receptors. *In* "Eosinophils: Biological and Clinical Aspects" (S. Makino and Fukuda, eds) pp. 95–123.

Capron, M., Grangette, C., Torpier, G. and Capron, A. (1989) The second receptor for IgE in eosinophil effector function. *Chem. Immunol.* **47**, 128–178.

Chihara, J., Plumas, J., Tavernier, J., Gruart, V., Prin, L., Capron, A. and Capron M. (1990). Characterization of a receptor for interleukin-5 (IL-5) on human eosinophils: Variable expression and induction by granulocyte/macrophage colony-stimulating factor (GM-CSF). *J. Exp. Med.* **172**, 1347–1351.

Desreumaux, P., Janin, A., Colombel, J.-F., Prin, L., Plumas, J., Emilie, D., Torpier, G., Capron, A. and Capron, M. (1992). Interleukin-5 messenger RNA expression by eosinophils in the intestinal mucosa of patients with coeliac disease. *J. Exp. Med.* **175**, 293–296.

Devos, R., Plaetinck, G., Van der Heyden, J., Cornelis, S., Vandekerckove, J., Fiers, W. and Tavernier, J. (1991). Molecular basis of a high affinity murine interleukin-5 receptor. *EMBO J.* **10**, 2133–2137.

Gleich, G.J. and Adolphson, C.R. (1986). The eosinophilic leukocyte. *Adv. Immunol.* **39**, 177–253.

Hamid, W., Azzawi, M., Ying, S., Moqbel, R., Wardlaw, A.J., Corrigan, C.J., Bradley, B., Durham, S.R., Collins, J.V., Jefery, P.K., Quint, D.J. and Kay, A.B. (1991). Expression of mRNA for interleukin-5 in mucosal bronchial biopsies from asthma. *J. Clin. Invest.* **87**, 1541–1546.

Ingley, E. and Young, I.G. (1991). Characterization of a receptor for interleukin-5 on human eosinophils and the myeloid leukemia line HL-60. *Blood* **78**, 339–344.

Kay, A.B., Ying, S., Vaarnney, V., Gaga, M., Durham, S.R., Moqbel, R., Wardlaw, A.J. and Hamid, Q. (1991). Messenger RNA expression of the cytokine gene cluster, interleukin-3 (IL-3), IL-4, IL-5 and granulocyte/macrophage colony-stimulating factor, in allergen induced late-phase cutaneous reactions in atopic subjects *J. Exp. Med.* **173**, 775–778.

Migita, M., Yamaguchi, N., Mita, S., Higuchi, S., Hitoshi, Y., Yoshida, Y., Tomonaga, M., Matsuda, I., Tominaga, A. and Takatsu, K. (1991). Characterization of the human IL-5 receptors on eosinophils. *Cell. Immunol.* **133**, 484–497.

Mita, S., Harada, N., Naomi, S., Hitoshi, Y., Sakamoto, K., Akagi, M., Tominaga, A. and Takatsu, K. (1988). Receptors for T cell-replacing factor/interleukin-5: Specificity, quantitation and its implication. *J. Exp. Med.* **168**, 863.

Owen, W.F., Rothenberg, M.E., Peterson, J., Weller, P.F., Silberstein, D., Sheffer, A.L., Stevens, R.J., Soberman, R.J. and Austen, K.F. (1989). Interleukin-5 and phenotypically altered eosinophils in the blood of patients with the idiopathic hypereosinophilic syndrome. *J. Exp. Med.* **170**, 343–348.

Plaetinck, G., Van der Heyden, J., Tavernier, J., Fache, I., Tuypens, T., Fischkoff, S., Fiers, W. and Devos, R. (1990). Characterization of interleukin-5 receptors on eosinophilic sublines from human promyelocytic leukemia (HL-60) *J. Exp. Med.* **172**, 683–691.

Plaut, M., Pierce, J.H., Watson, C.J., Hanley-Hyde, J., Nordan, R.P. and Paul, W.E. (1989). Mast cell lines produce lymphokines in response to cross-linkage of FcϵR1 or to calcium ionophores. *Nature* **339**, 64–67.

Samoszuck, M. and Nansen, L. (1990). Detection of interleukin-5 messenger RNA in Reed-Sternberg cells of Hodgkin's disease with eosinophils. *Blood* **1**, 13.

Tavernier, J., Devos, R., Cornelis, S., Tuypens, T., Van der Heyden, J., Fiers, W. and Plaetinck, G. (1991). A human high affinity interleukin-5 receptor (IL-5R) is composed of an IL-5 specific α chain and a β chain shared with the receptor for GM-CSF. *Cell* **66**, 1175–1184.

Tomassini, M., Tsicopoulos, A., Tai, P.C., Gruart, V., Tonnel, A.B., Prin, L., Capron, A. and Capron, M. (1991). Release of granule proteins by eosinophils from allergic and other hypereosinophilic patients upon immunoglobulin dependent activation. *J. Allergy Clin. Immunol.* **88**, 365–375.

Yamaguchi, Y., Suda, T., Suda, J., Eguchi, M., Miura, Y., Harada, N., Tominaga, A. and Takatsu, K. (1988a). Purified interleukin-5 supports the terminal differentiation and proliferation of murine eosinophilic precursors. *J. Exp. Med.* **167**, 43–56.

Yamaguchi, Y., Hayashi, Y., Miura, Y., Kasahara, T., Kitamura, S., Torisu, M., Mita, S., Tominaga, A., Takatsu, K. and Suda, T. (1988b). Highly purified murine interleukin-5 (IL-5) stimulates eosinophil function and prolongs in vitro survival. *J. Exp. Med.* **167**, 1737–1742.

Discussion

P. Venge

Has this IL-5 messenger RNA been found in normal cells, and do you know what would induce this message in normal eosinophils?

M. Capron
We have found, in particular, very strong messenger RNA (mRNA) by *in situ* hybridization in other diseases, such as bladder biopsies of patients with cystitis, in skin biopsies of patients with *dermatitis herpetiformis*, and also in gastroenteritis with eosinophils, but other patients are negative, for example, with systemic mastocytosis. We have not yet looked at normal eosinophils.

S.T. Holgate
The presence of message by *in situ* hybridization was shown very clearly in your slide but in the human mast cell, by direct immunostaining using two different monoclonal antibodies to IL-5, one to the secreted form and one to the non-secreted form, we can actually localize the product to the cell. It looks as though it is pre-formed in the granules. Have you done direct immunostaining of human eosinophils with monoclonal antibodies to the cytokines?

M. Capron
Immunostaining is being done now. It is rather difficult to have 99% pure eosinophils in order to be sure that the secreted IL-5 comes from eosinophils, so we took the alternative approach and try to label the cells with anti-IL-5.

S.T. Holgate
So you do *in situ* hybridization and look for the product in the same cell?

Could the correlation found by Dr Kay between *in situ* hybridization signals in bronchial biopsies and the number of eosinophils that he counts (I think using EG2), be explained on the basis that some of the message seen was in fact not originating from T cells but from the eosinophils themselves?

A.B. Kay
I showed a slide in which we could count the T cells and CD2 in lavage. [**Prof. Holgate** I am thinking of the tissue rather than lavage.] No, we do not have information on that.

M. Capron
In Dr Kay's experiments I think they also have very intense labelling, and it is very difficult to identify eosinophils or other cells because the morphology is slightly altered by the *in situ* hybridization.

P.F. Weller
The finding that eosinophils have the potential capacity to release their own IL-5 is intriguing. One corollary of this has to do with assays of IL-5 activity in the serum or plasma of patients with eosinophilic diseases such as the hypereosinophilic syndrome. It is possible that some of the IL-5 activity that has been detected is really eosinophil-derived.

M. Capron
It is difficult to know the source of IL-5 *in vivo*. I did not mention that if there is a lot of soluble IL-5 receptor α-chain, which is produced *in vivo* by the cells, it is possible that it might interfere with the titration of IL-5 because IL-5 can be blocked and inhibited by the IL-5 receptor α-chain.

R. Moqbel
In our studies we have confirmed the presence of IL-6 mRNA in peripheral blood eosinophils that have either been cultured with interferon-γ or ionophore, as well as in 20% of cells that are cultured in medium alone. This suggests that the gene may in fact be expressed to a considerable extent. Unfortunately, we have not been able to show IL-5 undergoing the same stimulation, at least in peripheral blood. It will be very interesting to see Dr Capron's results when *in situ* hybridization is done on eosinophils outside the tissue.

M. Capron
With all these results in peripheral blood and tissues there was no *in vitro* stimulation. They were spontaneously expressing the mRNA. We have not looked – although we must – to see whether we can induce, for instance, the expression of mRNA for IL-5 from cord blood cells.

R. Moqbel
It would be interesting to determine the amount of IL-5 produced by the eosinophil compared to the T-lymphocyte.

M. Capron
We found 3 units/ml, which is enough to induce eosinophil differentiation *in vitro* for 2×10^6 cells – which is significant. These results have to be confirmed.

8

The Mobilization and Activation of Eosinophils

P.F. WELLER

Harvard Thorndike Laboratory, Charles A. Dana Research Institute, Department of Medicine, Beth Israel Hospital and Harvard Medical School, Boston, MA 02215, USA

Introduction

Eosinophilic leukocytes are prominent cellular participants in allergic diseases and asthma. While increases in the circulating blood pool of eosinophils may accompany these diseases, it is within tissue sites, where eosinophils are characteristically present (Beasley *et al.*, 1989; Azzawi *et al.*, 1990), that these leukocytes function and contribute to the immunopathogenesis of allergic diseases. Many studies have aimed at delineating the mechanisms underlying the preferential accumulation of eosinophils within the tissue sites of allergic diseases. Although specific eosinophil chemoattractant factors have been sought, the most potent currently known eosinophil chemoattractants, platelet-activating factor (PAF) and C5a, are equally active as neutrophil chemoattractants (Wardlaw *et al.*, 1986) and by themselves would not account for a preferential tissue accumulation of eosinophils. To evaluate the mobilization and recruitment of eosinophils from the bloodstream, we have investigated mechanisms by which eosinophils adhere to cytokine-stimulated vascular endothelial cells and respond to lymphocyte-derived cytokines. These studies have identified mechanisms of leukocyte recruitment that are utilized by eosinophils but not neutrophils. Further, we have evaluated functional roles of eosinophils that may be pertinent to their participation in the chronic airway inflammatory responses that

T-Lymphocyte and Inflammatory Cell Research in Asthma
ISBN 0-12-388170-6

characterize asthma. These roles of eosinophils include their functioning as HLA-DR-dependent, major histocompatibility complex (MHC)-restricted antigen presenting cells and the capacities of eosinophils to elaborate the cytokines, transforming growth factor-α (TGF-α) and transforming growth factor-β (TGF-β), that might contribute to airway epithelial hyperplasia and subepithelial fibrosis.

Eosinophil Mobilization

Pathways of Eosinophil Adherence to Cytokine-Stimulated Endothelial Cells

Eosinophil adherence to ELAM and VCAM

The adherence of human eosinophils to cytokine-stimulated human endothelial cells is only partially due to CD18-dependent pathways and is also mediated by binding to endothelial leukocyte adhesion molecule-1 (ELAM) and vascular cell adhesion molecule-1 (VCAM) (Weller *et al.*, 1991b). Utilizing recombinant adhesion molecules, we have shown that eosinophils bind specifically to both recombinant soluble ELAM and recombinant soluble VCAM (Weller *et al.*, 1991b). Eosinophil binding to ELAM was inhibited by a monoclonal antibody (BB11) against ELAM. Eosinophil binding to recombinant soluble VCAM as well as to CHO cells expressing VCAM-1 was inhibited with a monoclonal antibody to VCAM (4B9) and by pretreatment of eosinophils with blocking monoclonal antibodies (HP1/2 or HP2/1) to the very late activation antigen-4 (VLA-4). VLA-4 is the β_1-integrin previously identified as the ligand expressed on lymphocytes and mononuclear cells that binds to VCAM-1 as well as fibronectin (Elices *et al.*, 1990, Freedman *et al.* 1990; Hemler *et al.*, 1990). In accord with the function of VLA-4 as a ligand for binding to VCAM and of the abilities of anti-VLA-4 monoclonal antibodies to inhibit eosinophil binding to VCAM, cytofluorographic studies demonstrated that human eosinophils, but not neutrophils, express VLA-4. VLA-4 expression was demonstrable on eosinophils from both normal donors and eosinophilic donors. Similar findings demonstrating eosinophil adherence via VLA-4 to VCAM have been presented by others (Bochner *et al.*, 1991, Dobrina *et al.*, 1991, Walsh *et al.*, 1991).

Eosinophil adherence to TNF-α-stimulated endothelial cells

Eosinophil binding to tumour necrosis factor-α (TNF-α)-stimulated human umbilical vein endothelial cells (HUVECs) utilized several adherence pathways (Weller *et al.*, 1991b). An anti-CD18 monoclonal antibody (60.3) only partially inhibited eosinophil adherence. Similarly, partial inhibition of eosinophil adherence was achieved with monoclonal antibodies that blocked ELAM (BB11) or VCAM (4B9) expressed on the stimulated HUVECs or that blocked eosinophil VLA-4 (HP2/1 or HP1/2). Combinations of monoclonal antibodies, blocking two or more of these adherence pathways, yielded greater inhibition of eosinophil adherence. Of note, blockade of CD18 and VLA-4 integrin pathways with monoclonal antibodies 60.3 and HP2/1 produced virtually complete inhibition of eosinophil adherence to TNF-α-treated HUVECs (Weller *et al.*, 1991b).

Thus, eosinophils, like neutrophils, monocytes and lymphocytes, can bind to intercellular adhesion molecule 1 (ICAM-1, CD54) by means of lymphocyte function-associated antigen 1 (LFA-1, CD11a–CD18 complex). In the leukocyte adhesion deficiency syndrome due to genetic deficiencies in CD18; in which the abilities of neutrophils to emigrate from the vasculature into sites of inflammation are impaired, both lymphocytes and eosinophils can be found in inflammatory lesions (Anderson *et al.*, 1985), indicating that *in vivo* these two cell types possess mechanisms of adherence independent of CD18. One non-CD18-dependent pathway involving binding to the selectin ELAM is utilized by both eosinophils and neutrophils. A non-CD18-dependent pathway utilized by eosinophils and not neutrophils involves binding to VCAM-1 mediated by VLA-4 expressed on eosinophils and not neutrophils (Weller *et al.*, 1991b).

In order for eosinophils to be mobilized from the bloodstream to enter tissues, these leukocytes must first adhere to vascular endothelial cells. This mobilization of eosinophils, therefore, can utilize at least three pathways to bind to adhesion molecules expressed on cytokine-stimulated human endothelial cells. In addition to binding via CD18-dependent integrins, eosinophils can bind to ELAM-1 and VCAM-1. Unlike neutrophils, eosinophils express VLA-4 and can bind to VCAM. Thus, VLA-4-mediated binding to VCAM expressed on endothelial cells at specific sites of inflammation would contribute to the accumulation of eosinophils, but not neutrophils. Since VCAM expression can be preferentially elicited by IL-4 (Masinovsky *et al.*, 1990, Thornhill and Haskard, 1990, Thornhill *et al.*, 1991) and VCAM can facilitate the adherence of lymphocytes and monocytes as well as eosinophils, adherence to endothelial cell-expressed VCAM could contribute to the concomitant recruitment of eosinophils and mononuclear leukocytes, without neutrophils, into specific sites of allergic and other immunologic reactions.

Human Eosinophil Chemoattractants

Lymphocyte chemoattractant factor and eosinophil CD4 function

Eosinophil CD4 expression

CD4, first recognized on helper T lymphocytes, is also expressed on cells of myeloid lineage, including monocytes and macrophages. We have shown that human eosinophils express CD4 (Lucey *et al.*, 1989a). By flow cytometric analyses with anti-CD4 monoclonal antibodies, human eosinophils express demonstrable CD4, albeit at lower levels than found on T helper cells (Lucey *et al.*, 1989a). CD4 is expressed on eosinophils from normal donors as well as hypereosinophilic donors, indicating that CD4 expression is not restricted to eosinophils with an activated phenotype, as present in the blood of eosinophilic patients (Weller, 1991). Eosinophil CD4, like CD4 expressed on other cell types, binds human immunodeficiency virus 1 (HIV) gp120 (Lucey *et al.*, 1989a). Moreover, eosinophils (>99% pure), when cultured with 3T3 fibroblasts and granulocyte–macrophage colony-stimulating factor (GM-CSF) and pulse-labelled with ^{35}S-methionine/cysteine, synthesized immunoprecipitable ^{35}S-labelled CD4 (Lucey *et al.*, 1989a). Thus, mature, blood-derived eosinophils not only express CD4 but also retain the capacity to synthesize CD4 protein.

Eosinophil CD4 function

To investigate the functions of CD4 expressed on eosinophils, we utilized three distinct ligands that interact with CD4 (Rand *et al.*, 1991a). The first of these is the lymphokine, lymphocyte chemoattractant factor (LCF), a 56 000 Da homotetrameric basic glycoprotein that is formed by CD8$^+$ human T-lymphocytes (Cruikshank *et al.*, 1987, 1991). Of note, an agonist that stimulates the synthesis and release of LCF from T cells is histamine, acting via H2 receptors (Center *et al.*, 1983). LCF acts on CD4$^+$ T-lymphocytes and CD4$^+$ monocytes (Cruikshank *et al.*, 1987). On these CD4-bearing mononuclear leukocytes, LCF stimulates cellular migration, augments expression of MHC class II antigens, increases interleukin-2 (IL-2) receptor expression and elicits fluxes in the intracellular messengers, calcium and inositol phosphates (Center and Cruikshank, 1982; Center *et al.*, 1983; Berman *et al.*, 1985; Cruikshank *et al.*, 1987, 1991). For CD4$^+$ T-lymphocytes and monocytes, several lines of evidence indicate that CD4 is the cell receptor for LCF. First, all LCF functional responses, as mentioned above, are blocked by Fab fragments of the anti-CD4 monoclonal antibody OKT4. Second, LCF binds to CD4 affinity columns. Third, anti-CD4 antibody (OKT4) inhibits LCF binding to $CD4^+$ cells. Fourth, all LCF functional responses are mediated by cloned recombinant LCF, and finally, responsiveness to LCF is conferred by transfection of human CD4 into recipient cells (Cruikshank *et al.*, 1987, 1991).

Since LCF is a chemoattractant for $CD4^+$ T cells and monocytes, we studied whether LCF similarly functions as a chemoattractant for $CD4^+$ human eosinophils (Rand *et al.*, 1991a). Eosinophil chemotaxis was assayed in modified Boyden chambers, using aniline blue fluorescence staining of eosinophils and automated image analysis quantitation of populations of eosinophils migrating at several depths within micropore filters (McCrone *et al.*, 1988). With eosinophils from both normal and hypereosinophilic donors, LCF uniformly elicited eosinophil migration. Since the concentrations of LCF exhibiting half-maximal chemoattractant responses, the ED_{50}, ranged from 1.0 ng/ml down to 0.03 ng/ml (10^{-11}–10^{-12} M) (Rand *et al.*, 1991a), LCF proved to be a potent chemoattractant for human eosinophils. In standard checkerboard analyses, LCF was both chemokinetic and chemotactic for eosinophils (Rand *et al.*, 1991a). To ascertain the comparative potency of LCF as an eosinophil chemoattractant, eosinophil migration studies were performed in parallel with the lipid, platelet activating factor (PAF), and the complement fragment, C5a. PAF and C5a are the most potent currently recognized eosinophil chemoattractants (Wardlaw *et al.*, 1986), although neither is specific for eosinophils and each will also potently stimulate neutrophil migration. In these comparative studies with several eosinophil donors, LCF was 100- to 1000-fold more potent than either C5a or PAF as an eosinophil chemoattractant (Rand *et al.*, 1991a). LCF did not stimulate migration of neutrophils, which lack CD4 expression, so that LCF differed from C5a and PAF not only in being appreciably more potent as an eosinophil chemoattractant but also in being specific for eosinophils in comparison with neutrophils (Rand *et al.*, 1991a). Thus, LCF, with ED_{50} values of between 10^{-11} and 10^{-12} M, is a markedly potent stimulus for eosinophil migration (Rand *et al.*, 1991a).

To determine whether LCF-induced migration responses of eosinophils were mediated by CD4, two experimental approaches were utilized (Rand *et al.*, 1991a). First, the activities of other ligands that bind to CD4 were evaluated to determine if these other CD4-binding ligands also stimulate eosinophil migration (Cruikshank *et al.*, 1987; Kornfeld *et al.*, 1988). OKT4, an anti-CD4 monoclonal antibody, stimulated eosinophil migration, whereas two control proteins, an immunoglobulin G (IgG) subclass control myeloma protein and a monoclonal antibody (W6/32) directed against other eosinophil cell-surface expressed proteins, MHC class I proteins, did not stimulate eosinophil migration (Rand *et al.*, 1991a). In addition, recombinant HIV gp120, which binds to CD4 on eosinophils (Lucey *et al.*, 1989a), elicited eosinophil migration (Rand *et al.*, 1991a). Second, the capacity of CD4-blocking antibodies to competitively inhibit LCF-induced eosinophil migration was tested (Rand *et al.*, 1991a). Monovalent Fab fragments of the anti-CD4 monoclonal antibody, OKT4, which themselves did not stimulate eosinophil migration, inhibited eosinophil migration elicited by LCF. Thus, LCF-induced eosinophil migration is mediated via binding to CD4 expressed on eosinophils.

As assessed by cytofluorographic immunofluorescence, CD4 expression on eosinophils is low in comparison to that on helper T-lymphocytes and overlaps background fluorescence of eosinophils analysed alone or after staining with IgG subclass control myeloma proteins (Lucey *et al.*, 1989a). Nevertheless, two experimental findings suggest that all eosinophils express functional CD4 (Rand *et al.*, 1991a). First, the pattern of CD4 expression found on eosinophils from all normal and eosinophilic donors, examined after staining with various anti-CD4 monoclonal antibodies, consistently yielded a single unimodal peak of CD4 staining. This unimodal staining was of greater fluorescence intensity than found with either background or control antibody fluorescent staining of eosinophils, although the magnitudes of anti-CD4 staining usually overlapped with the histogram of control eosinophil fluorescence. There was never a bimodal pattern of staining indicative of separate $CD4^+$ and $CD4^-$ subpopulations of eosinophils (Lucey *et al.*, 1989a; Rand *et al.*, 1991a). The second line of evidence that virtually all eosinophils expressed CD4 was obtained from analyses of the eosinophil migratory responses elicited by the CD4-binding lymphokine, LCF (Rand *et al.*, 1991a). Eosinophils from all donors, regardless of the mean level of eosinophil CD4 expression, migrated in response to LCF. Specific enumeration and analysis of the numbers of eosinophils migrating at different levels into chemotactic filters in response to LCF provided no evidence that only subpopulations of eosinophils were responding to LCF. Moreover, with cells from six donors the net numbers of eosinophils migrating in response to LCF were comparable to the net eosinophil migration elicited by PAF and C5a. Since receptors for C5a (Gerard *et al.*, 1989) and probably PAF are expressed in large numbers on all eosinophils, the quantitatively comparable migration of eosinophils elicited by LCF and by C5a or PAF further indicates that functional CD4 is expressed on all, or virtually all, human eosinophils.

While LCF was a potent eosinophil chemoattractant, it did not by itself stimulate some other effector functions of eosinophils (Rand *et al.*, 1991a). LCF itself neither stimulated eosinophil respiratory burst activity nor primed for heightened respiratory burst activity in response to other agonists. LCF did not elicit eosinophil degranulation. Further, LCF neither directly stimulated eosinophil leukotriene C_4 release nor did it enhance the capacity of eosinophils to generate leukotriene C_4 in response to stimulation by submaximal concentrations of calcium inophore A23187.

Thus, these findings document that CD4 expressed on human eosinophils functions as a signal-transducing transmembrane protein and that three ligands binding to CD4, namely LCF, HIV gp120 and anti-CD4 monoclonal antibodies, are capable of stimulating eosinophil migratory responses (Rand *et al.*, 1991a). The lymphokine LCF, therefore, is capable of stimulating migration of $CD4^+$ eosinophils as well as of $CD4^+$ lymphocytes and $CD4^+$ monocytes.

LCF utilizes CD4 as its receptor on eosinophils as well as lymphocytes and monocytes and stimulates the migration of all three $CD4^+$ cell types. Since histamine, as released at sites of IgE-mediated mast cell responses, elicits LCF release from $CD4^-$ lymphocytes (Center *et al.*, 1983; Berman *et al.*, 1985) elaboration of LCF at sites of allergic responses may contribute to the recruitment and activation of both eosinophils and mononuclear cells. In chronic asthma, airway tissues are infiltrated with eosinophils and $CD4^+$ mononuclear cells, with many IL-2 receptor-bearing mononuclear cells (Azzawi *et al.*, 1990). Analogously, in cutaneous (Frew and Kay 1988) and pulmonary (Diaz *et al.*, 1989; Frew *et al.*, 1989) late phase reactions, eosinophils and $CD4^+$ lymphocytes are prominent in the elicited cellular infiltrate. Thus, LCF, perhaps elaborated in response to locally released histamine, would be a candidate mediator to contribute to the preferential tissue influx of eosinophils, lymphocytes and mononuclear cells.

Interleukin-2 and eosinophil function

Eosinophil IL-2 receptor expression

On lymphocytes and monocytes, interleukin-2 (IL-2) receptors are composed of two non-covalently associated subunits, p55 (CD25) and p75. Association of both subunits is required to constitute a high-affinity IL-2 receptor, whereas individually, p55 and p75 bind IL-2 with only low and intermediate affinities, respectively. We (Rand *et al.*, 1991b) and others (Riedel *et al.*, 1990; Plumas *et al.*, 1991), have shown that eosinophils express CD25 detectable by flow cytometry with anti-CD25 monoclonal antibodies. Moreover, CD25 is demonstrable on eosinophils, without requiring *in vitro* activation, by immunoprecipitation of cell-surface radioiodinated CD25 (Rand *et al.*, 1991b). Northern blotting established that eosinophils contain mRNA for p55 (Rand *et al.*, 1991b). In contrast, binding of anti-p75 antibody to eosinophils was not detectable by flow cytometry; and in IL-2 ligand-binding assays, high-affinity IL-2 receptors were below the limits of detection on eosinophils from individuals with eosinophilia (Rand *et al.*, 1991b). Thus, the p55 component of the IL-2 receptor is expressed on eosinophils, whereas the p75 subunit is not detectable by flow cytometry.

Eosinophils respond to interleukin-2

Eosinophils have the capacity to respond to IL-2 as evidenced by their responses in migration assays. Recombinant human IL-2 was a potent chemoattractant for eosinophils with an ED_{50} for migration of about 10^{-12} M (Rand *et al.*, 1991b). Although the p55 subunit, but not the p75 subunit, of the heterodimeric high-affinity IL-2 receptor is detectable on eosinophils by flow cytometry, two findings indicate that migratory responses of eosinophils are apparently mediated by high-affinity IL-2 receptors. First, the molar potency of IL-2 as an eosinophil chemoattractant, with responses elicited by 10^{-12} M IL-2, is compatible with responses being mediated by a high-affinity receptor (Rand *et al.*, 1991b). Second, IL-2-induced eosinophil migration is competitively inhibited by monoclonal antibodies to either the p55 or p75 IL-2 receptor subunits (Rand *et al.*, 1991b). IL-2, which is principally chemokinetic and not chemotactic for eosinophils, is about 100- to 1000-fold more potent as an eosinophil chemoattractant than either PAF or C5a. Thus, while it is possible that IL-2 may stimulate other as yet unrecognized responses in eosinophils, IL-2 constitutes another lymphokine with potent activity in eliciting eosinophil migration.

Eosinophil Activation

Eosinophil MHC Class II-Dependent Antigen Presentation

Eosinophil HLA-DR expression

Although immature eosinophils developing within the marrow, like other immature myeloid cells, express MHC class II proteins, peripheral blood eosinophils express little of the MHC class II proteins (Lucey *et al.*, 1989b). Even phenotypically activated eosinophils, obtained from the blood of patients with eosinophilia, do not display elevated amounts of these MHC proteins (Lucey *et al.*, 1989b). Mature eosinophils, however, can be induced to express the MHC class II protein HLA-DR. When

HLA-DR$^-$, peripheral blood-derived eosinophils are maintained in culture with 3T3 fibroblasts and GM-CSF, eosinophils uniformly express heightened levels of HLA-DR (Lucey *et al.*, 1989b). This heightened expression of HLA-DR, detectable by flow cytometry, increases in magnitude over a week in culture on eosinophils derived from both normal and eosinophilic donors. This increased cell-surface expression of HLA-DR is not attributable solely to mobilization of latent, intracellular pools of HLA-DR, since eosinophils, cultured at ~100% purity with GM-CSF and 3T3 fibroblasts, synthesize new ^{35}S-methionine/cysteine-labelled heterodimeric HLA-DR. Thus, mature eosinophils have the capacity to express HLA-DR and, as also demonstrated with CD4, retain the capacity to synthesize new immunologically pertinent cell-surface proteins (Lucey *et al.*, 1989b).

Eosinophil HLA-DR function

To determine if eosinophil HLA-DR expression is functionally important, we have evaluated whether eosinophils can serve as antigen-presenting cells in stimulating lymphocyte proliferative responses. Our findings indicate that eosinophils, induced *in vitro* to express HLA-DR by incubation with GM-CSF, can function as HLA-DR-dependent, MHC-restricted antigen presenting cells (Weller *et al.*, 1991a). Eosinophils can process antigen and present it to CD4$^+$ lymphocytes in the context of the MHC class II protein HLA-DR and specifically stimulate lymphocyte proliferation. Expression of HLA-DR on eosinophils *in vivo* has been noted with eosinophils recovered from the sputum of asthmatics (Hansel *et al.*, 1991) and from the peritoneal cavity (Roberts *et al.*, 1991). Thus, eosinophils in airway tissues have the potential capability to process and present locally encountered antigens to CD4$^+$ lymphocytes and to initiate antigen-dependent lymphocyte responses.

Eosinophil-Derived Transforming Growth Factor Cytokines

Eosinophils recruited into tissue sites may have multiple functional capabilities including the ability to elaborate cytokines. The capacity of human eosinophils to elaborate cytokines was first demonstrated for transforming growth factor-α (TGF-α) (Wong *et al.*, 1990). Human eosinophils, in both tissue lesions and in peripheral blood, were shown to contain mRNA transcripts for the TGF-α. In addition, expression of TFG-α protein by eosinophils was demonstrated by both immunocytochemistry and radioimmunoassay. Since not all eosinophils, either in tissue lesions or in the blood of normal and eosinophilic donors, contained

TGF-α mRNA by *in situ* hybridization, it is likely that TGF-α expression in eosinophils is regulated by exposure of eosinophils to other activating stimuli. These findings that human eosinophils elaborate TGF-α are corroborated by our findings that hamster eosinophils likewise elaborate TGF-α and the findings that the eosinophil is the cellular source of TGF-α in healing cutaneous wounds in rabbits (Todd *et al.*, 1991).

Moreover, we have shown that human eosinophils are capable of expressing transforming growth factor-β (TGF-β) transcripts and protein (Wong *et al.*, 1993). TGF-β is capable of stimulating fibroblasts and contributing to the formation of extracellular matrix components (Barnard *et al.*, 1990; Pelton and Moses 1990). Thus, this eosinophil-derived cytokine might have a role in contributing to the development of the subepithelial fibrosis that develops in asthma (Roche *et al.*, 1989; Brewster *et al.*, 1990) TGF-α with its multiple effects (Lyons and Moses, 1990, Massagué, 1990) may contribute to airway epithelial cell hyperplasia.

Conclusions

Eosinophils are recruited into sites of early and late phase immediate hypersensitivity reactions as well as into tissue sites associated with other immunologically mediated diseases. While eosinophils are present to varying extents with other cell types, including neutrophils, lymphocytes and monocytes, the mechanisms whereby eosinophils, a minority of the circulating blood leukocytes, are recruited in large numbers into tissue sites have been uncertain. Mechanisms whereby eosinophils are mobilized from the vasculature into sites of inflammatory reactions can involve the adherence of eosinophils to vascular endothelial cells and the migration of eosinophils in response to specific lymphokines. In addition to utilizing CD18-dependent mechanisms for adherence to cytokine-stimulated endothelial cells, eosinophils adhere via CD18-independent mechanisms by binding to either endothelial leukocyte adhesion molecule-1 (ELAM) or vascular cell adhesion molecule-1 (VCAM). Eosinophils, but not neutrophils, express the integrin very late activation antigen-4 (VLA-4), the ligand involved in mediating adhesion to VCAM. Although many eosinophil chemoattractants have been reported over the years, the most potent ones presently known are C5a and PAF, which are equipotent as neutrophil chemoattractants. In contrast, two of the cytokines active on eosinophils, IL-3 and GM-CSF, are active at lower concentrations as eosinophil chemoattractants ($ED_{50} \sim 10^{-8}$ M) but also stimulate neutrophil migration (Warringa *et al.*, 1991). IL-5 is active at a similar concentration of about 10^{-8} M as an eosinophil chemoattractant. Both LCF and IL-2, however, are active as eosinophil chemoattractants with ED_{50} values of $10^{-12} - 10^{-11}$ M, making them the most potent currently known eosinophil chemoattractants.

The roles of eosinophils in the pathogenesis of allergic inflammation may be multiple. In addition to the well-recognized effector functions of eosinophils that are mediated by degranulation or by the elaboration of lipid mediators, eosinophils may be able to engage in dynamic interactions with other cells. Eosinophils respond to T-lymphocyte-derived cytokines, including LCF (Rand *et al.*, 1991a), IL-5 (Sanderson *et al.*, 1988) and IL-2 (Rand *et al.*, 1991b). Eosinophils can utilize the VLA-4–VCAM adhesion pathway that would also be involved in the recruitment of lymphocytes and monocytes. Since both LCF and IL-2 are potent eosinophil chemoattractants, eosinophils would be recruited along with mononuclear cells by those lymphokines that stimulate CD4-bearing and IL-2 receptor-expressing lymphocytes and monocytes, respectively. Conversely, eosinophils have the capacity to stimulate lymphocyte responses by acting as MHC-restricted, HLA-DR-dependent antigen processing and presenting cells (Weller *et al.*, 1991a). Thus, in many ways eosinophils are akin to macrophages in their immunologic functions (Weller, 1991). Eosinophils have effector functions based on their capacities to elaborate lipid products and to degranulate. Moreover, eosinophils have other capabilities (Weller, 1991), including elaborating cytokines, such as the fibrogenic cytokines, TGF-α (Wong *et al.*, 1990) and TGF-β (Wong *et al.*, 1993), and collaboratively stimulating lymphocyte responses. The functioning of eosinophils with their multiple functional capabilities, including their interactions with lymphocytes, is intimately involved in the pathogenesis of allergic inflammation.

Acknowledgements

The author's studies have been supported in part by grants (AI20241, AI22571) from the National Institutes of Health and the MWV Leukocyte Research Fund. The collaborative assistance of many colleagues and co-investigators, including Sandra W. Ryeom, Claudia Cabral, Tonya Barrett, Janet Buhlmann and Drs Ann M. Dvorak, David T.W. Wong, Daniel R. Lucey, Thomas H. Rand, Craig Gerard, Norma P. Gerard, David S. Silberstein, Hardy Kornfeld, Susan E. Goelz, Anne Nicholson-Weller and Stephen J. Calli, is gratefully acknowledged.

References

Anderson, D.C., Schmalstieg, F.C., Finegold, M.J., Hughes, B.J., Rothlein, R., Miller, L.J., Kohl, S., Tosi, M.F., Jacobs, R.L., Waldrop, T.C., Goldman, A.S., Shearer, W.T. and Springer, T.A. (1985). The severe and moderate phenotypes of heritable Mac-1, LFA-1 deficiency: their quantitative definition and relation to leukocyte dysfunction and clinical features. *J. Infect. Dis.* **152**, 668–689.

Azzawi, M., Bradley, B., Jeffrey, P.K., Frew, A.J., Wardlaw, A.J., Knowles, G., Assoufi, B., Collins, J.V., Durham, S. and Kay, A.B. (1990). Identification of activated T lymphocytes and eosinophils in bronchial biopsies in stable atopic asthma. *Am. Rev. Respir. Dis.* **142**, 1407–1413.

Barnard, J.A., Lyons, R.M. and Moses, H.L. (1990). The cell biology of transforming growth factor beta. *Biochim. Biophys. Acta* **1032**, 79–87.

Beasley, R., Roche, W.R., Roberts, J.A. and Holgate, S.T. (1989). Cellular events in the bronchi in mild asthma and after bronchial provocation. *Am. Rev. Respir. Dis.*

Berman, J.S., Beer, D.J., Cruikshank, W.W. and Center, D.M. (1985). Chemoattractant lymphokines specific for the helper/inducer T-lymphocyte subset. *Cell. Immunol.* **95**, 105–112.

Bochner, B.S., Luscinskas, F.W., Gimbrone, M.A.J., Newman, W., Sterbinsky, S.A., Derse-Anthony, C.P., Klunk, D. and Schleimer, R.P. (1991). Adhesion of human basophils, eosinophils, and neutrophils to interleukin 1-activated human vascular endothelial cells: contributions of endothelial cell adhesion molecules. *J. Exp. Med.* **173**, 1553–1557.

Brewster, C.E.P., Howarth, P.H., Djukanovic, R., Wilson, J., Holgate, S.T. and Roche, W.R. (1990). Myofibroblasts and subepithelial fibrosis in bronchial asthma. *Am. J. Respir. Cell. Molec. Biol.* **3**, 507–511.

Center, D.M. and Cruikshank, W. (1982). Modulation of lymphocyte migration by human lymphokines I. Identification and characterization of chemoattractant activity for lymphocytes from mitogen-stimulated mononuclear cells. *J. Immunol.* **128**, 2569–2571.

Center, D.M., Cruikshank, W.W., Berman, J.S. and Beer, D.J. (1983). Functional characteristics of histamine receptor-bearing mononuclear cells. I. Selective production of lymphocyte chemoattractant lymphokine utilizing histamine as a ligand. *J. Immunol.* **131**, 1854–1859.

Cruikshank, W.W., Berman, J.S., Theodore, A.C., Bernardo, J. and Center, D.M. (1987). Lymphokine activation of $T4^+$ lymphocytes and monocytes. *J. Immunol.* **138**, 3817–3823.

Cruikshank, W.W., Berman, J.S., Theodore, A.C., Bernardo, J. and Center, D.M. (1991). Lymphocyte chemoattractant factor (LCF) induces CD4-dependent intracytoplasmic signalling in lymphocytes. *J. Immunol.* **146**, 2928–2934.

Diaz, P., Gonzalez, M.C., Galleguillos, F.R., Ancic, P., Cromwell, O., Shepherd, D., Durham, S.R., Gleich, G.J. and Kay, A.B. (1989). Leukocytes and mediators in bronchoalveolar lavage during allergen-induced late-phase asthmatic reactions. *Am. Rev. Respir. Dis.* **139**, 1383–1389.

Dobrina, A., Menegazzi, R., Carlos, T.M., Nardon, E., Cramer, R., Zacchi, T., Harlan, J.M. and Patriarca, P. (1991). Mechanisms of eosinophil adherence to cultured vascular endothelial cells. Eosinophils bind to the cytokine-induced ligand vascular cell adhesion molecule-1 via the very late activation antigen 4 integrin receptor. *J. Clin. Invest.* **88**, 20–26.

Elices, M.J., Osborn, L., Takada, Y., Crouse, C., Luhowskyj, S., Hemler, M.E. and Lobb, R.R. (1990). VCAM-1 on activated endothelium interacts with the leukocyte integrin VLA-4 at a site distinct from the VLA-4/fibronectin binding site. *Cell* **60**, 577–584.

Freedman, A.S., Munro, J.M., Rice, G.E., Bevilacqua, M.P., Morimoto, C., McIntyre, B.W., Rhynhart, K., Pober, J.S. and Nadler, L.M. (1990) Adhesion of human B cells to germinal centers *in vitro* involves VLA-4 and INCAM-110. *Science* **249**, 1030–1033.

Frew, A.J. and Kay, A.B. (1988). The relationship between infiltrating $CD4^+$ lymphocytes, activated eosinophils, and the magnitude of the allergen-induced late phase cutaneous reaction in man. *J. Immunol.* **141**, 4158–4164.

Frew, A.J., Corrigan, C.J., Maestrelli, P., Tsai, J.J., Kurihara, K., O'Hehir, R.E., Hartnell, A., Cromwell, O. and Kay, A.B. (1989). T lymphocytes in allergen-induced late-phase reactions and asthma. *Int. Arch. Allergy Appl. Immunol.* **88**, 63–67.

Gerard, N.P., Hodges, M.K., Drazen, J.M., Weller, P.F. and Gerard, C. (1989). Characterization of a receptor for C5a anaphylatoxin on human eosinophils. *J. Biol. Chem.* **264**, 1760–1766.

Hansel, T.T., Braunstein, J.B., Walker, C., Blaser, K., Bruijnzeel, P.L.B., Virchow, J.-C. Jr. and Virchow, C. (1991). Sputum eosinophils from asthmatics express ICAM-1 and HLA-DR. *Am. Rev. Respir. Dis.* **143**, A431.

Hemler, M.E., Elices, M.J., Parker, C. and Takada, Y. (1990). Structure of the integrin VLA-4 and its cell-cell and cell-matrix adhesion functions. *Immunol. Rev.* **114**, 45–65.

Kornfeld, H., Cruikshank, W.W., Pyle, S.W., Berman, J.S. and Center, D.M. (1988). Lymphocyte activation by HIV-1 envelope glycoprotein. *Nature* **335**, 445–448.

Lucey, D.R., Dorsky, D.I., Nicholson-Weller, A. and Weller, P.F. (1989a). Human eosinophils express CD4 protein and bind HIV-1 GP120. *J. Exp. Med.* **169**, 327–332.

Lucey, D.R., Nicholson-Weller, A. and Weller, P.F. (1989b). Mature human eosinophils have the capacity to express HLA-DR. *Proc. Natl. Acad. Sci. U.S.A.* **86**, 1348–1351.

Lyons, M. and Moses, H.L. (1990). Transformining growth factors and the regulation of cell proliferation. *Eur. J. Biochem.* **187**, 467–473.

Masinovsky, B., Urdal, D. and Gallatin, W.M. (1990). IL-4 acts synergistically with IL-1 beta to promote lymphocyte adhesion to microvascular endothelium by induction of vascular cell adhesion molecule-1. *J. Immunol.* **145**, 2886–2895.

Massagué, J. (1990). Transforming growth factor-α *J. Biol. Chem.* **265**, 21393–21396.

McCrone, E.L., Lucey, D.R. and Weller, P.F. (1988). Fluorescent staining for leukocyte chemotaxis: Eosinophil-specific staining with aniline blue. *J. Immunol. Meth.* **114**, 79–88.

Pelton, R.W. and Moses, H.L. (1990). The beta-type transforming growth factor. Mediators of cell regulation in the lung. *Am. Rev. Respir. Dis.* **142**, S31–S35.

Plumas, J., Gruart, V., Aldebert, D., Truong, M.J., Capron, M., Capron, A.

and Prin, L. (1991). Human eosinophils from hypereosinophilic patients spontaneously express the p55 but not the p75 interleukin-2 receptor subunit. *Eur. J. Immunol.* **21**, 1265–1270.

Rand, T.H., Cruikshank, W.W., Center, D.M. and Weller, P.F. (1991a). CD4-mediated stimulation of human eosinophils: Lymphocyte chemoattractant factor and other CD4-binding ligands elicit eosinophil migration. *J. Exp. Med.* **173**, 1521–1528.

Rand, T.H., Silberstein, D.S., Kornfeld, H. and Weller, P.F. (1991b). Human eosinophils express functional interleukin-2 receptors. *J. Clin. Invest.* **88**, 825–832.

Riedel, D., Lindemann, A., Brach, M., Mertelsmann, R. and Hermann, F. (1990). Granulocyte-macrophage colony-stimulating factor and interleukin-3 induce surface expression of interleukin-2 receptor p55 chain and CD4 by human eosinophils. *Immunology* **70**, 258–261.

Roberts, R.L., Ank, B.J., Salusky, I.B. and Stiehm, E.R. (1990). Purification and properties of peritoneal eosinophils from pediatric dialysis patients. *J. Immunol. Meth.* **126**, 205–211.

Roche, W.R., Beasley, R., Williams, J.H. and Holgate, S.T. (1989). Subepithelial fibrosis in the bronchi of asthmatics. *Lancet* **1**, 520–524.

Sanderson, C.J., Campbell, H.D. and Young, I.G. (1988). Molecular and cellular biology of eosinophil differentiation factor (interleukin-5) and its effects on human and mouse B cells. *Immunol. Rev.* **102**, 29–50.

Thornhill, M.H. and Haskard, D.O. (1990). IL-4 regulates endothelial cell activation by IL-1, tumor necrosis factor, or IFN-γ. *J. Immunol.* **145**, 865–872.

Thornhill, M.H., Wellicome, S.M., Mahiouz, D.L., Lanchbury, J.S.S., Kyan-Aung, U. and Haskard, D.O. (1991). Tumor necrosis factor combines with IL-4 or IFN-γ to selectively enhance endothelial cell adhesiveness for T cells. The contribution of vascular cell adhesion molecule-1-dependent and -independent binding mechanisms. *J. Immunol.* **146**, 592–598.

Todd, R., Donoff, B.R., Chiang, T., Chou, M.Y., Elovic, A., Gallagher, G.T. and Wong, D.T. (1991). The eosinophil as a cellular source of transforming growth factor alpha in healing cutaneous wounds. *Am. J. Pathol.* **138**, 1307–1313.

Walsh, G.M., Mermod, J.J., Hartnell, A., Kay, A.B. and Wardlaw, A.J. (1991). Human eosinophil, but not neutrophil, adherence to IL-1 stimulated human umbilical vascular endothelial cells is alpha 4 beta 1 (very late antigen-4) dependent. *J. Immunol.* **146**, 3419–3423.

Wardlaw, A.J., Moqbel, R., Cromwell, O. and Kay, A.B. (1986). Platelet activating factor. A potent chemotactic and chemokinetic factor for human eosinophils *J. Clin. Invest.* **78**, 1701–1706.

Warringa, R.A., Koenderman, L., Kok, P.T., Kreukniet, J. and Bruijnzeel, P.L. (1991). Modulation and induction of eosinophil chemotaxis by granulocyte-macrophage colony-stimulating factor and interleukin-3. *Blood* **77**, 2694–2700.

Weller, P.F. (1991). The immunobiology of eosinophils. *New Engl. J. Med.* **324**, 1110–1118.

Weller, P.F., Rand, T.H. and Finberg, R.W. (1991a). Human eosinophils function as HLA-DR dependent, MHC-restricted antigen-presenting cells. *FASEB J.* **5**, A640.

Weller, P.F., Rand, T.H., Goelz, S.E., Chi-Rosso, G. and Lobb, R.J. (1991b).

Human eosinophil adherence to vasclar endothelium mediated by binding to VCAM-1 and ELAM-1. *Proc. Natl. Acad. Sci. U.S.A.* **88**, 7430–7433.

Wong, D.T.W., Weller, P.F., Galli, S.J., Rand, T.H., Elovic, A., Chiang, T., Chou, M.Y., Gallagher, G.T., Matossian, K., McBride, J. and Todd, R. (1990). Human eosinophils express transforming growth factor α. *J. Exp. Med.* **172**, 673–681.

Wong, D.T.W., Elovic, A., Matossian, K., Nagura, N., McBridge, J., Gordon, J.R., Rand, T.H., Galli, S.J. and Weller, P.F. (1991). Eosinophils from patients with blood eosinophilia express transforming growth factors B_1. *Blood* **70**, 272–277.

Discussion

M. Capron

With regard to the expression of IL-2 receptor CD25 on the eosinophils, do you know whether eosinophils could release soluble CD25?

P.F. Weller

We have not looked at that. The only data I have bearing on that are the intriguing findings you published demonstrating elevated levels of IL-2 receptor in the serum of patients with hypereosinophilic syndrome. This raises the possibility that they might have been derived from eosinophils. The levels of IL-2 receptors demonstrable in all cells are relatively low as assessed by flow cytometry so, although the eosinophil levels are low, I think they are biologically active.

A.B. Kay

Do the lymphocyte-derived and IL-2 chemoattractants which have such high potency, have activity *in vivo*? Have they, in fact, been administered to the skin of man?

P.F. Weller

Lymphocyte chemoattractant factor (LCF) has not been administered to individuals to see whether local accumulation of eosinophils can be demonstrated.There is a literature on administering IL-2 to patients, many of whom will develop eosinophilia. I cannot find any descriptions of the histopathology of lesions looking early after giving IL-2 intradermally. People have looked late, at 24 or 47 h or even days later, but not early.

A.B. Kay

You mentioned that these factors do not cause degranulation, but do they prime the cell in the same way as platelet-activating factor (PAF) or C5A? Is there upregulation of CR3? Do they make the cell hyperadhesive? Do they have the same sort of actions as secretagogues and chemoattractants?

P.F. Weller

We have evaluated some of these possiblities. They do not prime the cells, say, for respiratory burst activity or alter the dose responsiveness of eosinophils to other stimuli for degranulation or respiratory burst activity. They are different in this regard.

A.B. Kay

It is curious, is it not, in that they make the cell move, but do nothing else to it?

P.F. Weller

It is curious, but causing the eosinophil to move clearly establishes its activity. It may well be acting in other ways to stimulate other responses of eosinophils, such as the production of cytokines that we have not evaluated.

VLA-4 is a protein that binds fibronectin, and it is a recognized mediator of co-stimulatory signals on lymphocytes, so that *perhaps*, in concert with eosinophils bound by means of VLA-4 to fibronectin, other responses can be elicited by some of these lymphokines that are not readily demonstrable in the test-tube by themselves.

A.B. Kay

According to your hypothesis, soluble vascular cell adhesion molecule (VCAM) would probably be a chemoattractant. [*P.F. Weller agreed.*]

J. Lamb

Does the binding of human immunodeficiency virus gp120 to eosinophils alter their function, phenotype or the cytokines that they release?

P.F. Weller

We have not looked at any of those possibilities yet, so I do not know. It is something that should be done.

J. Lamb

I was thinking of this in the context of your suggestion that CD4 on the membrane is involved in signal transduction.

P. Venge

For many years we have tried to identify the chemoattractant activities *in vivo*, looking in the bronchoalveolar lavage (BAL) fluid and in serum. Every time we come up with something that seems to be a good chemoattractant for the eosinophils it is always also a chemoattractant for the neutrophils. There are no selective eosinophil chemoattractants in the BAL fluid. I cannot recognize the specificity you describe, for example, in the BAL fluid from asthmatics. What are we doing wrong, or have you been able to show that this is actually an *in vivo* phenomenon?

P.F. Weller

You have assayed activities in BAL fluid and found activity both for neutrophils and eosinophils? [*P. Venge assented.*] I am sure that is true. We still have to come back to *in vivo* situations, though, where within the tissues there may be a preferential accumulation of eosinophils without neutrophils. There have to be mechanisms operable within the tissue environment that would cause the eosinophils to be recruited. However, this may not be reflected on assaying in the BAL fluid, and it may be that in that soup a multitude of factors are present and are contributing to the concomitant migration of eosinophils and neutrophils.

P. Venge

Have you tried to inhibit this activity? Have you taken the BAL fluid and tried to inhibit the activity by means of antibodies to IL-2 or the LCF?

P.F. Weller

No, we have not.

9

Eosinophil-Derived Pro-inflammatory Mediators

P. VENGE

Laboratory for Inflammation Research, Department of Clinical Chemistry, University Hospital, Uppsala, Sweden

Introduction

Accumulation and activation of eosinophil granulocytes in tissues is a common finding in a variety of human diseases. The best-studied disease is bronchial asthma but eosinophil activation is observed in almost any inflammatory disease (Spry, 1988; Hällgren and Venge, 1991). The role of these cells in the tissues is, however, still somewhat enigmatic. This is not to say that we do not have a number of ideas. Thus, in patients infected by parasites it is likely that the accumulation of eosinophils reflects the parasite-killing potential of the eosinophil and that the eosinophil presence in tissues is part of the normal defence reaction. Their role in allergic reactions has long been disputed and according to some hypotheses may be regarded as a defence reaction towards products produced by the mast cell, since some of the substances released by these cells may be neutralized by eosinophil-derived products. A common histopathological finding is also the presence of eosinophils in fibrotic processes and diseases, which has led to the hypothesis of a role for eosinophils in tissue repair processes. The most popular hypothesis today, however, is related to the spectacular cytotoxic potential of the human eosinophil (Venge and Peterson, 1989). Thus, the eosinophil has the potential to destroy almost any cell in the body by virtue of the release of cytotoxic granule proteins or by the production of oxygen-derived radicals.

T-Lymphocyte and Inflammatory Cell Research in Asthma
ISBN 0-12-388170-6

My own view of the human eosinophil is that it probably has the capacity to do all the things discussed above but that the activity of the cell is dependent on the circumstances under which it is attracted and activated. The eosinophil, therefore, appears to be an extremely versatile cell with many potential activities. Although I believe that one important physiological role of the eosinophil is to defend the body against parasites, we may not yet have discovered the major physiological role of this cell. Since the most likely role of the eosinophil is determined by the functions of the secreted products, either the functions of the molecules stored in the granules or of those produced upon activation, I will in this chapter briefly review our present knowledge of these products.

Granule Proteins of Human Eosinophils

The granule proteins of human eosinophil granulocytes are distributed between two major populations of granules. One is peroxidase-positive (Peterson *et al.*, 1987) and characterized by crystalloids, which contain one of the four major proteins of the human eosinophil, i.e. the major basic protein (MBP) (Gleich and Adolphson, 1986). The other granule population is peroxidase-negative which due to its lack of crystalloids is of lower density. Both granule populations seem to contain eosinophil cationic protein (ECP) (Olsson *et al.*, 1977) and eosinophil protein X/eosinophil-derived neurotoxin (EPX/EDN) (Durack *et al.*, 1981; Peterson and Venge, 1983; Slifman *et al.*, 1989) whereas the more dense and crystalloid-containing granules, in addition, contain eosinophil peroxidase (EPO) (Carlson *et al.*, 1985) in their matrix. A fifth major protein of the eosinophil is the Charcot–Leyden crystal (CLC) protein (Gleich *et al.*, 1976; Weller *et al.*, 1984), which presumably is a plasma membrane protein and shed from the eosinophil. The CLC protein forms the typical extracellular needle-like crystals found in tissues of heavy eosinophil infiltration. The biological role of the CLC protein may be related to its lysophospholipase activity.

One of the characteristic features of the four granule proteins are their high isoelectric points, which in the case of ECP and EPO exceeds pH 11. The proteins of the eosinophil granules are some of the most basic proteins in the human body. The biological meaning of this is not known but could be related to their cytotoxic activities described below. The molecular weights of the four granule proteins vary from 14 kDa for MBP to 67 kDa for EPO. Cloning of the proteins have revealed large amounts of the basic amino acid arginine in their sequences (Rosenberg *et al.*, 1989a,b; Barker *et al.*, 1989, 1990; Hamann *et al.*, 1989, 1990b; Ten *et al.*, 1989b).

The amino acid sequence of EPO showed a large degree of homology with myeloperoxidase of the neutrophil granulocytes. In spite of this, however, polyclonal antibodies produced against EPO and MPO showed no cross-reactivity (Öberg *et al.*, 1983; Carlson *et al.*, 1985). The amino acid sequence of ECP and EPX/EDN showed a large degree of homology, about 70%, with each other. Also a homology to pancreatic ribonuclease and angiogenin was shown and indeed both proteins have ribonuclease activities with EPX/EDN being the most active (Gullberg *et al.*, 1986; Gleich *et al.*, 1986). The close relationship between ECP and EPX/EDN is also indicated by the monoclonal antibody EG2, which recognizes a common epitope on the two proteins (Tai *et al.*, 1984). The relative content of the four major proteins in normal human eosinophil granules is similar and in the range of 10–15 $\mu g/10^6$ eosinophils. The number of eosinophils from patients with various causes of eosinophilia, however, may vary quite considerably.

Eosinophil Cationic Protein (ECP)

ECP is a one-chain zinc-containing protein with a molecular weight varying from 18 to 21 kDa. The heterogeneity is due to differences in glycosylation of the protein molecule (Peterson *et al.*, 1988). ECP is a potent cytotoxic molecule with the capacity to kill mammalian (Ding-E Young *et al.*, 1986) as well as non-mammalian cells such as parasites (Venge and Peterson, 1989; McLaren *et al.*, 1981, 1984, 1985).

One of the most conspicuous targets for the action of ECP is the brain with vast and non-selective destruction of brain tissue at very low concentrations. In order to achieve destruction of the Purkinje cells in the cerebellum of experimental animals within 3 weeks with resulting severe symptoms of ataxia, it was found that only 60 ng needed to be injected into the cerebrospinal fluids of the animals (Fredens *et al.*, 1982, 1985).

In a number of human diseases, ECP has been detected by immunohistochemical techniques in tissues of tissue injury, which suggest that ECP may be involved in the destruction of the cells. These diseases include asthma, myocarditis and colitis to mention a few (Dahl *et al.*, 1988; Fredens *et al.*, 1988; Venge *et al.*, 1988; Hällgren *et al.*, 1989b, 1991; Tottrup *et al.*, 1989; Gustafsson *et al.*, 1991).

The non-cytotoxic activities of ECP include the alteration of proteoglycan production by human embryonic fibroblasts (Särnstrand *et al.*, 1988) and stimulation of airway mucus secretion (Lundgren *et al.*, 1991). The former finding may point to a role in tissue repair processes and may have a bearing on the findings of the eosinophil presence in fibrotic processes (Rennard *et al.*, 1984). The latter may be of importance for the understanding of the role of the eosinophil in diseases such as asthma, since one characteristic of this disease is airways hypersecretion.

Another non-cytotoxic activity of potential interest is the capacity of ECP to inhibit T-lymphocyte proliferation, not only as a response to mitogens, but also in mixed leukocyte reactions (Peterson *et al.*, 1986). This effect is seen *in vitro* at concentrations as low as 10^{-8} mol/litre. Hence, by virtue of its granule proteins, the eosinophil may be active in the regulation of T cell-mediated reactions. ECP also shortens the coagulation time of plasma by mechanisms related to the enhancement of the activity of Factor XII (Venge *et al.*, 1979). These findings may be of relevance not only in the hypereosinophilic syndrome in which thromboembolic phenomena are very common (Spry, 1988; Liesveld and Abboud, 1991), but also in allergic reactions where activation of Factor XII has been demonstrated concomitant to the activation of the eosinophil (Dahl and Venge, 1981). Another study showed an effect on fibrinolysis due to preactivation of plasminogen and the consequent enhancement of plasminogen activator activation of plasminogen (Dahl and Venge, 1979).

It should be emphasized that most of the described effects of ECP *in vitro* take place at concentrations which are comparable to those found *in vivo*, i.e. 10^{-9}–10^{-6} mol/litre. Locally, these concentrations may even be exceeded. Thus in sputum of asthmatics and in the synovial fluid of patients with rheumatoid arthritis (Hällgren *et al.*, 1984a) concentrations as high as 10^{-5} mol/litre have been found. One important question, therefore, is how the cytotoxic activity of these proteins is regulated extracellularly. So far two potential mechanisms have been described: First, it has been proposed that ECP binds to heparin as a 1:1 complex and this binding neutralizes the activity of ECP (Fredens *et al.*, 1991). No *in vivo* data exist, however, which support this potential mechanism. Second, it has been suggested that ECP binds to α_2-macroglobulin (Peterson and Venge, 1987), probably at the site of the binding of proteolytic enzymes. ECP binding requires the prior exposure of α_2-macroglobulin to limited proteolytic attack by proteases such as cathepsin G or thrombin. Active proteases, which could accomplish this phenomenon, are generated in the inflammatory process not only from neutrophils, mast cells or macrophages, but also as a consequence of protease formation during activation of the complement and coagulation cascades. The binding of ECP to α_2-macroglobulin *in vivo* is indicated by the existence of high molecular weight forms of ECP in serum of patients with eosinophilia who also have very high levels of ECP in serum (Venge *et al.*, 1977). This interaction with α_2-macroglobulin may be an important mechanism of neutralizing the actions of ECP, since it is the only obvious interaction of ECP with any plasma component.

Sensitive immunoassays have been developed for ECP, which allow the measurement of ECP in most body fluids as an indicator of eosinophil activation and turnover (Venge *et al.*, 1977; Reimert *et al.*, 1991; Peterson *et al.*, 1991). This approach has been used extensively not only in asthma and allergic diseases (Venge and Carlson, 1990; Bousquet *et al.*, 1990; Venge, 1990; Venge and Håkansson, 1991) but also in inflammatory diseases of the gut, skin, joints, brain, etc. (Schmekel *et al.*, 1982, 1990; Hällgren *et al.*, 1983, 1984a,b, 1985, 1987, 1989a,b; Lundin *et al.*, 1985; Colombel *et al.*, 1988; Lavö *et al.*, 1989). The data derived from these studies have been of vital importance in the definition of the eosinophil as one of the major inflammatory cells (Venge, 1990).

Eosinophil Protein X or Eosinophil-Derived Neurotoxin (EPX/EDN)

EPX and EDN are the same protein (Slifman *et al.*, 1989), so the provisional name EPX/EDN is used, since no agreement has been reached on how to name it. EPX/EDN is a single-chain protein, which is less basic than ECP but with a similar size, i.e. a molecular weight of 18 kDa (Durack *et al.*, 1981; Ackerman *et al.*, 1983b; Peterson and Venge, 1983; Hamann *et al.*, 1989, 1990b; Rosenberg *et al.*, 1989b; Slifman *et al.*, 1989). EPX/EDN is a potent ribonuclease and about 100 times more active than ECP (Gullberg *et al.*, 1986). It also has some cytotoxic properties and the name EDN is, in fact, a reflection of its neurotoxic activities. Thus, when injected into the brains of experimental animals EPX/EDN produced damage to the tissues reminiscent of the so-called Gordon phenomenon with destruction, among other things, of Purkinje cells of the cerebellum and the development of ataxia (McNaught, 1938; Durack *et al.*, 1979, 1981; Fredens *et al.*, 1982, 1985; Perez *et al.* 1989). As described above, however, ECP seems to be a far more potent neurotoxin (Fredens *et al.*, 1982), producing the Gordon phenomenon at concentrations about 100 times lower than EPX/EDN. Like ECP, EPX/EDN inhibits T-lymphocyte proliferation in a non-cytotoxic fashion and at concentrations similar to those of ECP (Peterson *et al.*, 1986).

EPX/EDN does not seem to kill parasites as efficiently as ECP. The effect of EPX/EDN on parasites, such as the larvae of *Schistosoma mansoni*, is very characteristic and differs from that produced by ECP. When the parasite is exposed to EPX/EDN it is reversibly paralysed (McLaren *et al.*, 1981, 1984, 1985). This phenomenon could be an important defence mechanism facilitating the eradication of the parasite.

Immunoassays for EPX/EDN have been developed and used to measure the concentrations of EPX/EDN in various body fluids as indicators of eosinophil turnover and activity (Peterson and Venge, 1983; Durham *et al.*, 1989; Griffin *et al.*, 1991; Wardlaw *et al.*, 1988).

Eosinophil Peroxidase (EPO)

EPO is a two-chain protein with a total molecular weight of 67 kDa (Carlson *et al.*, 1985). The molecular weights of the light and heavy chains are 15 kDa and 52 kDa, respectively. The main function of EPO is to act as a peroxidase and together with a halide or thiocyanate and H_2O_2, EPO is a potent cytotoxic principle (Jong *et al.*, 1980, 1984; Jong and Klebanoff, 1980; Klebanoff *et al.*, 1989; Ayars *et al.*, 1989; Hamann *et al.*, 1990a; Slungaard and Mahoney, 1991a,b).

Examples of the cytotoxic activity and possibly important pathophysiologic mechanisms are the damage by EPO of nasal sinus mucosa (Hisamatsu *et al.*, 1990) and endothelial cells of the heart (Slungaard and Mahoney, 1991b). EPO also has a number of non-cytotoxic effects of mammalian cells of considerable interest. Thus, EPO induces degranulation of mast cells (Chi and Henderson, 1984; Henderson *et al.*, 1980) and causes platelet aggregation (Rohrbach *et al.*, 1990). In addition, EPO may be involved in the inactivation of lipid mediators such as the leukotrienes (Henderson *et al.*, 1982). EPO is taken up by the neutrophil granulocytes through a specific and probably receptor-related mechanism (Zabucchi *et al.*, 1986, 1990). This uptake might constitute an important scavenger mechanism, which neutralizes the toxic effects of EPO. The interaction with neutrophils also leads to an increased adhesiveness of the neutrophil. EPO can be measured in several body fluids including plasma by sensitive immunoassays (Carlson *et al.*, 1985).

Major Basic Protein (MBP)

The name major basic protein derives from the fact that in guinea-pig eosinophils this protein seems to be the dominating protein, making up about 50% of the protein content of the granule proteins (Gleich *et al.*, 1973). As mentioned above, MBP is stored in the granules in the typical crystalloids. The molecular weight of MBP is about 13.9 kDa (Barker *et al.*, 1990). It is also found in other cells such as the basophil and some placenta cells (Ackerman *et al.*, 1983a; Maddox *et al.*, 1984). The major biological function of the eosinophilic MBP is related to its cytotoxic activities which involves the killing and damage of parasites and mammalian cells such as pneumocytes, nasal mucosa, etc. (Wassom and

Gleich, 1979; Zheutlin *et al.*, 1984, 1985; Ayars *et al.*, 1985, 1989; Hastie *et al.*, 1987; Hamann *et al.*, 1990a; Hisamatsu *et al.*, 1990). The localization of MBP at sites of tissue injury has been demonstrated in the same diseases as ECP, i.e. in asthma, myocarditis, etc., and suggests a role for MBP in these diseases (Filley *et al.*, 1982; Peters *et al.*, 1983; Trocme *et al.*, 1989; Ten *et al.*, 1989a, 1990; Hisamatsu *et al.*, 1990; DeMello *et al.*, 1990). *In vivo*, the release of all four granule proteins seems to occur simultaneously, the demonstration of one protein being indicative of the secretion of all. To what extent these proteins have different or similar targets or whether they potentiate the cytotoxicity of each other is not known at present but is an important question for future research.

As with the other eosinophil granule proteins, MBP also has a number of non-cytotoxic effects on various cells. These include degranulation of basophils and mast cells, platelet aggregation (Zheutlin *et al.*, 1984; Butterfield *et al.*, 1990; Rohrbach *et al.*, 1990), induction of neutrophil superoxide production, contraction of airway smooth muscle and inhibition of airway mucus production (Zheutlin *et al.*, 1984; Rohrbach *et al.*, 1990; White *et al.*, 1990; Moy *et al.*, 1990, Lundgren *et al.*, 1991). Interesting

Table 9.1
Non-cytotoxic effects of human eosinophil granule proteins

Granule protein	Effects
ECP	Inhibits T cell proliferation Inhibits delayed hypersensitivity to PPD Alters proteoglycan production by fibroblasts Stimulates airway mucus secretion Causes basophil histamine release
EPO	Causes basophil and mast cell histamine release Causes platelet aggregation Causes increased neutrophil adhesiveness Inhibits receptor-mediated events on neutrophils, e.g. phagocytosis, chemotaxis
EPX/EDN	Inhibits T cell proliferation
MBP	Causes basophil and mast cell histamine release Inhibits airways mucus secretion Contracts airways smooth muscle Causes platelet aggregation Induces neutrophil superoxide production

Table 9.2
The effects of human eosinophil granule proteins on coagulation

Granule protein	Effects
ECP	Shortens coagulation time at low doses Prolongs coagulation time at high doses Preactivates plasminogen Inhibits streptokinase Heparin antagonist
EPO	Causes platelet aggregation
MBP	Heparin antagonist Causes platelet aggregation

functions of MBP are the effects on respiratory epithelium (White *et al.*, 1990), which may partly explain the development of the hyperresponsiveness in the airways of asthmatics (Gleich *et al.*, 1988).

The physiological control of the activities of MBP is not well understood. The binding of MBP to acidic polyamines and the identification of a ProMBP were recently demonstrated (Barker *et al.*, 1991). The binding and neutralization of the activities by heparin comprise an alternative control mechanism (Gleich and Adolphson, 1986). An interesting observation is the finding that mast cells are able to sequester MBP (Butterfield *et al.*, 1990). MBP may also be measured in various body fluids by means of a sensitive immunoassay (Wassom *et al.*, 1979; Ackerman *et al.*, 1981; Gleich and Adolphson, 1986; Gleich, 1990; Durham *et al.*, 1989).

Other Granule Proteins

In addition to the four major proteins, the granules of human eosinophils contain several other enzymatic activities (Spry, 1988; Weller, 1991), some of which have been characterized. These include collagenolytic activity, histaminase, phospholipase and arylsulphatase B activities (Weller and Austen, 1983). Even transforming growth factor-α (Wong *et al.*, 1990) and granulocyte–macrophage colony-stimulating factor (GM-CSF) have been shown to be expressed in human eosinophils. The relevance of these enzymatic activities to the specific actions of the human eosinophil is uncertain, although previous hypotheses have related some of these to the possible regulatory role of eosinophils in allergy. Thus, by means of these activities, the eosinophil has potential to inactivate a number of the putative mediators of the allergic inflammation such as histamine, platelet-activating factor (PAF) and leukotrienes.

Newly-Formed Mediators

An important factor in defining the role of the eosinophil in inflammation has been the demonstration of the eosinophil as a potent producer of several mediators of inflammation. Thus, the eosinophil is an efficient generator of oxygen-derived toxic metabolites such as O_2-, H_2O_2 and $OH^{\cdot}$. In this respect the eosinophil is, in fact, comparable to the neutrophil (DeChatelet *et al.*, 1977; Pincus *et al.*, 1981, 1982). The eosinophil is also a potent producer of a number of lipid mediators including prostaglandins (PGE_2), leukotrienes (LTC_4) (Verhagen *et al.*, 1984; Shaw *et al.*, 1984; Bruynzeel *et al.*, 1985) and platelet-activating factor (PAF) (Lee *et al.*, 1984). Both LTC_4 and PAF are potent spasmogenic lipids (Barnes, 1989; Townley *et al.*, 1989). In addition, PAF is a potent and fairly selective chemotactic signal for eosinophils themselves (Morita *et al.*, 1989; Sigal *et al.*, 1987; Håkansson *et al.*, 1987; Wardlaw *et al.*, 1986). In addition, PAF induces secretion of eosinophil granule proteins (Kroegel *et al.*, 1988, 1989). These findings indicate that the eosinophil through its capacity to produce various mediators, may act as a potent pro-inflammatory cell by affecting a number of cells in the body, including itself. Taken together these findings emphasize the hypothesis that one role of the eosinosphil is that of a potent pro-inflammatory cell.

Conclusion

Upon stimulation the eosinophil will release a number of potentially potent substances. One family of such substances are the four major proteins of human eosinophils, ECP, EPO, EPX/EDN and MBP. All these four proteins have both cytotoxic and non-cytotoxic biological activities. Although much focus has been directed recently towards the cytotoxic capacity of these proteins, it is quite obvious that they have many more exciting activities, which may be of relevance to the role of the eosinophil *in vivo*. These activities are summarized in Tables 9.1 and 9.2 and include non-cytotoxic activities such as the modulation of T-lymphocyte activities, induction and alteration of proteoglycan production by fibroblasts, regulation of mucus secretion and a variety of effects on haemostatic mechanisms. In addition to these activities, the recent demonstration that the eosinophil may produce various cytokines adds to the impression that this cell is a multifaceted and versatile cell. It is my belief that the true role of the eosinophil has yet to be discovered.

References

Ackerman, S.J., Gleich, G.J., Weller, P.F. and Ottesen, E.A. (1981). Eosinophilia and elevated serum levels of eosinophil major basic protein and charcot-leyden crystal protein (lysophospholipase) after treatment of patients with Bancroft's filariasis. *J. Immunol.* **127**, 1093–1098.

Ackerman, S.J., Kephart, G.M., Habermann, T.M., Greipp, P.R. and Gleich, G.J. (1983a). Localization of eosinophil granule major basic protein in human basophils *J. Exp. Med.* **158**, 946–961.

Ackerman, S.J., Loegering, D.A., Venge, P., Olsson, I., Harley, J.B., Fauci, A.S. and Gleich, G.J. (1983b). Distinctive cationic proteins of the human eosinophil granule: major basic protein, eosinophil cationic protein and eosinophil-derived neutrotoxin. *J. Immunol.* **131**, 2977–2982.

Ayars, G.H., Altman, L.C., Gleich, G.J., Loegering, D.A. and Baker, C.B. (1985). Eosinophil and eosinophil granule-mediated pneumocyte injury. *J. Allergy Clin. Immunol.* **76**, 595–604.

Ayars, G.H., Altman, L.C., McManus, M.M., Agosti, J.M., Baker, C., Luchtel, D.L., Loegering, D.A. and Gleich, G.J. (1989). Injurious effect of the eosinophil peroxide-hydrogen peroxide-halide system and major basic protein on human nasal epithelium *in vitro*. *Am. Rev. Respir. Dis.* **140**, 125–131.

Barker, R.L., Loegering, D.A., Ten, R.M., Hamann, K.J., Pease, L.R. and Gleich, G.J. (1989). Eosinophil cationic protein cDNA: Comparison with other toxic cationic proteins and ribonucleases. *J. Immunol.* **143**, 952–955.

Barker, R.L., Loegering, D.A., Arakawa, K.C., Pease, L.R. and Gleich, G.J. (1990). Cloning and sequence analysis of the human gene encoding eosinophil major basic protein *Gene.* **86**, 285–289.

Barker, R.L., Gundel, R.H., Gleich, G.J., Checkel, J.L., Loegering, D.A., Pease, L.R. and Hamann, K.J. (1991). Acidic polyamino acids inhibit human eosinophil granule major basic protein toxicity. Evidence of a functional role for ProMBP. *J. Clin. Invest.* **88**, 798–805.

Barnes, P.J. (1989). New concepts in the pathogenesis of bronchial hyperrresponsiveness and asthma. *J. Allergy Clin. Immunol.* **83**, 1013–1026.

Bousquet, J., Chanez, P., Lacoste, J.Y., Barnéon, G., Ghavanian, N., Enander, I., Venge, P., Ahlstedt, S., Simony-Lafontaine, J., Godard, P. and Michel, F.-B. (1990). Eosinophilic inflammation in asthma. *New Engl. J. Med.* **323**, 1033–1039.

Bruynzeel, P.L., Kok, P.T., Hamelink, M.L., Kijne, A.M. and Verhagen, J. (1985). Exclusive leukotriene C4 synthesis by purified human eosinophils induced by opsonized zymosan. *FEBS Letts* **189**, (2), 350–354.

Butterfield, J.H., Weiler, D., Peterson, E.A., Gleich, G.J. and Leiferman, K.M. (1990). Sequestration of eosinophil major basic protein in human mast cells. *Lab. Invest.* **62**, 77–86.

Carlson, M.G., Peterson, C.G. and Venge, P. (1985). Human eosinophil peroxidase: purification and characterization. *J. Immunol.* **134**, 1875–1879.

Chi, E.Y. and Henderson, W.R. (1984). Ultrastructure of Mast Cell Degranulation Induced by Eosinophil Peroxidase. *J. Histochem. Cytochem.* **32**, 332–341.

Colombel, J.F., Hällgren, R., Venge, P., Mesnard, B. and Rambaud, J.C. (1988). Neutrophil and eosinophil involvement of the small bowel affected by chronic alcoholism. *Gut* **29**, 1656–1660.

Dahl, R. and Venge, P. (1979). Enhancement of urokinase-induced plasminogen activation by the cationic protein of human granulocytes. *Thromb. Res.* **14**, 599–608.

Dahl, R. and Venge, P. (1981). Activation of blood coagulation during inhalation challenge tests. *Allergy* **36**, 129–133.

Dahl, R., Venge, P. and Fredens, K. (1988). The eosinophil. *In* "Asthma: Basic Mechanisms and Clinical Management" (P.J. Barnes, I. Rodger and N. Thomson), eds pp. 115–130. Academic Press, London.

DeChatelet, L.R., Shirley, P.S., McPhail, L.C., Huntley, C.C., Muss, H.B. and Bass, D.A. (1977). Oxidative metabolism of the human eosinophil. *Blood* **50**, (3), 525–535.

DeMello, D.E., Liapis, H., Jureidini, S., Nouri, S., Kephart, G.M. and Gleich, G.J. (1990). Cardiac localization of eosinophil-granule major basic protein in acute necrotizing myocarditis. *New Engl. J. Med.* **323**, 1542–1545.

Ding-E Young, J., Peterson, C.G., Venge, P. and Cohn, Z.A. (1986). Mechanism of membrane damage mediated by human eosinophil cationic protein. *Nature* **321**, 613–616.

Durack, D.T., Sumi, S.M. and Klebanoff, S.J. (1979). Neurotoxicity of human eosinophils. *Proc. Natl. Acad. Sci. U.S.A.* **76**, 1443–1447.

Durack, D.T., Ackerman, S.J., Loegering, D.A. and Gleich, G.J. (1981), Purification of human eosinophil-derived neurotoxin. *Proc. Natl. Acad. Sci. U.S.A.* **78**, 5165–5169.

Durham, S.R., Loegering, D.A., Dunnette, S., Gleich, G.J. and Kay, A.B. (1989). Blood eosinophils and eosinophil-derived proteins in allergic asthma. *J. Allergy Clin. Immunol.* **84**, 1–14.

Filley, W.V., Kephart, G.M., Holley, K.E. and Gleich, G.J. (1982). Identification by immunofluorescence of eosinophil granule major basic protein in lung tissues of patients with bronchial asthma. *Lancet* **3**, 11–16.

Fredens, K., Dahl, R. and Venge, P. (1982). The Gordon phenomenon induced by the eosinophil cationic protein and eosinophil protein-X. *J. Allergy Clin. Immunol.* **70**; 361–366.

Fredens, K., Dahl, R. and Venge, P. (1985). Eosinophils and cellular injury: the Gordon phenomeon as a model. *Allergy. Proc.* **6**, 346–351.

Fredens, K., Dybdahl, H., Dahl, R. and Baandrup, U. (1988). Extracellular deposit of the cationic proteins ECP and EPX in tissue infiltrations of eosinophils related to tissue damage. *APMIS* **96**, 711–719.

Fredens, K., Dahl, R. and Venge, P. (1991). In vitro studies of the interaction between heparin and eosinophil cationic protein. *Allergy* **46**, 27–29.

Gleich, G.J. (1990). The eosinophil and bronchial asthma: Current understanding. *J. Allergy Clin. Immunol.* **85**, (2), 422–436.

Gleich, G.J. and Adolphson, C.R. (1986). The eosinophil leukocyte: structure and function. *Adv. Immunol.* **39**; 177–253.

Gleich, G.J., Loegering, D.A. and Maldonado, J.E. (1973). Identification of a major basic protein in guinea pig eosinophil granules. *J. Exp. Med.* **137**, 1459–1471.

Gleich, G.J., Loegering, D.A., Mann, K.G. and Maldonado, J.E. (1976). Comparative properties of the charcot-leyden crystal protein and the major basic protein from human eosinophils. *J. Clin. Invest.* **57**, 633–640.

Gleich, G.J., Loegering, D.A., Bell, M.P., Checkel, J.L., Ackerman, S.J. and Kean, D.J. (1986). Biochemical and functional similarities between human eosinophil derived neurotoxin and eosinophil cationic protein: Homology with ribonuclease. *Proc. Natl. Acad. Sci. U.S.A.* **83**, 3146–3150.

Gleich, G.J., Flavahan, N.A., Fujisawa, T. and Vanhoutte, P.M. (1988). The eosinophil as a mediator of damage to respiratory epithelium: A model for bronchial hyperreactivity. *J. Allergy Clin. Immunol.* **81**, 776–781.

Griffin, E., Håkansson, L., Formgren, H., Jörgensen, K., Peterson, C. and Venge, P. (1991). Blood eosinophil number and activity in relation to lung function in asthmatic patients with eosinophilia. *J. Allergy Clin. Immunol.* **87**, 548–557.

Gullberg, U., Widegren, B., Arnason, U., Egesten, A. and Olsson, I. (1986). The cytotoxic eosinophil cationic protein (ECP) has ribonuclease activity. *Biochem. Biophys. Res. Commun.* **139**, 1239–1242.

Gustafsson, R., Fredens, K., Nettelbladt, O. and Hällgren, R. (1991). Eosinophil activation in systemic sclerosis. *Arthr. Rheum.* **34**,(4), 414–422.

Håkansson, L., Westerlund, D. and Venge, P. (1987). A new method for the measurement of eosinophil migration. *J. Leukocyte Biol.* **42**, 689–696.

Hällgren, R. and Venge, P. (1991). The eosinophil in inflammation. *In* "Clinical Impact of the Monitoring of Allergic Inflammation" (P. Matsson, S. Ahlstedt, P. Venge, J. Thorell and J. London, eds), pp. 119–140. Academic Press, New York.

Hällgren, R., Terent, A. and Venge, P. (1983). Eosinophil cationic protein (ECP) in the cerebrospinal fluid. *J. Neurol. Sci.* **58**, 57–71.

Hällgren, R., Bjelle, A. and Venge, P. (1984a). Eosinophil cationic protein in inflammatory synovial effusions as evidence of eosinophil involvement. *Ann. Rheum. Dis.* **43**, 556–562.

Hällgren, R., Borg, T., Venge, P. and Modig, J. (1984b). Signs of neutrophil and eosinophil activation in adult respiratory distress syndrome. *Crit. Care Med.* **12**, 14–18.

Hällgren, R., Feltelius, N., Svensson, K. and Venge, P. (1985). Eosinophil involvement in rheumatoid arthritis as reflected by elevated serum levels of eosinophil cationic protein. *Clin. Exp. Immunol.* **59**, 539–546.

Hällgren, R., Samuelsson, T., Venge, P. and Modig, J. (1987). Eosinophil activation in the lung is related to lung damage in adult respiratory distress syndrome. *Am. Rev. Respir. Dis.* **135**, 639–642.

Hällgren, R., Bjermer, L., Lundgren, R. and Venge, P. (1989a). The eosinophil component of the alveolitis in idiopathic pulmonary fibrosis. Signs of eosinophil activation in the lung are related to lung function. *Am. Rev. Respir. Dis.* **139**, 373–377.

Hällgren, R., Colombel, J.F., Dahl, R., Fredens, K., Kruse, A., Jacobsen, S., Venge, P. and Rambaud, J.C. (1989b). Neutrophil and eosinophil involvement of the small bowel in patients with celiac disease and Crohn's disease. Studies on the secretion rate and immunohistochemical localization of the granulocyte granule constituents in jejunum. *Am. J. Med.* **86**, 56–64.

Hällgren, R., Bohman, S.-O. and Fredens, K. (1991). Activated eosinophil infiltration and deposits of eosinophil cationic protein in renal allograft rejection. *Nephron* **59**, 266–270.

Hamann, K.J., Barker, R.L., Loegering, D.A., Pease, L.R. and Gleich, G.J. (1989). Sequence of human eosinophil-derived neurotoxin cDNA: Identity of deduced amino acid sequence with human nonsecretory ribonucleases. *Gene* **83**, 161–167.

Hamann, K.J., Gleich, G.J., Checkel, J.L., Loegering, D.A., McCall, J.W. and Barker, R.L. (1990a). In vitro killing of microfilariae of *Brugia pahangi* and *Brugia malayi* by eosinophil granule proteins. *J. Immunol.* **144**, 3166–3173.

Hamann, K.J., Ten, R.M., Loegering, D.A., Jenkins, R.B., Heise, M.T., Schad, C.R., Pease, L.R., Gleich, G.J. and Barker, R.L. (1990b). Structure and chromosome localization of the human eosinophil-derived neurotoxin and eosinophil cationic protein genes: Evidence for intronless coding sequences in the ribonuclease gene superfamily. *Genomics* **7**, 535–546.

Hastie, A.T., Loegering, D.A., Gleich, G.J. and Kueppers, F. (1987). The effect of purified human eosinophil major basic protein on mammalian ciliary activity. *Am. Rev. Respir. Dis.* **135**, 848–853.

Henderson, W.R., Chi, E.Y. and Klebanoff, S.J. (1980). Eosinophil peroxidase-induced mast cell secretion. *J. Exp. Med.* **152**, 265–279.

Henderson, W.R., Jörg, A. and Klebanoff, S.J. (1982). Eosinophil peroxidase-mediated inactivation of leukotrienes B4, C4 and D4. *J. Immunol.* **128**, 2609–2613.

Hisamatsu, K., Ganbo, T., Nakazawa, T., Murakami, Y., Gleich, G.J., Makiyama, K. and Koyama, H. (1990). Cytotoxicity of human eosinophil granule major basic protein to human nasal sinus mucosa in vitro. *J. Allergy Clin. Immunol.* **86**, 52–63.

Jong, E.C. and Klebanoff, S.J. (1980). Eosinophil-mediated mammalian tumor cell cytotoxicity: Role of the peroxidase system. *J. Immunol.* **124**, 1949–1953.

Jong, E.C., Henderson, W.R. and Klebanoff, S.J. (1980). Bactericidal activity of eosinophil peroxidase. *J. Immunol.* **124**, 1378–1382.

Jong, E.C., Chi, E.Y. and Klebanoff, S.J. (1984). Human neutrophil-mediated killing of schistosomula of schistosomal binding of eosinophil peroxidase. *Am. J. Trop. Med. Hyg.* **33**, 104–115.

Klebanoff, S.J., Agosti, J.M., Jörg, A. and Waltersdorph, A.M. (1989). Comparative toxicity of the horse eosinophil peroxidase-H_2O_2 halide system and granule basic proteins. *J. Immunol.* **143**, 239–244.

Kroegel, C., Yukawa, T., Dent, G., Chanez, P., Chung, K.F. and Barnes, P.J. (1988). Platelet-activating factor induces eosinophil peroxidase release from purified human eosinophils. *Immunology* **64**, 559–562.

Kroegel, C., Yukawa, T., Dent, G., Venge, P., Fan Chung, K. and Barnes, P.J. (1989). Stimulation of degranulation from human eosinophils by platelet-activating factor. *J. Immunol.* **142**, 3518–3526.

Lavö, B., Knutson, L., Lööf, L., Odlind, B., Venge, P. and Hällgren, R. (1989). Challenge with gliadin induces eosinophil and mast cell activation in the jejunum of patients with celiac disease. *Am. J. Med.* **87**, 655–660.

Lee, T.C., Lenihan, D.J., Malone, B., Roddy, L.L. and Wasserman, S.I. (1984). Increased biosynthesis of platelet-activating factor in activated human eosinophil. *J. Biol. Chem.* **259**, 5526–5530.

Liesveld, J.L. and Abboud, C.N. (1991). State of the art: The hypereosinophilic syndromes. *Blood Rev.* **5**, 29–37.

Lundgren, J.D., Davey, R.T., Jr., Lundgren, B., Mullol, J., Marom, Z., Logun,

C., Baraniuk, J., Kaliner, M.A. and Shelhamer, J.H. (1991). Eosinophil cationic protein stimulates and major basic protein inhibits airway mucus secretion. *J. Allergy Clin. Immunol.* **87**, 689–698.

Lundin, A., Håkansson, L., Hällgren, R., Michaelsson, G. and Venge, P. (1985). Increased in vivo secretory activity of neutrophil granulocytes in patients with psoriasis and palmoplantar pustulosis. *Acta Dermatol. Res.* **277**, 179–184.

Maddox, D.E., Kephart, G.M., Coulam, C.B., Butterfield, J.H., Benirschke, K. and Gleich, G.J. (1984). Localization of a molecule immunochemically similar to eosinophil major basic protein in human placenta. *J. Exp. Med.* **160**, 29–41.

McLaren, D.J., McKean, J.R., Olsson, I., Venge, P. and Kay, A.B. (1981). Morphological studies on the killing of schistosomula of Schistosoma Mansoni by eosinophil and neutrophil cationic proteins in vitro. *Parasite Immunol.* **3**, 359–373.

McLaren, D.J., Peterson, C.G. and Venge, P. (1984). Schistosoma Mansoni: further studies of the interaction between schistosomula and granulocyte-derived cationic proteins in vitro. *Parasitology*. **88**, 491–503.

McLaren, D.J., McKean, J.R., Peterson, C.G., Kay, A.B. and Venge P. (1985). *In* "Inflammation Basic Mechanisms, Tissue Injuring Principles and Clinical Models" (P. Venge and A. Lindbom, eds), pp. 341–345. Almqvist & Wiksell International, Stockholm.

McNaught, J.B. (1938). The Gordon test for Hodgkin's disease. A reaction to eosinophils. *J. Am. Med. Assoc.* 1280–1284.

Morita, E., Schröder, J.-M. and Christophers, E. (1989). Differential sensitivities of purified human eosinophils and neutrophils to defined chemotaxins. *Scand. J. Immunol.* **29**, 709–716.

Moy, J.N., Gleich, G.J. and Thomas, L.L. (1990). Noncytotoxic activation of neutrophils by eosinophil granule major basic protein: Effect on superoxide anion generation and lysosomal enzyme release. *J. Immunol.* **145**, 2626–2632.

Öberg, G., Lindmark, G., Moberg, L. and Venge, P. (1983). The peroxidase activity and cellular content of granule proteins in PMN during pregnancy. *Brit. J. Haematol.* **55**, 701–708.

Olsson, I., Venge, P., Spitznagel, J.K. and Lehrer, R. (1977). Arginine-rich Cationic proteins of human eosinophil granules. Comparison of the constituents of eosinophilic and neutrophilic leukocytes. *Lab. Invest.* **36**, 493–500.

Perez, O., Capron, M., Lastre, M., Venge, P., Khalife, J. and Capron, A. (1989). *Angiostrongylus cantonensis*: Gordon-like phenomenon (neurotoxic syndrome) in experimental infections. Role of eosinophils and IgE antibodies. *Exp. Parasitol.* **68**, 403–413.

Peters, M.S., Schroeter, A.L., Kephart, G.M. and Gleich, G.J. (1983). Localization of eosinophil granule major basic protein in chronic urticaria. *J. Invest. Dermatol.* **81**, 39–43.

Peterson, C.G. and Venge, P. (1983). Purification and characterization of a new cationic protein – eosinophil protein X(EPX) – from granules of human eosinophils. *Immunology* **50**, 19–26.

Peterson, C.G. and Venge, P. (1987). Interaction and complex formation between the eosinophil cationic protein (ECP) and alpha-2-macroglobulin. *Biochem. J.* **245**, 781–787.

Peterson, C.G., Skoog, V. and Venge, P. (1986). Human eosinophil cationic proteins (ECP and EPX) and their suppressive effects on lymphocyte proliferation. *Immunobiology* **171**, 1–13.

Peterson, C.G., Garcia, R.C., Carlson, M.G. and Venge, P. (1987). Eosinophil cationic protein (ECP), eosinophil protein x (EPX) and eosinophil peroxidase (EPO): Granule distribution, degranulation and characterization of released proteins. *In* "Eosinophil Granule Proteins. Biochemical and Functional Studies" (C. Peterson, ed.), pp. 1–19. Doctoral Thesis of Uppsala University, Uppsala.

Peterson, C.G., Jörnvall, H. and Venge, P. (1988). Purification and characterization of eosinophil cationic protein from normal human eosinophils. *Eur. J. Haematol.* **40**, 415–423.

Peterson, C.G., Enander, I., Nystrand, J., Anderson, A-S., Nilsson, L. and Venge, P. (1991). Radioimmunoassay of human eosinophil cationic protein (ECP) by an improved method. Establishment of normal levels in serum and turnover in vivo. *Clin. Exp. Allergy*.

Pincus, S.H., Schooley, W.R., DiNapoli, A.M. and Broder, S. (1981). Metabolic heterogeneity of eosinophils from normal and hypereosinophilic patients. *Blood* **58**, 1175–1181.

Pincus, S.H., DiNapoli, A.M. and Schooley, W.R. (1982). Superoxide production by eosinophils: Activation by histamine. *J. Clin. Invest.* **79**, 53–57.

Reimert, C.M., Venge, P., Kharazmi, A. and Bendtzen, K. (1991). Detection of eosinophil cationic protein (ECP) by an enzyme-linked immunosorbent assay. *J. Immunol. Meth.* **138**, 285–290.

Rennard, S.I., Bitterman, P.B. and Crystal, R.G. (1984). IV. Mechanisms of fibrosis. *Am. Rev. Respir. Dis.* **130**, 492–496.

Rohrbach, M.S., Wheatley, C.L., Slifman, N.R. and Gleich, G.J. (1990). Activation of platelets by eosinophil granule proteins. *J. Exp. Med.* **172**, 1271–1274.

Rosenberg, H.F., Ackerman, S.J. and Tenen, D.G. (1989a). Human eosinophil cationic protein. Molecular cloning of a cytotoxin and helminthotoxin with ribonuclease activity. *J. Exp. Med.* **170**, 163–176.

Rosenberg, H.F., Tenen, D.G. and Ackerman, S.J. (1989b). Molecular cloning of the human eosinophil-derived neurotoxin: A member of the ribonuclease gene family. *Proc. Natl. Acad. Sci. U.S.A.* **86**, 4460–4464.

Särnstrand, B., Westergren-Thorsson, G., Hernäs, J., Peterson, C.G., Venge, P. and Malmström, A. (1988). Eosinophil cationic protein and transforming growth factor-A stimulates synthesis of hyaluronan and proteoglycan in human fibroblast cultures. *In* "5th International Colloquium on Pulmonary Fibrosis" (abst.).

Schmekel, B., Hällgren, R., Stålenheim, G. and Venge, P. (1982). Indices of inflammatory cell activity and pulmonary function in different stages of sracoidosis. *Acta Med. Scand.* **211**, 393–399.

Schmekel, B., Wollmer, P., Venge, P., Linden, M. and Blom-Bülow, B. (1990). Transfer of 99mTcDTPA and bronchoalveolar lavage findings in patients with asymptomatic extrinsic allergic alveolitis. *Thorax* **45**, 525–529.

Shaw, R.J., Cromwell, O. and Kay, A.B. (1984). Preferential generation of leukotriene C4 by human eosinophils. *Clin. Exp. Immunol.* **56**, 716–722.

Sigal, C.E., Valone, F.H., Holtzman, M.J. and Goetzl, E.J. (1987). Preferential human eosinophil chemotactic activity of the platelet-activating factor (PAF) 1-0-hexadecyl-2-acetyl-sn-glyceryl-3-phosphocholine (AGEPC). *J. Clin. Immunol.* **7**, 179–184.

Slifman, N.R., Peterson, C.G., Gleich, G.J., Dunette, S.L. and Venge, P. (1989). Human eosinophil-derived neurotoxin and eosinophil protein x are likely the same protein. *J. Immunol.* **143**, 2317–2322.

Slungaard, A. and Mahoney, J.R. Jr. (1991a). Thiocyanate is the major substrate for eosinophil peroxidase in physiologic fluids. Implications for cytotoxicity. *J. Biol. Chem.* **266**, 4903–4910.

Slungaard, A. and Mahoney, J.R. Jr. (1991b). Bromide-dependent toxicity of eosinophil peroxidase for endothelium and isolated working rat hearts: A model for eosinophilic endocarditis. *J. Exp. Med.* **173**, 117–126.

Spry, C.J. (1988) "Eosinophils. A comprehensive Review and Guide to the Scientific and Medical Literature". Oxford University Press, Oxford.

Tai, P.-C., Spry, C.J., Petterson, C., Venge, P. and Olsson, I. (1984). Monoclonal antibodies distinguish between storage and secreted forms of eosinophil cationic protein. *Nature* **309**, 182–184.

Ten, R.M., Gleich, G.J., Holley, K.E., Perkins, J.D. and Torres, V.E. (1989a). Eosinophil granule major basic protein in acute renal allograft rejection. *Transplantation* **47**, 959–963.

Ten, R.M., Pease, L.R., McKean, D.J., Bell, M.P. and Gleich, G.J. (1989b). Molecular cloning of the human eosinophil peroxidase. Evidence for the existence of a peroxidase multigene family. *J. Exp. Med.* **169**, 1757–1769.

Ten, R.M., Kephart, G.M., Posada, M., Abaitua, I., Soldevilla, L., Kilbourne, E.M., Dunnette, S.L. and Gleich, G.J. (1990). Participation of eosinophils in the toxic oil syndrome. *Clin. Exp. Immunol.* **82**, 313–317.

Tottrup., A., Fredens, K., Funch-Jensen, P., Aggestrup, S. and Dahl, R. (1989). Eosinophil infiltration in primary esophageal achalasia. A possible pathogenic role. *Dig: Dis. Sci.* **34**, 1894–1899.

Townley, R.G., Hopp, R.J., Agrawal, D.K. and Bewtra, A.K. (1989). Platelet-activating factor and airway reactivity. *J. Allergy Clin. Immunol.* **83**, 997–1010.

Trocme, S.D., Kephart, G.M., Allansmith, M.R., Bourne, W.M. and Gleich, G.J. (1989). Conjunctival deposition of eosinophil granule major basic protein in vernal keratoconjunctivitis and contact lens-associated giant papillary conjunctivitis. *Am. J. Ophthalmol.* **108**, 57–63.

Venge, P. (1990). What is the role of the eosinophil? *Thorax* **45**, 161–163.

Venge, P. and Peterson, C.G. (1989). Eosinophil biochemistry and killing mechanisms. *In* "Eosinophils in Asthma" (J. Morley and I. Colditz, eds), pp. 163–177. Academic Press, New York, London.

Venge, P. and Carlson, M. (1990). Eosinophil granule proteins in bronchial asthma. *In* "Eosinophils, Allergy and Asthma" (A.B. Kay, ed.), pp. 96–105. Blackwell Scientific, Oxford.

Venge, P. and Håkansson, L. (1991). The eosinophil and asthma. *In* "Asthma. Its Pathology and Treatment" (M. Kaliner, P.J. Barnes and C.G. Persson, eds), pp. 477–502. Marcel Dekker, New York.

Venge, P., Roxin, L.-E. and Olsson, I. (1977). Radioimmunoassay of human eosinophil cationic protein. *Brit. J. Haematol.* **37**, 331–335.

Venge, P., Dahl, R. and Hällgren, R. (1979). Enhancement of factor XII dependent reactions by eosinophil cationic protein. *Thromb. Res.* **14**, 641–649.

Venge, P., Dahl, R. and Fredens, K. (1988). Epithelial injury by human eosinophils. *Am. Rev. Respir. Dis.* **138**, s54–s57.

Verhagen, J., Bruynzeel, P.L.B., Koedam, J.A., Wassink, G.A., de Boer, M., Terpstra, G.K., Kreukniet, J., Veldink, G.A. and Vliegenthart, J.F.G. (1984). Specific leukotriene formation by purified human eosinophils and neutrophils. *FEBS Letts* **168**(1), 23–28.

Wardlaw, A.J., Moqbel, R., Cromwell, O., and Kay, A.B. (1986). Platelet-activating factor A potent chemotactic and chemokinetic factor for human eosinophils. *J. Clin. Invest.* **78**, 1701–1706.

Wardlaw, A.J., Dunnette, S., Gleich, G.J., Collins, J.V. and Kay, A.B. (1988). Eosinophils and mast cells in bronchoalveolar lavage in subjects with mild asthma. *Am. Rev. Respir. Dis.* **137**, 62–69.

Wassom, D.L. and Gleich, G.J. (1979). Damage to *Trichinella spiralis* newborn larvae by eosinophil major basic protein. *Am. J. Trop. Med. Hyg.* **28**, 860–863.

Wassom, D.L., Loegering, D.A. and Gleich, G.J. (1979). Measurement of guinea pig eosinophil major basic protein by radioimmunoassay. *Molec. Immunol.* **16**, 711–719.

Weller, P.F. (1991). The immunobiology of eosinophils. *New Engl. J. Med.* **324**, 1110–1118.

Weller, P.F. and Austen, K.F. (1983). Human eosinophil arylsulfatase B Structure and activity of the purified tetrameric lysosomal hydrolase. *J. Clin. Invest.* **71**, 114–123.

Weller, P.F., Bach, D.S. and Austen, K.F. (1984). Biochemical characterization of human eosinophils charcot-leyden crystal protein lysophospholipase. *J. Biol. Chem.* **259**, 15100–15105.

White, S.R., Ohno, S., Munoz, N.M., Gleich, G.J., Abrahams, C., Solway, J. and Leff, A.R. (1990). Epithelium-dependent contraction of airway smooth muscle caused by eosinophil. MBP. *Am. J. Physiol. Lung Cell. Molec. Physiol.* **259**, L294-L303.

Wong, D.T., Weller, P.F., Galli, S.J., Elovic, A., Rand, T.H., Gallagher, G.T., Chiang, T., Chou, M.Y., Matossian, K., McBride, J. and Todd, R. (1990). Human eosinophils express transforming growth factor alpha. *J. Exp. Med.* **172**, 673–681.

Zabucchi, G., Menegazzi, R., Soranzo, M.R. and Patriarca, P. (1986). Uptake of human eosinophil peroxidase by human neutrophils. *Am. J. Pathol.* **124**, 510–518.

Zabucchi, G., Menegazzi, R., Cramer, R., Nardon, E. and Patriarca, P. (1990). Mutual influence between eosinophil peroxidase (EPO) and neutrophils: neutrophils reversibly inhibit EPO enzymatic activity and EPO increases neutrophil adhesiveness. *Immunology* **69**, 580–587.

Zheutlin, L.M., Ackerman, S.J., Gleich, G.J. and Thomas, L.L. (1984). Stimulation of basophil and rat mast cell histamine release by eosinophil granule-derived cationic proteins. *J. Immunol.* **133**, 2180–2185.

Zheutlin, L.M., Ackerman, S.J., Gleich, G.J. and Thomas, L.L. (1985). Donor sensitivity to basophil activation by eosinophil granule major basic protein. *Int. Arch. Allergy Appl. Immunol.* **77**, 216–217.

Discussion

S.T. Holgate

May I bring Dr Venge back to some of his and other people's earlier work relating to the effect of these arginine-rich proteins on the bronchial epithelium, which is obviously of interest for an asthma group. From our work on bronchial biopsies we have been singularly unimpressed by the deposition of major basic protein (MBP) and cationic protein in relation to the epithelial injury in what we consider clinical asthma, rather than the deaths that have been featured in Gleich's and other people's publications.

We are also singularly unimpressed by the *in vitro* work showing for MBP and, to a lesser or greater degree, your cationic protein, a selectivity against particular types of epithelial cells. The lesion in asthma that we see in our biopsies is a very specific lesion. It involves both the suprabasal cells (not the basal cells) and also disturbance to the desmosomal plaque proteins that hold the epithelium together. It appears that there is weakening of this structure, with a loss of permeability through the epithelium as a result. Yet, if MBP is put in these culture systems, either in epithelium or amniotic tissue cells, there is a cytotoxic death of the epithelial cell, with the cell often still attached to its neighbour cells through the desmosomal attachment proteins. I find it increasingly difficult to support the hypothesis that release of these proteins as cytotoxic agents explains the epithelial injury in asthma.

In the *British Journal of Pharmacology* (October 1991) Clive Robinson and co-workers report a novel effect of eosinophils on the epithelium which involves a cognate interaction between the eosinophil and the suprabasal cell. This results in the secretion by the suprabasal cell of neutral proteases, in particular, endoproteases, and by the epithelial cell, including gelatinase and stromolysin. Using blot techniques, they have shown that these enzymes have quite a wide range of substrate specificity. The most recent work suggests that they are able to hydrolyse the plaque proteins of desmosomes.

I wonder, therefore, whether there is not a much more subtle lesion involved in the eosinophil-directed damage to the epithelium, rather than the fairly blunt injury of basic protein- or cationic protein-induced cytotoxicity.

P. Venge

I think you have almost answered your own question. It is not very easy, as you suggest, and is one of the reasons why I put some emphasis on these non-cytotoxic effects. It is also clear that many of these cytotoxic effects shown especially on epithelial cells in the airways have been obtained at very high concentrations, which may raise some doubts about the relevance of these results. I completely agree with you.

C. Page

Professor Holgate, have you ever found deposits of MBP or eosinophil cationic protein (ECP) around ganglionic structures in airways? Recent work presented to the British Pharmacological Society by Alison Fryer, at Johns Hopkins, has shown that there is, as it were, not injury but antagonism of muscarinic M2 receptors and upregulation of ganglionic transmission.

S.T. Holgate
We do see the proteins there. We have to be much more imaginative now about these cells rather than taking what I consider rather an old-fashioned view.

B.B. Vargaftig
In epithelial cell cultures of guinea-pig trachea we had tons of eosinophils, with or without different activators, and could never see any chromium or indium release under conditions in which polyarginine or different complement-derived substances, for instance, are very effective. We have added a cathepsin G and elastase, either purified from or co-liberated by neutrophils, and they induce a very marked lesion of the epithelial cells.

Can you really talk about platelet aggregation with MBP and eosinophil peroxidase or is it agglutination, a simple charge sort of effect?

P. Venge
I do not know, although it is most likely. These are the results of Gleich and co-workers.

G.J. Laurent
Is there any evidence on how the activation of fibroblast proteoglycan production is acting? Is it a direct effect on the cells or is it inducing release and activation via some sort of autocrine leap via another growth factor?

P. Venge
It seems to be a direct effect, although it is diffcult to rule out some indirect effect since these cultures were made in the presence of small amounts of serum – but the conclusion (again in collaboration with the group in Lund) is that this is probably a direct effect.

G.J. Laurent
Secondly, the two negative findings: neither evidence of stimulation of collagen production by ECP nor convincing evidence of fibroblast replication in response to ECP could be found. Was this done with a

variety of cell types, and were any sort of synergy experiments tried to see whether ECP could perhaps activate another growth factor?

P. Venge

No, these were done only with the embryonic human fibroblasts, and there were no synergy experiments.

G.J. Laurent

I think those experiments need to be done with a variety of fibroblast cell lines because they are very varied in response. Because they have not responded in these experiments does not mean that ECP may not play a role.

P. Venge

Fibroblasts from different sources have been used, but only human embryonic fibroblasts. It is not restricted to one cell line.

A.R. Leff

You mentioned the non-cytotoxic effects of MBP and that it contracts airway smooth muscle. At least in all the experiments that I know, this requires an intact epithelium, and part of looking for the defect depends upon having a bioassay system. The effect with an intact epithelium is a very acute effect and precedes any cytotoxic activity.

Incidentally, no other eosinophil protein applied to the intact epithelium of an animal model (in this case, the guinea-pig) contracts airway smooth muscle or does anything acutely; so much of the effect has to do with time, and then of course with the intermediate cell interactions.

A.B. Kay

I think this conversation is extremely interesting, and perhaps should have come sooner, in a sense. After probably nearly 100 bronchial biopsies from asthmatics of varying degrees of severity, I am certainly convinced that the eosinophil or its products are always there. Coming back to my brief exchange with Dr Leff, the eosinophil is always there in asthma. I do not think there is any record, even from the autopsy work, of there not being a florid eosinophilia. I think Gleich has one anecdote, an exception rather than the rule.

I agree with Professor Holgate that in these biopsies the epithelial damage does not seem to go together with a pattern of deposition of either an EG2-positivity or anti-MBP. They seem to be little islands and blocks of staining which do not go together with the damage above. If there is a direct cause and effect, I agree it is likely to be more subtle.

The cells which are damaged do not look as if it is a cytotoxic phenomenon but as if there really is something else.

As I have suggested several times, you have pointed to what really are functions of the eosinophil in the sense of it possibly being a repair cell: it inhibits T cell proliferation and mucus hypersecretion (which is very interesting), and also stimulates the fibroblasts to lay down collagen. We have the cell there, it goes together with all the clinical correlates, but there is still the possibility that its repair role has been seriously underestimated. [*P. Venge agreed.*]

10

Mechanisms of Immediate Hypersensitivity and Hyperresponsiveness: Mediators, Antagonists and Role of Interleukins

M. BUREAU, E. COËFFIER, S. DESQUAND,
J. LEFORT, M.A. MARTINS*, M. PRETOLANI,
P. SILVA*, D. VINCENT and B.B. VARGAFTIG

Unité de Pharmacologie cellulaire, Unité Associée Institut Pasteur-INSERM 285, 25 Rue du Dr Roux, 75015, Paris, France

**FIOCRUZ, Rio de Janeiro, Brazil*

Introduction: The Hypothesized Role of PAF

The story of platelet-activating factor (PAF) involvement in asthma and allergy differs from that of other mediators. PAF was discovered in the early 1970s (Benveniste *et al.*, 1972) and for many years was studied within the frame of cell immunology, until we showed that it displays *in vivo* effects compatible with a proposed role in allergy in guinea-pigs (Vargaftig *et al.*, 1980) and McManus *et al.* (1980) did the same using rabbits. PAF activates inflammatory cells and induces systemic hypotension, pulmonary hypertension, increased vasopermeability, bronchoconstriction, leukopenia and thrombocytopenia (see Braquet *et al.*, 1987). Since, contrary to those of other mediators, the effects of PAF are not blocked by cyclooxygenase inhibitors nor by histamine antagonists,

T-Lymphocyte and Inflammatory Cell Research in Asthma
ISBN 0-12-388170-6

it was logical to hypothesize that it plays a role in allergy in the guinea-pig, where a role for histamine and prostanoids had been ruled out. Nevertheless, extensive investigations using different antagonists led to a reappraisal of the role of PAF. Indeed, different types of antagonists, including compounds BN 52021 or WEB 2086, suppressed *in vitro* and *in vivo* bronchoconstriciton by allergen in passively sensitized guinea-pigs, as well as the accompanying release of mediators from guinea-pig perfused lungs (Pretolani *et al.*, 1987; Lagente *et al.*, 1987). When tested against allergen-induced bronchoconstriction in actively sensitized animals or against mediator release from isolated lungs, both antagonists were inactive (Pretolani *et al.*, 1987; Desquand *et al.*, 1990, 1991), even though other investigators (Casals-Stenzel, 1987) had demonstrated some effectiveness, but only in the presence of anti-histamines. The variable activity of PAF antagonists against allergen in guinea-pigs depends rather on the crucial role of the booster injection of antigen, than on the distinction between active and passive shock or on the presence of anti-histamine agents. Work in progress suggests that the booster induces a micro-shock, leading to inflammation and then to cytokine production.

The Model of Acute Hypersensitivity in Guinea-Pigs

Anaphylactic bronchoconstriction in sensitized guinea-pigs is the most commonly used test for studying anti-asthmatic agents. Guinea-pigs possess a developed respiratory smooth muscle, which contracts markedly in response to the intravenous or intratracheal injection of antigen. The resulting acute bronchoconstriction is partially antagonized by histamine H_1 receptor antagonists which are, however, not very useful in human asthma. In fact, the anaphylactic bronchoconstriction in the guinea-pig is essentially histamine-dependent, and may involve additional mediators according to the inflammatory status of the animal. Even though there is strong evidence for the involvement of lipoxygenase-dependent derivatives of arachidonic acid, the exact role of these derivatives is unclear: do they only participate in acute bronchoconstriction and/or in the increased vascular permeability or do they also account for eosinophil recruitment and/or activation and if so, at which level? This question is still unresolved. The additional involvement of other mediators can be shown by manoeuvres such as antibody transfer or enhanced antibody production, the use of downregulating agents (antihistamines) or upregulating agents (β-adrenoceptor antagonists). In fact, the direct demonstration that 5-lipoxygenase inhibitors or leukotriene antagonists are effective against immediate hypersensitivity reactions requires that endogenous histamine, originating mostly from the liver, is antagonized. In addition, cyclooxygenase is easily activated in the guinea-pig lung and most of the arachidonic acid that becomes available is transformed into thromboxane A_2 (TxA_2), a powerful bronchoconstrictor agent. Thus, in order to tailor a model to study the effectiveness of a 5-lipoxygenase inhibitor, animals and isolated preparations must be exposed to a histamine antagonist and to a cyclooxygenase inhibitor. Under those conditions, the intravenous injection of the antigen induces a moderate and protracted bronchoconstriction which can be enhanced with the non-selective adrenoceptor antagonist propranolol.

In addition to bronchoconstriction, the guinea-pig model of immediate hypersensitivity is characterized by an increased bronchopulmonary vascular permeability, which can be visualized with tracers or dyes. The lung vascular permeability and the accompanying leukocyte recruitment induced by the secretagogue f-L-methionyl-L-leucyl-L-phenylalanine (fMLP) in the guinea-pig are not inhibited by aspirin (Bureau *et al.*, submitted), even though the bronchoconstriction is (Boukili *et al.*, 1986). All *in vivo* effects of fMLP in the guinea-pig are inhibited by the systemic administration of pertussis toxin (Arreto *et al.*, 1991), but whether granulocytes are needed for the expression of the enhanced permeability is not known. Since antigen-induced increase of the guinea-pig bronchial vascular permeability is suppressed by antihistamines, it is likely that histamine is centrally involved. Indeed, histamine augments powerfully the bronchial and tracheal vascular permeability, but so does PAF. A marked recruitment of leukocytes follows the intratracheal administration of antigen to passively sensitized guinea-pigs, but paradoxically, a lowered recruitment followed shock in actively sensitized lungs, otherwise more responsive to antigen (Bureau *et al.*, unpublished). In fact, the combination of antagonists mepyramine (anti-H_1) and cimetidine (anti-H_2) uncover a very consistent leukocyte recruitment, probably by preventing the marked vascular effects of antigen.

The Evolution of Specific Hypersensitivity Towards Non-specific Hyperresponsiveness

Hyperresponsiveness *in vivo* is expressed as a lowered threshold and/or an enhanced response to standard bronchoconstrictor agents, in terms of airway resistance and/or lung compliance. The demonstration that PAF primes for enhanced responsiveness *in vivo* to the chemically unrelated bronchoconstrictor agent 5-HT (Vargaftig *et al.*, 1983), extended its proposed role to the late phase response in asthma.

Modulation of the establishment or of the expression of hyperresponsiveness can be attempted by treating the animal before and/or together with the antigen or just before the administration of the unspecific agonist. This procedure allows the hyperresponsiveness to be correlated to different expressions of cell stimulation, including the enrichment of lymphocytes, eosinophils or other cells, or detached epithelial cells in bronchoalveolar lavage (BAL) fluid. To be completed, the *in vivo* approach requires some correlation between mediator formation/release and hyperresponsiveness, such as we have been providing for a few years using the guinea-pig isolated, perfused lungs (Pretolani *et al.*, 1988, 1989a,b, 1990, 1991; Pretolani and Vargaftig, 1991). Indeed, the evaluation of the content of mediators in the BAL, which can be performed *in vivo*, is hindered by metabolism and removal and by intrinsic difficulties of collection during bronchoconstriction and enhanced vascular permeability. In the *ex vivo* approach, lungs are collected after different *in vivo* manoeuvres (cell depletion, drug administration, etc.) to correlate antigenic or other challenges, by the intravascular (intra-arterial) or intratracheal routes, drug addition to the perfusing medium or their introduction into the airways, to dynamic processes (effects on intrapulmonary airway resistance, lung weight as expression of water gain) and finally to the release of mediators. According to the quantity and nature of the mediators involved, inferences can be made on the kinetics of the release, the cell sources and the specificity of the different interferences. Using this system we have shown important differences between sensitized and boosted guinea-pigs, including an enhanced bronchoconstriction, release of larger amounts of eicosanoids and of histamine, as compared with lungs from non-immunized or from passively sensitized animals. These modifications of the responsiveness in sensitized lungs result from the booster injection of the antigen administered, in our protocol, 14 days after the first sensitizing injection. The number of eosinophils found in the BAL fluid more than doubles in boosted guinea-pigs. It is likely that repeated exposures to the allergen induce acute allergic inflammation, unperceived clinically because of the low amounts of antigen delivered in the presence of $Al(OH)_3$. This acute inflammation may nevertheless be traced by markers, such as the acute phase protein haptoglobin.

Prophylactic anti-asthmatic drugs may be effective by preventing the development of hyperresponsiveness, even if they do not interfere with the acute manifestations of experimental asthma. Nedocromil sodium and cetirizine, administered to guinea-pigs from the day of the booster injection until the day of lung removal, reduce hyperresponsiveness and the increased numbers of eosinophils in the BAL (Pretolani *et al.*, 1990 and unpublished). Interestingly, lungs collected from the treated guinea-pigs behaved almost as those from non-boosted animals (Pretolani *et al.*, 1990), since the enhanced responsiveness to PAF was back to basal values.

Eosinophils

As stated above, eosinophils may play an important role in asthma, and their mechanism of recruitment is a potential target for drug modulation. Lungs and BAL cells of guinea-pigs (Lellouch-Tubiana *et al.*, 1988) and mice (unpublished) are enriched in eosinophils after systemic or intrapulmonar challenge with antigen.

Eosinophils are found in the bronchial submucosa of asthmatic patients (Djukanovic *et al.*, 1990) and of guinea-pigs after challenge with PAF or antigen (Lellouch-Tubiana *et al.*, 1988). PAF stimulates markedly the migration of guinea-pig eosinophils *in vivo* and *in vitro* (Coëffier *et al.*, 1991) and eosinophils may be involved in the transition between the early manifestations of immediate hypersensitivity and its protracted and delayed phase. Once activated, eosinophils release cytotoxic basic proteins which are claimed to detach and lyse the respiratory epithelium, thus exposing the submucosal structures, including the nerve terminals, which are otherwise protected from the environment (Gleich *et al.*, 1979; Venge, 1990). A rapid transvascular migration of mature cells should account for the early enrichment, but other mechanisms are likely to explain the marked and delayed late phase. These mechanisms include local differentiation of circulating precursors and proliferation/differentiation mechanisms at distance, particularly at the bone marrow compartment. Indeed, we found an increased number of mature eosinophils in the bone marrow of guinea-pigs 7 days after the antigen booster (Pretolani *et al.*, 1991). Allergen-induced migration of eosinophils into the airways is a potentially relevant drug target and up to now only few studies have been performed using potential inhibitors. We developed two models for *in vivo* migration, one using guinea-pigs and the other using mice. In both instances, ovalbumin-sensitized animals are challenged with the allergen, guinea-pigs by the intravenous or intranasal route, in the presence of the antihistamine mepyramine to protect against immediate death, and mice by intranasal instillation. Within 24 h, the BAL population is markedly enriched in eosinophils, as compared with controls. The increase in BAL eosinophils is inhibited by dexamethasone and nedocromil sodium. PAF antagonists may be effective in guinea-pigs but not in mice, suggesting species-dependent mechanisms. Since it is likely that more than one mediator (PAF, eicosanoids, and/or cytokines such as IL-5?)

could account for the complexities of eosinophil recruitment into the allergic lung, these models could be used to dissect the role of various cells in the perpetuation of asthma.

Eosinophil recruitment to the lungs requires the upregulation of adhesion proteins at the level of the endothelium and is expected to be followed by epithelial shedding which may contribute to airway hyperresponsiveness. Nevertheless, it is important to recognize that the presence of eosinophils by itself does not explain epithelial shedding or hyperresponsiveness, which are not found in humans or animals infected with parasites and showing intense hypereosinophilia. In addition, a marked eosinophil invasion into lungs and BAL follows the intranasal administration of antigen to sensitized mice, without signs of toxicity to the epithelium. In addition, cationic proteins other than those from eosinophils also induce hyperresponsiveness in rats (Coyle *et al.*, submitted). It is thus likely that, in addition to recruitment, other mechanisms are required for the full expression of the capacity of eosinophils to intensify and perpetuate asthma and allergy in general. Indeed, Lapa e Silva *et al.* (unpublished) noted that eosinophils migrated to antigen-challenged guinea-pig lungs in the absence of epithelial damage, as if an additional component is missing to complete the eosinophil-induced damage. In this context, we have demonstrated that the intradermal injection of PAF to allergic humans induces a marked eosinophilic infiltration, whereas non-allergic controls show only non-specific (neutrophil) infiltration (Hénocq and Vargaftig, 1986, 1988). In general, sensitized guinea-pigs respond more intensively to PAF or LTB_4 than their non-immunized counterparts. Guinea-pig peritoneal eosinophils exposed to rhIL-5 are markedly primed for migration and calcium translocation induced by PAF (Coëffier *et al.*, 1991) and finally, eosinophils collected from the BAL of sensitized and boosted guinea-pigs are primed *ex vivo* for an enhanced migration by LTB_4, PAF and C5a, indicating that they have been probably activated *in vitro*. These results support the concept that the allergic potential ("atopy") is essential for the expression of the activity of the different mediators of inflammation.

Eosinophil recruitment and activation are attributed to the production of chemoattractant mediators. Silva *et al.* (1991) demonstrated that 6–24 h after the short-lasting pleurisy which follows the intrapleural injection of PAF to rats, the number of eosinophils in the pleural cavity more than doubles. In addition, the transfer of the cell-free pleural washing from the PAF-injected cavity to that of a naive animal induced a pure eosinophilia, demonstrating that a target present in the pleural cavity of the PAF-injected rat produces an eosinophil chemoattractant. The formation of this potential mediator was suppressed by the co-injection of PAF with low amounts of specific antagonists, with dexamethasone and nedocromil sodium. Also co-injected with PAF to the donor rat, the protein synthesis inhibitors cyclohexemide and actinomycin D suppressed eosinophilia in the donor as well as in the recipient animals. In contrast, the co-injection to a recipient animal of nedocromil sodium or of dexamethasone, of the PAF antagonists or the protein synthesis inhibitors together with the chemoattractant material generated in the PAF-injected pleural cavity, failed to interfere with eosinophil recruitment. Eosinophilia following the injection of the pleural washing generated in the donor to the recipient rat was blocked with cetirizine, which suppressed eosinophilia when administered to the donor and to the recipient rats, but failed to prevent the formation of the chemoattractant activity when injected to the donor rat together with PAF (Martins *et al.*, 1992). Cetirizine does not act as an inhibitor of the formation of the chemoattractant substance, but rather as an antagonist of the generated activity.

Endotoxin-Induced Neutrophil Recruitment, Increased Vascular Permeability and Hyperresponsiveness

The intratracheal instillation of endotoxin lipopolysaccharide (LPS) to guinea-pigs is followed within 2–3 h by bronchopulmonary hyperresponsiveness to serotonin or acetylcholine, accompanied by neutrophil migration to the airways and by an augmented tracheobronchial vascular permeability (Vincent *et al.*, 1991). LPS-induced hyperresponsiveness in dogs or sheep requires the presence of intact circulating neutrophils, but, in the guinea-pig, neutrophil depletion did not reduce hyperresponsiveness, unless platelets were also depleted. In fact, specific platelet depletion or their inhibition with prostacyclin suppressed hyperresponsiveness. It is noteworthy that dexamethasone and a 5-lipoxygenase inhibitor suppressed the LPS-induced increased vascular permeability as well as neutrophil migration into the airways, but failed to modify hyperresponsiveness. PAF antagonists and mepyramine blocked the permeability effects of LPS but were inactive against neutrophil migration and hyperresponsiveness. Indomethacin had no effect. Accordingly, LPS-induced hyperresponsiveness in the guinea-pig is not histamine- or arachidonate-dependent, even if suppression of neutrophil migration to the BAL by the lipoxygenase inhibitor indicates its efficacy on the non-hyperresponsiveness process of cell migration to the airways. The platelet-dependent mechanism responsible for LPS-induced hyperresponsiveness has not been identified as yet.

Conclusions

Recent developments concerning the physiopathology of bronchopulmonary hyperresponsiveness and the related recruitment of inflammatory cells into the airway provide novel and potentially important targets for drug modulation. This is particularly important for cytokine (IL-5, GM-CSF and other) generation and activity and for their interaction (synergism) with lipid mediators. Of course, anti-allergic drugs may also antagonize the mediators involved or behave as so-called "cell-stabilizing agents", but presently no research project on asthma/allergy should be undertaken without a complete overview of these novel mechanisms.

References

Arreto, C.D., Kadiri, C., Bureau, M.F., Lefort, J., Leduc, D. and Vargaftig, B.B. (1991). Selective modulation by pertussis toxin of the fMLP-induced bronchospasm, leucocyte recruitment and increase of pulmonary vaso-permeability. *Fund. Clin. Pharmacol.* **5**, 404 (abst).

Benveniste, J., Henson, P.M. and Cochrane, C.G. (1972). Leucocyte-dependent histamine release from rabbit platelets: the role of IgE, basophils and a platelet-activating factor. *J. Exp. Med.* **136**, 1356.

Boukili, M.A., Bureau, M., Lagente, V., Lefort, J., Lellouch-Tubiana, A., Malanchère, E. and Vargaftig, B.B. (1986). Pharmacological modulation of the effects of N-formyl-L-methionyl-L-leucyl-L-phenylalanine in guinea-pigs: involvement of the arachidonic acid cascade. *Brit. J. Pharmacol.* **89**, 349.

Braquet, P., Touqui, L., Shen, T.Y. and Vargaftig, B.B. (1987). Perspectives in platelet-activating factor research. *Pharmacol. Rev.* **39**, 97.

Bureau, M., De Clerck, F., Lefort, J., Arreto, C.D. and Vargaftig, B.B. (1993). Thromboxane A2 accounts for bronchoconstriction but not for platelet sequestration and microvascular albumin exchanges induced by fMLP in the guinea-pig lung. *J. Pharmacol. Exp. Ther.* (submitted).

Casals-Stenzel, J. (1987). Effects of WEB 2086, a novel antagonist of platelet-activating factor, in active and passive anaphylaxis. *Immunopharmacology* **13**, 117.

Coëffier, E., Joseph, D. and Vargaftig, B.B. (1991). Activation by recombinant human interleukin-5 (rh-IL5) of guinea-pig eosinophils: selective priming to PAF-acether and interference of its antagonists. *J. Immunol.* **147**, 2295.

Desquand, S., Lefort, J., Dumarey, C. and Vargaftig, B.B. (1990). The booster injection of antigen during active sensitization of guinea-pigs modulated the antigen-anaphylactic activity of the PAF antagonist compound WEB 2086. *Brit. J. Pharmacol.* **100**, 217.

Desquand, S., Lefort, J., Dumarey, C. and Vargaftig, B.B. (1991). Interference of BN 52021, an antagonist of PAF with different forms of active anaphylaxis in the guinea-pig; importance of the booster injection. *Brit. J. Pharmacol.* **102**, 687.

Djukanovic, R., Roche, W.R., Wilson, J.W., Beasley, C.R.W., Twentyman,

O.P., Howarth, P.H. and Holgate, S.T. (1990). Mucosal inflammation in asthma. *Am. Rev. Respir. Dis.* **142**, 434.

Gleich, G.J., Frigas, E., Loegering, D.A., Wasson, D.L. and Steinmuller, D. (1979). Cytotoxic properties of the eosinophil major basic protein. *J. Immunol.* **123**, 2925.

Hénocq, E. and Vargaftig, B.B. (1986). Accumulation of eosinophils in response to intracutaneous PAF-acether and allergens in man. *Lancet* **ii**, 1378.

Hénocq, E. and Vargaftig, B.B. (1988). Skin eosinophilia in atopic patients. *J. Allergy Clin. Immunol.* **81**, 691.

Lagente, V., Touvay, C., Randon, J., Desquand, S., Cirino, M., Vilain, B., Lefort, J., Braquet, P. and Vargaftig, B.B. (1987). Interference of the PAF-acether antagonist BN 52021 with passive anaphylaxis in the guinea-pig. *Prostaglandins* **33**, 265.

Lellouch-Tubiana, A., Lefort, J., Simon, M.T., Pfister, A. and Vargaftig, B.B. (1988). Eosinophil recruitment into guinea pig lungs after PAF-acether and allergen administration. Modulation by prostacyclin, platelet depletion, and selective antagonists. *Am. Rev. Respir. Dis.* **137**, 948.

Martins, M.A., Pasquale, C.P., Silva, P.M.R., Pires, A.L.A., Ruffie, C., Cordeiro, R.S.B. and Vargaftig, B.B. (1992). Interference of cetirizine with the late eosinophil accumulation induced by either PAF-acether or compound 48/80. *Brit. J. Pharmacol.* **105**, 176.

McManus, L., Hanahan, D.J., Demopoulos, C.A. and Pinckard, R.N. (1980). Pathobiology of the intravenous infusion of acetyl glyceryl ether phosphorylcholine (AGEPC), a synthetic platelet-activating factor (PAF), in the rabbit. *J. Immunol.* **124**, 2919.

Pretolani, M. and Vargaftig, B.B. (1991) Rôle des médiateurs lipidiques dans les réactions allergiques. *C.R. Soc. Biol.* **185**, 37.

Pretolani, M., Lefort, J., Malanchère, E. and Vargaftig, B.B. (1987). Interference by novel PAF-acether antagonist WEB 2086 with the bronchopulmonary responses to PAF-acether and to active and passive anaphylactic shock in guinea-pigs. *Eur. J. Pharmacol.* **140**, 311.

Pretolani, M., Lefort, J. and Vargaftig, B.B. (1988). Active immunization induces lung hyperresponsiveness in the guinea pig. *Am. Rev. Respir. Dis.* **138**, 1572.

Pretolani, M., Lefort, J., Dumarey, C. and Vargaftig, B.B. (1989a). Role of lipoxygenase metabolites for the hyper-responsiveness to platelet-activating factor of lungs from actively sensitized guinea pigs. *J. Pharmacol. Exp. Ther.* **248**, 353.

Pretolani, M., Lefort, J. and Vargaftig, B.B. (1989b). Limited interference of specific Paf antagonists with hyperresponsiveness to PAF itself of lungs from actively sensitized guinea-pigs. *Brit. J. Pharmacol.* **97**, 433.

Pretolani, M., Lefort, J., Silva, P.M.R., Malanchère, E., Dumarey, C., Bachelet, M. and Vargaftig, B.B. (1990). Protection by nedocromil sodium of active immunization induced bronchopulmonary alterations in the guinea-pig. *Am. Rev. Respir. Dis.* **141**, 1259.

Pretolani, M., Lefort, J., Boukili, M.A., Bachelet, C.M. and Vargaftig, B.B. (1991). Potential involvement of eosinophils and of rh interleukin-5 (IL-5) in the *ex vivo* lung hyperresponsiveness in the guinea-pig. *Am. Rev. Respir. Dis.* **143**, A14 (abst.).

Silva, P.M.R., Martins, M.A., Castro-Faria-Neto, H.C., Cordeiro, R.S.B. and Vargaftig, B.B. (1991). Generation of an eosinophilotactic activity in the pleural cavity of PAF-acether injected rats. *J. Pharmacol. Exp. Ther.* **257**, 1039.

Vargaftig, B.B., Lefort, J., Chignard, M. and Benveniste, J. (1980). Platelet-activating factor induces a platelet-dependent bronchoconstriction unrelated to the formation of prostaglandin derivatives. *Eur. J. Pharmacol.* **65**, 185.

Vargaftig, B.B., Lefort, J. and Rotilio, D. (1983). Route-dependent interactions between PAF-acether and guinea-pig broncho-pulmonary smooth muscle: relevance of cyclooxygenase mechanisms. *In* "INSERM Symposium: Platelet-Activating Factor and Structurally Relative Ether Lipids", vol. 23, p. 307. Elsevier Sciences Publishers, New York.

Venge, P. (1990). The human eosinophil in inflammation. *Agents Actions* **29**, 122.

Vincent, D., Lefort, J., Bureau, M., Dry, J. and Vargaftig, B.B. (1993). Dissociation between LPS-induced bronchial hyperreactivity and airway edema in the guinea-pig. *J. Appl. Physiol.*, **74**, 1027.

Discussion

C. Page

Do sensitized animals treated with IL-5 become hyperresponsive *in vivo*?

B.B. Vargaftig

It is erratic: from time to time they do. We think there is a problem of catabolism. We have introduced IL-5 directly into the trachea by instillation but sometimes it works and sometimes it does not.

A.B. Kay

We have had an ongoing interest in chemotactic responsiveness of the guinea-pig eosinophil. Recently, in my group, we went back to a very old story about the activity released in the anaphylactic diffusate from sensitized guinea-pig lung which attracts the eosinophil. We were able to establish, perhaps not surprisingly after all these years, that using purified cell suspensions of eosinophils and neutrophils, the chemotactic responsiveness is very similar between the two cell types, and that the activity that we used to call ECFA, therefore, is a neutrophil chemo-attractant as well.

It turns out that following methanol extraction and the usual purification procedures for lipid mediators, the activity can be accounted for on the basis of leukotriene B_4 (LTB_4) and 8,15-dihydroperoxy-eicosatetraenoic acid (diHETE). The 8,15-diHETE has about a third of the chemotactic activity of LTB_4, which is quite interesting. The activity from the antigen-challenged lung can be inhibited by 5-lipoxygenase inhibitors.

M.T. Withnall
Priming is manifest in a number of different ways. I am interested in the priming that Dr Vargaftig sees, which is a selective increase in response to PAF itself. When an increase in responsiveness is seen only to one mediator like this, it is often associated with an increase in the number of receptors. Do you know whether that is so in this case?

B.B. Vargaftig
No, but it must be determined.

M.T. Withnall
Secondly, priming often requires protein synthesis. That is not the case in your situation where it is seen after 10 min. If the cells are exposed to IL-5 for a longer time period, are there any changes to the characteristics of the hyperresponsiveness to PAF?

B.B. Vargaftig
Under many conditions it is possible to have very short priming with acute reactants. Priming requires protein synthesis with lipopolysaccharide, of course, but with fMLP, for instance, not much time is needed.

F.B. de Brito
Your priming really concerns recruitment of the eosinophils into the lung. What do these eosinophils look like? Have they degranulated, and do they appear to be functionally normal?

B.B. Vargaftig
This is a very interesting question. The electron microscopy is being done now. There is a change in the pattern of normodense to hypodense towards hypodense. In our hands at least, what would be called hypodense in the guinea-pig bronchoalveolar lavage (BAL) fluid – and to that extent also for the peritoneal cavity – does not look under electronmicroscopy like what would be expected as hypodense. The eosinophils are less dense, but they do not seem to have been activated.

S.T. Holgate
We hope that these models in animals reflect a situation in humans, since it is the rationale in many ways for developing them. If I understood the data correctly, administration of IL-5 leads to an enhanced response to PAF in this model. Yet in human beings with bronchial asthma, a disease where we have been hearing impressively that IL-5 is a major player as a cytokine, notably, PAF responsiveness is not upregulated but

is almost identical in normal individuals and asthmatics. Could you explain this discrepancy?

B.B. Vargaftig
You are right with respect to the asthma studies, but (as we have published) when PAF is injected into the human skin in different conditions there is a huge recruitment of eosinophils, provided that the donor is an allergic patient, whereas with controls there is only neutrophil recruitment.

S.T. Holgate
The point I wish to emphasize is in thinking of animal models to understand the basis of this disease, we have to come back all the time to the human situation, if indeed we want to do medicine rather than veterinary science.

B.B. Vargaftig
This is a philosophical approach with which I fully disagree.

11

The Role of Cytokines in Eosinophilia and Modulatory Effects of Glucocorticoids

F.B. DeBRITO, C.E. LAWRENCE and J.-A. KARLSSON

Rhône-Poulenc Rorer, Rainham Road South, Dagenham, Essex RM10 7XS, UK

Introduction

Eosinophilic granulocytes, which normally comprise less than 5% of the total white cell population in the peripheral blood of healthy subjects, are characteristically increased in certain diseases such as parasite infections and allergies. The stimuli and mechanisms behind this increase are obscure and there is even debate about the exact role of the eosinophil. Eosinophil granules contain cytotoxic proteins and are also capable of synthesizing and releasing a range of mediators with pro-inflammatory actions. It is generally assumed that granule-derived cytotoxic proteins mediate parasite killing (Butterworth, 1984) and contribute to myocardial tissue damage, and eventually death, in idiopathic hypereosinophilia (Fauci, 1982; Liesveld and Abboud, 1991). Large numbers of mature eosinophils accumulate in respiratory tissue of subjects with asthma or rhinitis (Ädelroth *et al.*, 1990; Pin *et al.*, 1992). A significant proportion of these cells appear to be activated (hypodense) and increased levels of eosinophil products, such as eosinophil cationic protein (ECP) and major basic protein (MBP), can be detected in tissue biopsies, bronchoalveolar lavage fluid (BAL) and sputum samples (Griffin

T-Lymphocyte and Inflammatory Cell Research in Asthma
ISBN 0-12-388170-6

et al., 1991, Venge *et al.*, 1991; Varney *et al.*, 1992). The contribution of eosinophil products to asthma symptoms, although widely accepted, however, remains hypothetical.

In recognition of the importance of mucosal inflammation for respiratory symptoms, inhaled glucocorticoid therapy is now being advocated for use also in mild asthma (British Thoracic Society, 1990). Glucocorticoids possess potent anti-inflammatory effects and they may act at several levels to reduce the eosinophilia: (1) suppression of eosinophil myelopoiesis in the bone marrow; (2) inhibition of adherence to endothelial cells; (3) inhibition of migration; (4) inhibition of survival of eosinophils in inflamed tissue, and (5) inhibition of release of pro-inflammatory mediators. It has been known for some time that T-lymphocytes are required for the development and maturation of eosinophils *in vivo* (Beeson and Bass, 1977) and recent studies have identified the haemopoietic growth factors granulocyte–macrophage colony-stimulating factor (GM-CSF), interleukin-3 (IL-3) and IL-5 as particularly important in this process (Whetton and Dexter, 1989; Silberstein *et al.*, 1989; Sanderson, 1990). Glucocorticoids could thus act either directly on the eosinophil or indirectly through inhibition of synthesis and release of select growth factors from immunocompetent cells.

The purpose of this review is to discuss cytokines involved in parasitic and allergic eosinophilia. Their actions have been extensively studied by various *in vitro* systems, but emerging animal and clinical data prompt a reappraisal of some of the proposed roles. A review of this topic would be incomplete without consideration of glucocorticoids, the most effective treatment of eosinophilic inflammation.

Eosinophil Myelopoiesis

The major site of eosinopoiesis in normal adult mammals is the bone marrow. In certain species such as rodents, the process can also be observed in the spleen. As with the development of other blood cells, several proliferation and differentiation steps are assumed to occur. Pluripotent haemopoietic stem cells give rise to eosinophil lineage committed progenitors which proliferate and differentiate into eosinophil precursors destined to become mature eosinophils. Little is known about constitutive haemopoiesis leading to the production of eosinophil progenitors. Studies of colony growth from blood-derived cells have, however, deduced that eosinophils and basophils arise from the same progenitors (Denburg *et al.*, 1989). Such studies have also led to the recognition of the importance of humoral factors in the growth and development of eosinophils such as the haemopoietic growth factors GM–CSF, IL-3 and IL-5 (see below). Relatively more is known about the individual stages of the terminal events of eosinopoiesis referred to generally as differentiation. These have been identified by nuclear segmentation, cell shape and size as well as synthesis and packaging of granule contents (e.g. eosinophil peroxidase; crystalloid product) (Bainton and Farquhar, 1970). The earliest morphologically distinct stage is the eosinophil promyelocyte which, through successive proliferations, gives rise sequentially to myelocytes and metmyelocytes. Proliferation then ceases and terminal maturation begins.

Eosinophil progenitor cells circulate in the peripheral blood of a number of species, including man, although their destination and further development remain unknown. The numbers of these progenitors may be increased in disease (Spry, 1988). In patients with asthma, an increase in circulating eosinophil progenitors has been reported during exacerbations, whereas the number falls during remission (Gibson *et al.*, 1990). More recently, a significant relationship between antigen-induced increases in airway hyperresponsiveness and blood eosinophil progenitor number has been reported (Gibson *et al.*, 1991). While the presence of these cells in lung tissue has yet to be established, their identification in human nasal polyps suggests that eosinopoiesis may additionally occur locally at sites of inflammation (Otsuka *et al.*, 1987).

Cytokines Implicated in Eosinophil Myelopoiesis

Among several cytokines that have been examined for eosinopoietic activity, GM–CSF, IL-3 and IL-5 appear to be the most important. Their presence in colony-forming assays or suspension cultures of bone marrow or blood-derived cells, causes an increased production of eosinophils (Whetton and Dexter, 1989; Sanderson, 1990). Furthermore, their administration to experimental animals or humans gives rise to an eosinophilia (Whetton and Dexter, 1989) and mice with enhanced transcriptions of these cytokines have elevated numbers of eosinophils (Lübbert *et al.*, 1990; Dent *et al.*, 1990; see also Chapter 6). Other cytokines like G–CSF, tumour necrosis factor-α (TNF-α), interferon-γ (IFN-γ), IL-1, IL-2, IL-4 and IL-6 do not display these features although some (e.g. IL-2, G–CSF) in combination with other eosinopoietins (IL-3, IL-5) are able to influence eosinophil growth *in vitro* and could thus be considered accessory regulators (Enokihara *et al.*, 1988; Warren and Moore, 1988; Lu *et al.*, 1990).

In vitro generation of eosinophils by these eosinopoietins requires prolonged (2–5 weeks) incubation with marrow cells. There is evidence to suggest that other factors such as the presence of fibroblast products (Rothenberg *et al.*, 1989) are additionally necessary for the rapid induction and commitment of haemopoietic tissues to selective and maintained overproduction of eosinophils. Studies have, therefore, attempted to identify these conditions by examining the effect of exposing marrow to a combination of growth factors. Synergistic effects on eosinophil growth have been observed with IL-1, IL-3, GM–CSF and IL-5 on marrow from mice (Warren and Moore, 1988) but these cytokines had only additive effects on human marrow (Clutterbuck *et al.*, 1989). Furthermore, IL-5, which exhibits activity in both liquid and semi-liquid medium cultures when human marrow cells are used, is only active in liquid cultures when murine cells are used (Sanderson, 1990). Thus, distinct species differences exist and, moreover, eosinophil growth stimulated by GM–CSF and IL-3 is not inhibited by an IL-5 antibody (Enokihara *et al.*, 1989), indicating that the effect by these cytokines is not mediated by IL-5.

Different eosinopoietins may support distinct stages of eosinophil growth. Early studies identified IL-5 as a factor that caused marked but transient production of eosinophils in liquid marrow cultures when cells were derived from parasite-induced hypereosinophilic mice (i.e. marrow have elevated eosinophil precursor numbers) (Sanderson *et al.*, 1985). This suggested a terminal differentiation function for the factor and was supported by observations that eosinophil colonies produced in semi-solid cultures by IL-5 were composed predominantly of mature eosinophils in contrast to those generated by GM–CSF and IL-3 which comprised myeloblasts, myelocytes and metmyelocytes (Sonoda *et al.*, 1989). Similarly, in human eosinophilic HL-60 cells GM–CSF and IL-5 stimulated proliferation and differentiation whereas IL-3 only enhanced proliferation (Fabian *et al.*, 1992).

Other experiments involving the pre-incubation of marrow with growth factor followed by a second exposure to the same or a different factor found IL-3 and GM–CSF to be better promoters of eosinophil precursor growth than IL-5 (Lu *et al.*, 1990; Ema *et al.*, 1990; Sanderson, 1990). Finally, the study by Clutterbuck and co-workers (1989), in which a combination of eosinopoietins resulted in additive effects on eosinophil production, also suggests that eosinophil precursor populations may be differentially targeted by the eosinopoietins. Thus the general view that has emerged from these observations is that IL-3 and GM–CSF promoted early and late stages of eosinophil growth while IL-5 supported mainly late stages and the sequential actions of these eosinopoietins resulted in eosinophilia. This hypothesis seems now rather too simplistic and is, for example, difficult to reconcile with the reported similarity in time-course of eosinopoietic activity of GM–CSF, IL-3 and IL-5 (Clutterbuck *et al.*,

1989). A further complication in assessing the eosinopoietic activity of GM–CSF and IL-3 also is the broad spectrum of growth-stimulating activity that the factors possess which impose on eosinophils the need to compete with other cells for growth and survival in *in vitro* culture systems.

In conducting studies on eosinophil growth using liquid cultures of bone marrow obtained from parasite-infected mice, we observed that while GM–CSF, IL-3 and IL-5 all increased mature eosinophil formation, IL-5 produced significantly more cells than GM–CSF or IL-3 (Fig. 11.1A). More detailed histological inspection of the haemopoietic growth factor-treated cultures found an eosinophilic staining mononucleated cell type whose numbers related to the cytokine concentration and amount of cell-associated eosinophil peroxidase present in the cultures (Fig. 11.1B). We have not as yet identified the cells but there are two possibilities. Either, these cells are immature eosinophils, possibly eosinophil myelocytes based on the "early-acting" growth activity of IL-3 and GM-CSF, or the cells are mononuclear phagocytes which have ingested granules from degenerating eosinophils, based on the ability of GM–CSF and IL-3 to promote also the growth and activity of these cells. If the cells were eosinophil myelocytes, it would suggest that the synthesis and packaging of granule peroxidase (and possibly other granule products) is complete at this stage of eosinophil development. Interestingly, an apparently

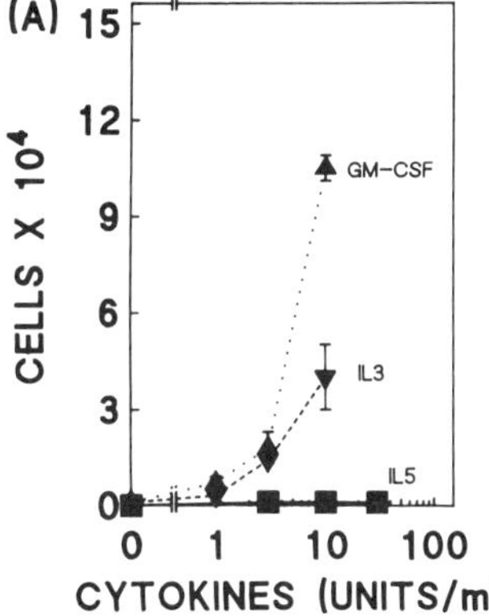

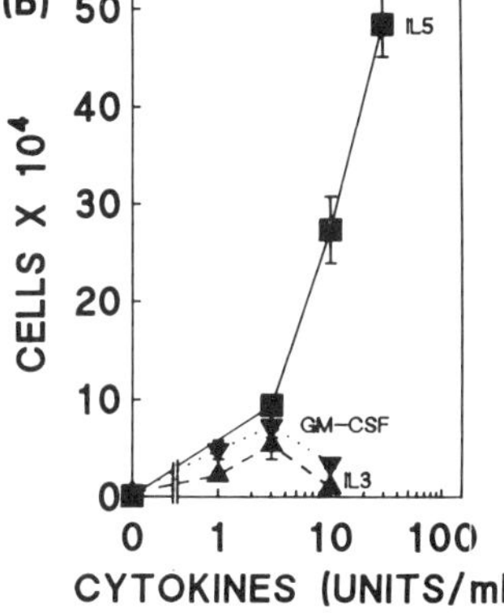

Fig. 11.1 Comparison of the eosinopoietic activity of haemopoietic growth factor with IL-5 in liquid cultures of murine bone marrow. Femoral bone marrow from 14-day *Mesocestoides corti* parasitized mice was cultured in the presence of recombinant murine IL-3, GM–CSF and IL-5 for 7 days. Eosinophils (A) and mononucleated eosinophilic cells (B) were determined by differential staining with neutral red and fast green. Each result represents the mean ± S.E.M. of quadruplicate cultures.

similar type of cell has been observed in tissues during the resolution of eosinophilia and identified as mononuclear phagocytes (Kawabori *et al.*, 1991).

IL-5 is unique among the known growth factors in that it appears to be rather specific for eosinophils (Sanderson *et al.*, 1985; Sonoda *et al.*, 1989; Clutterbuck *et al.*, 1989). Progress awaits the development of methods for the study of the growth of discrete subpopulations of eosinophil precursors before qualitative and quantitative differences in activity of the eosinopoietins can be fully established. An important step has been taken in this direction by Ema *et al.* (1990), who have described the production of eosinophils from CD34-positive cells isolated from human bone marrow.

Cytokine-Induced Survival and Activation of Mature Eosinophils

In addition to having eosinopoietic activity, GM–CSF, IL-3 and IL-5 increase the longevity and biological activity of mature eosinophils. Human eosinophils have a lifespan of a few days *in vitro* unless co-cultured with, for example, endothelial cell-conditioned media (Rothenberg *et al.*, 1987; Her *et al.*, 1991). This activity is mediated by GM–CSF (Her *et al.*, 1991) but also IL-3 and IL-5 markedly prolongs eosinophil survival *in vitro* (Begley *et al.*, 1986; Owen *et al.*, 1987; Rothenberg *et al.*, 1988; Yamaguchi *et al.*, 1988; Burke *et al.*, 1991; Hallsworth *et al.*, 1992). These cytokines also potentiate the effect of co-culture with 3T3 fibroblasts (Owen *et al.*, 1987; Rothenberg *et al.*, 1989) and inhibit apoptosis (Her *et al.*, 1991).

Culture of normodense human eosinophils with GM–CSF (Owen *et al.*, 1987), IL-3 (Rothenberg *et al.*, 1988) or IL-5 (Rothenberg *et al.*, 1989) produce a conversion to largely hypodense cells and prime the eosinophil for enhanced mediator release (Lopez *et al.*, 1988; Yamaguchi *et al.*, 1988; Howell *et al.*, 1989; Rothenberg *et al.*, 1989; Silberstein *et al.*, 1989; Coëffier *et al.*, 1991; Kita *et al.*, 1991a). IL-5 has been shown to potentiate platelet-activating factor (PAF)-induced guinea-pig eosinophil chemotaxis and superoxide production (Coëffier *et al.*, 1991) and to enhance the effects of PAF in a guinea-pig isolated lung preparation (Pretolani *et al.*, 1992).

GM–CSF, IL-3 and IL-5 are encoded for and synthesized by $CD4^+$ T-lymphocytes. Based on pioneering work on cytokine profiles of murine T-lymphocyte clones, Mosmann and co-workers have proposed the existence of different T helper subtypes (see Chapter 2). $CD4^+$ T-lymphocyte clones derived from human subjects seem to suggest the presence of similar subtypes as in the mouse (Wierenga *et al.*, 1991;

Parronchi *et al.*, 1991; see also Chapter 3). Endothelial cells (Her *et al.*, 1991), epithelial cells (Churchill *et al.*, 1992), monocytes/macrophages (Thorens *et al.*, 1987) and even eosinophils (Ohno *et al.*, 1991) are alternative sources of GM–CSF. IL-3 mRNA and/or protein have been detected in mast cells, epidermal keratinocytes and thymic epithelial cells (Frendl, 1992) as well as in supernatants from eosinophils and neutrophils (Kita *et al.*, 1991). IL-5 mRNA, apparently, can be found in mast cells (Plaut *et al.*, 1989) and eosinophils (Desreumaux *et al.*, 1992; see also Chapter 7). These three cytokines, together with IL-4, are clustered on the short arm of the human chromosome 5 (Van Leeuwen *et al.*, 1989). Little appears to be known, however, of the transcription factors involved in their production and whether the synthesis of these cytokines is individually controlled. These cytokines are all intimately involved in the allergic response and knowledge about their production and release no doubt will further our understanding about immediate hypersensitivity reactions.

Subsequent to release, the cytokines interact with their respective receptors on target cells. GM–CSF and IL-3 have wide ranging actions whereas IL-5 receptors are present mainly in human eosinophils and basophils (Chihara *et al.*, 1990; Lopez *et al.*, 1990). The receptors consist of an α- and a β-chain which, when combined form the high-affinity receptor (Tavernier *et al.*, 1991; see also Chapter 6). The α-chain is unique to each cytokine, whereas the β-chain is common and shared. Post-receptor events are largely unknown but may involve various protein phosphorylation steps (Murata *et al.*, 1990).

Taken together, these *in vitro* observations suggest an important additional role for these haemopoeitic growth factors, namely in prolongation of eosinophil viability in blood and tissue and in priming for enhanced mediator release and cytotoxicity. Furthermore, co-ordinated gene expression and common cell-signalling pathways may be the molecular basis for the induction and expression of eosinophilia.

In Vivo Studies Suggest a Major Role for IL-5 in Eosinopoiesis

The importance of the murine eosinopoietins, and in particular IL-5, in the development of eosinophilia, has been examined recently by the use of anti-cytokine antibodies. The administration of a single injection of 2 mg of the monoclonal anti-murine IL-5 antibody TRFK-5, intraperitoneally to mice at the time of infection with *Nippostrongylus brasiliensis*, was first shown to completely abolish the eosinophil response in the blood and lungs of these animals (Coffman *et al.*, 1989). The same antibody has been used to demonstrate a similar effect on the eosinophilias caused by infections with *Schistosoma mansoni* (Sher *et al.*, 1990), *Schistosoma japonicum* (Cheever *et al.*, 1991), *Heligmosomoides polygyrus* (Urban *et al.*, 1991), *Strongyloides venezuelensis* (Korenaga *et al.*, 1991) and *Mesocestoides corti* (Estes and Teale, 1991) in mice. Another monoclonal anti-IL-5 antibody, TRF, inhibited blood eosinophilia caused by *Toxocara canis* infection (Yamaguchi *et al.*, 1990a). Despite the substantial depletion of eosinophils caused by the anti-IL-5 treatment, there was little change to the parasite burden of mice, challenging the long-held view that eosinophils function as host-defence cells in immunity against parasite invasion (Butterworth, 1984). Our studies with the TRFK-5 antibody have further shown that as little as 10 μg given intraperitoneally to mice and as late as 4 days before the peak of the eosinophil response (day 14–21) to *M. corti*, was adequate to cause a virtual elimination of eosinophilia in the bone marrow and peritoneal cavity of these animals (De Brito *et al.*, unpublished data). The antibody-induced depletion of eosinophils was temporary and eosinophilia reappeared 2–3 weeks after administration. Taken together, these data demonstrate a critical role for IL-5 in parasite-induced eosinophilia in mice. In addition, we have observed that rats infected with *M. corti* mount a poor eosinophilic response after treatment with TRFK-5, suggesting that an IL-5-like factor is also critical for parasite-induced eosinophilia in this species.

The possible involvement of IL-5 in non-parasite-induced eosinophilia is beginning to receive attention. Eosinophil accumulation in the peritoneal cavity of mice following challenge with allergen (ragweed antigen) has been shown to be inhibited by anti-IL-5 treatment (Kaneko *et al.*, 1991). TRFK-5 administered parenterally to sensitized guinea-pigs before antigen challenge dose-dependently reduced the number of eosinophils in lung lavage (Gulbenkian *et al.*, 1992; Sanjar *et al.*, 1992; Chand *et al.*, 1992; De Brito *et al.*, unpublished data) and IL-5 appears to be selectively involved in the eosinophilia since lipopolysaccharide-induced neutrophil accumulation in the lungs of guinea-pigs was unaffected by TRFK-5 (Sanjar *et al.*, 1992). A chemoattractant activity by IL-5 has been demonstrated *in vitro* (Wang *et al.*, 1989; Coëffier *et al.*, 1991) and *in vivo* (Fattah *et al.*, 1990) and in these acute studies it seems likely that the anti-IL-5 antibody-inhibited migration of eosinophils into the tissue. The eosinophilia produced by repeated injections of IL-2 in mice, similarly could be inhibited by an anti-IL-5 antibody (Yamaguchi *et al.*, 1990b). This may be of clinical interest since administration of IL-2 to man also results in eosinophilia which is associated with IL-5 hypersecretion by T-lymphocytes (Macdonald *et al.*, 1990).

With regard to IL-3, one study found that treatment of *Nippostrongylus brasiliensis*-infected mice with specific antibody caused little change to blood eosinophilia but reduced intestinal mastocytosis by 40% (Madden *et al.*, 1991). The administration of a combination of anti-IL-3 and anti-IL-4 antibody was required to completely prevent intestinal mastocytosis but again there was little effect on attendant eosinophilia (Madden *et al.*, 1991). Whether IL-3 is involved in parasite-induced eosinophilia of other causes remains to be shown. As yet, there are no reported studies of the effects of GM–CSF-specific antibodies in experimental eosinophilias. Taken together, these experimental findings support a crucial role for IL-5 in animal models of parasite- and antigen-induced eosinophilia.

Is IL-5 Critically Involved also in Human Eosinophilia?

In man, increased levels of an IL-5-like activity have been detected in the blood and BAL fluid of hypereosinophilic patients with angio-oedema (Butterfield *et al.*, 1992), idiopathic hypereosinophilia (Owen *et al.*, 1989; Enokihara *et al.*, 1990), parasite infection (Limaye *et al.*, 1990), tryptophan-induced eosinophil myalgia syndrome (Owen *et al.*, 1990), IL-2 infusions (Macdonald *et al.*, 1990) and asthma (Walker *et al.*, 1992). Correlations between IL-5 levels and blood eosinophil counts were not attempted in these studies. Sedgwick and co-workers (1991) have found that BAL IL-5-levels were increased concomitantly with a pronounced eosinophilia, 48 h after segmental antigen challenge. In a study in which patients with onchocerciasis were treated with diethylcarbamazine, serum levels of IL-5 were found to rise to a peak in 24 h, remained elevated over the next 2–3 days and declined thereafter to baseline levels by day 6 (Limaye *et al.*, 1991). Eosinophil counts began to increase on the fourth day of treatment, peaked on day 7 and remained elevated for at least another week, indicating that increased numbers of circulating eosinophils were preceded by elevated levels of serum IL-5. Recombinant human IL-5 was recently applied topically to the nasal mucosa of rhinitic subjects (Terada *et al.*, 1992). IL-5 produced eosinophilia, and increased epithelial cells, ECP and immunoglobulin A (IgA) in nasal washings and the subjects became hyperresponsive to intranasal histamine.

An alternative approach to investigating the possible role of IL-5 in human disease has been to probe cells for IL-5 gene expression. Increased IL-5-specific mRNA has been reported in cells derived from Hodgkins disease (Samoszuk and Nansen, 1990) and Kimura's disease (Inoue *et al.*, 1990). In a study involving ten asthmatic patients, IL-5 transcripts were observed in mucosal bronchial biopsies of six patients (Hamid *et al.*, 1991). Within this group there was a significant correlation between the numbers of IL-5-positive cells and the total number of infiltrating eosinophils, activated eosinophils and activated T-lymphocytes (Hamid *et al.*, 1991). Similar correlations have been made for antigen challenge in the skin (Kay *et al.*, 1991) and nose (Durham *et al.*, 1992). BAL cells from asthmatic subjects, likewise have increased levels of mRNA for GM–CSF, IL-3, IL-4 and IL-5 when compared with cells from normal subjects (Robinson *et al.*, 1992). The data obtained from experimental studies thus support the hypothesis that IL-5 is important in mediation of human eosinophilia.

Glucocorticoids Suppress Tissue and Peripheral Blood Eosinophilia

The ability to reduce the number of eosinophils in peripheral blood is a well-recognized feature of glucocorticoid treatment. Although the underlying mechanisms of this effect are not known, two types of actions are generally thought to contribute to the effect. The first, readily demonstrated after oral or parenteral administration of a single dose is an immediate loss of eosinophils from the peripheral circulation within 4–5 h and which lasts for about 72 h (Kellgren and Janus, 1951; Dunsky *et al.*, 1979). Suppression of eosinophilia occurs without a change in numbers of resident eosinophils in the bone marrow and tissues but can lead to decreased recruitment of eosinophils into inflammatory lesions (Beeson and Bass, 1977; Butterfield and Gleich, 1989). Radiolabelling studies in the rat have indicated that the eosinophils are temporarily sequestered into a marginal pool and later return to the circulation (Anderson, 1969). The second type of action exhibited by glucocorticoids occurs after prolonged dosing and coincides with a progressive depletion of eosinophils from the bone marrow and tissues (Beeson and Bass, 1977; Butterfield and Gleich, 1989). It is not known whether glucocorticoids act on eosinophil progenitor cells or on later stages of eosinophil differentiation and maturation or even on the mature eosinophil when used in long-term treatment. Reduced adherence to the endothelium and migration of eosinophils may also contribute to fewer cells in the tissue (Altman *et al.*, 1981; Butterfield and Gleich, 1989). Recently it has been reported that a single high dose of dexamethasone to rats during infection with *Nippostrongylus brasiliensis* resulted in eosinophil degeneration in tissues within 24 h (Kawabori *et al.*, 1991). Glucocorticoids thus would appear to affect the growth, maturation and survival of eosinophils *in vivo*, but the contribution of these different actions to reduced numbers of eosinophils in blood and tissue requires further investigation.

Glucocorticoid Effects on Eosinophil Growth

The production of eosinophil colonies in human bone marrow cultures has been reported to be inhibited in some (Bjornson *et al.*, 1985; Slovick *et al.*, 1985; Liesveld *et al.*, 1988) but not all studies (Suda *et al.*, 1983; Butterfield *et al.*, 1986) by hydrocortisone (10 nM to 10 μM). Dexamethasone has been shown to inhibit eosinophil colony growth when present at a high concentration (3 μM) (Butterfield *et al.*, 1986). In these studies, conditioned medium or accessory cells were used as a source of growth factor and the responsible eosinopoietin (Liesveld *et al.*, 1988) was identified as GM–CSF in one of these studies. However, while the inhibitory effect of hydrocortisone was shown to be due to a direct action on eosinophil growth (Bjornson *et al.*, 1985), an indirect effect has also been noted (Slovick *et al.*, 1985; Liesveld *et al.*, 1988). In the latter studies, depletion of macrophages and T-lymphocytes from the marrow cells reversed the inhibition by hydrocortisone, suggesting that growth factor production rather than the progenitor itself was the target for the glucocorticoid. In support of this view it was found that addition of exogenous IL-1, IL-2 or GM-CSF to the cultures could overcome the inhibitory effect of hydrocortisone (Slovick *et al.*, 1985; Liesveld *et al.*, 1988).

From studies in man it seems that glucocorticoids are more effective in reducing eosinophil growth in patients with elevated levels of eosinophils than in healthy subjects. Thus, while prednisolone for 3 days (10 mg qid) had little effect on eosinophil colony formation (as assessed in agar cultures of bone marrow and blood) in healthy subjects there was a marked suppression in a hypereosinophilic individual even though the peripheral eosinophil count was reduced in all subjects (Butterfield *et al.*, 1986). The susceptibility of hypereosinophilic bone marrow to glucocorticoids has been confirmed in a study by Liesveld *et al.* (1988) who found that the incubation of marrow from three hypereosinophilic patients with 1 μM hydrocortisone resulted in the formation of significantly fewer eosinophil colonies. Gibson *et al.* (1990) recently reported that the prior inhalation of glucocorticoid by asthmatics, reduced the antigen-induced increase in eosinophil colony-forming cells in peripheral blood. Since the glucocorticoids most likely acted in the airways, these investigators suggested that factor(s) produced in airway tissues are responsible for the mobilization, recruitment and local development of eosinophils and that glucocorticoids inhibit the generation of these factors.

We have examined whether glucocorticoids can inhibit IL-5-induced eosinophil growth. Liquid cultures of bone marrow obtained from *M. corti*-infected mice were established in the presence and absence of recombinant murine IL-5 and varying concentrations of glucocorticoids. Following a 7-day incubation period, cultures maintained by IL-5 showed a 16-fold increase in eosinophil numbers (Ebsworth *et al.*, 1991). Hydrocortisone and dexamethasone inhibited this increase in a dose-dependent manner (Fig. 11.2). The inhibitory concentrations of these glucocorticoids (and their relative potency) corresponded to their affinity for the rat skeletal glucocorticoid receptor (Table 11.1). In the IL-5-stimulated liquid bone marrow cultures the presence of glucocorticoids also resulted in an elevation of the numbers of mononucleated type eosinophilic cells. These, as mentioned earlier, could be immature eosinophilic myelocytes or mononuclear phagocytes.

Glucocorticoid Effects on Eosinophil Survival

Recently, there have been a number of studies into the effects of glucocorticoids on the prolongation of survival of human peripheral blood eosinophils by eosinopoietins *in vitro*. Eosinophil viability maintained by either GM–CSF, IL-3 or IL-5 was inhibited by glucocorticoid in a time- and dose-dependent manner (Lamas *et al.*, 1991; Her *et al.*, 1991; Wallen *et al.*, 1991; Hallsworth *et al.*, 1992). Eosinophil viability was already reduced by the second day of incubation and was maximal on the fourth day. However, there was wide variation in the concentrations reported to be effective. In one study the concentration causing 50% reduction of GM–CSF-mediated survival was 50 nM (Lamas *et al.*, 1991) and in another this was as high as 10 μM (Hallsworth *et al.*, 1992). This variation could be related to the concentration of eosinopoietin present in the cultures as it has been observed that increasing the concentration of GM–CSF can overcome the inhibitory effect (Lamas *et al.*, 1991). This observation suggests that the mechanism of reduction in eosinophil viability is more than a direct cytotoxic action of glucocorticoids on eosinophils and that eosinophil survival *in vivo* would be governed by the concentration of glucocorticoid as well as by the type and concentration of eosinopoietin present in the tissue. Evidence has been obtained recently that the loss of viability of eosinophils in culture is due to endonuclease-specific DNA fragmentation (i.e. apoptosis) and that presence of eosinopoietin inhibits this process (Her *et al.*, 1991; Yamaguchi *et al.*, 1991). Glucocorticoids are known to activate apoptosis in, for example, thymocytes (Cohen, 1989) and it would be of interest to examine if these compounds reduce eosinophil survival by directly inducing apoptosis.

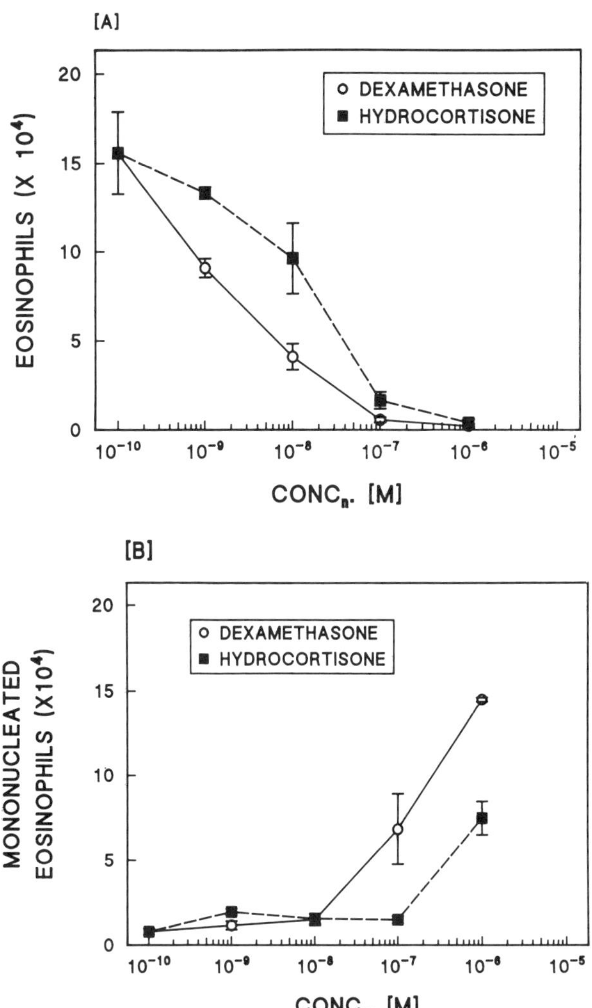

Fig. 11.2 Effect of dexamethasone and hydrocortisone on IL-5-induced growth of eosinophils (A) and mononucleated cells (B). Femoral bone marrow from 14-day *Mesocestoides corti* parasitized mice was cultured in the presence of recombinant murine IL-5 (2 units/ml) in the presence and absence of varying concentrations of dexamethasone and hydrocortisone for 7 days. Mature eosinophils and mononucleated eosinophilic cells were determined by differential staining with neutral red and fast green. Each result represents the mean ± S.E.M. of quadruplicate cultures.

Table 11.1
IC_{50} values of glucocorticoid effects on eosinophil growth

	IC_{50} (nM)	
	Dexamethasone	Hydrocortisone
Myelocyte (elevation)	100	300
Eosinophil (reduction)	2	20
Glucocorticoid receptor binding (rat skeletal muscle)	9	44

Glucocorticoid Effects on Eosinophil Adherence and Migration

Tissue eosinophilia depends not only on the production of eosinophils by the bone marrow but also on the functional ability of the cells to adhere to vascular endothelium and respond to chemotactic signals that direct their migration into tissues. These features of eosinophil function are also stimulated by GM–CSF, IL-3 and IL-5 (Silberstein *et al.*, 1989) so that inhibition of their production and/or action would manifest as reduced functional competence. Indeed, markers of eosinophil activation (ECP, EPX and MBP) have been shown to be reduced in allergic subjects treated by glucocorticoids (Venge *et al.*, 1991; Griffin *et al.*, 1991; Varney *et al.*, 1992). Eosinophils obtained from subjects treated with glucocorticoids have been reported to show an inability to adhere to nylon fibres and migrate in response to chemotactic stimuli (Altman *et al.*, 1981). There is currently little evidence *in vitro* for a direct effect of glucocorticoids on eosinophil function (Schleimer, 1990) and it therefore seems likely that the reduced eosinophil development and function is a consequence of glucocorticoid inhibition of cytokine release from T-lymphocytes, monocytes, macrophages, endothelial cells, etc.

Can Glucocorticoid-Mediated Regulation of Eosinophilia be Explained by Control of Cytokine Secretion?

T helper lymphocytes are critical for the development of eosinophilia (Beeson and Bass, 1977) and are a major source of eosinophil growth factors (Street and Mosmann, 1991). The activity of these cells is suppressed by glucocorticoids as evident from the clinical effectiveness of these agents in treating a wide variety of immunologically mediated conditions, including autoimmune diseases, hypersensitivity reactions, organ transplantation and graft versus host disease (Schleimer *et al.*, 1989). The synthesis and release of IL-2 (Gillis *et al.*, 1979), IL-3 (Culpepper and Lee, 1985), IL-4 (Wu *et al.*, 1991), IFN-γ (Arya *et al.*, 1984), GM–CSF (Culpepper and Lee, 1985) and IL-5 (Mirza and DeBrito, 1992; Hughes *et al.*, 1992) have been shown to be inhibited by glucocorticoids. These effects are independent of IL-2 (T cell growth factor) synthesis inhibition.

We have therefore investigated whether the reduced number of circulating eosinophils after prolonged glucocorticoid treatment is associated with diminished production of IL-5 *in vivo*. Using the *Mesocestoides corti* infection model of eosinophilia in mice in which serum levels of IL-5 can be observed to rise after infection and precede the development of eosinophilia (Fig. 11.3), mice were treated daily with dexamethasone for 7 days beginning 7 days after infection, and, serum IL-5 and marrow eosinophil counts determined at the end of treatment (i.e. day 14 post-

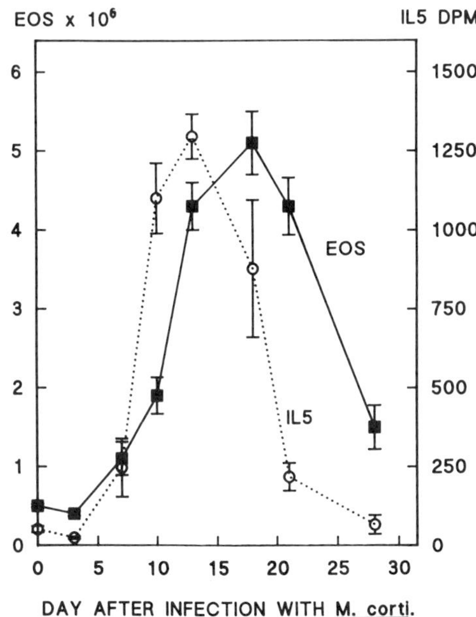

Fig. 11.3 Time-course of the development of marrow eosinophilia and relationship with serum IL-5 in *Mesocestoides corti*-infected mice. Eosinophil counts were determined in pair femurs by Discombes fluid and serum IL-5 by proliferation of Ly.H7.B13 cells. Each result represents the mean ± S.E.M. of six mice.

infection). Dexamethasone-treated mice showed a dose-related reduction in marrow eosinophil counts and a parallel reduction in serum IL-5 levels (Fig. 11.4). Since eosinophila in this model is critically dependent on IL-5 (Estes and Teale, 1991; authors' unpublished observations) the eosinopenia produced after prolonged glucocorticoid treatment most likely is a consequence of reduced production of IL-5.

Since we described earlier that dexamethasone could also inhibit the activity of IL-5, it was of interest to compare the sensitivity of this effect with that of the inhibition of IL-5 secretion to establish which of the two effects was the dominant *in vivo*. IC_{50} values were determined for both effects – inhibition of IL-5-induced eosinophil growth in bone marrow cultures and inhibition of ConA-induced lymphocyte secretion of IL-5 in spleen cell cultures, the cells being derived from 14-day *M. corti*-parasitized mice thus enabling a more meaningful comparison. The values obtained were 2 nM and 0.4 nM respectively, showing that the secretion

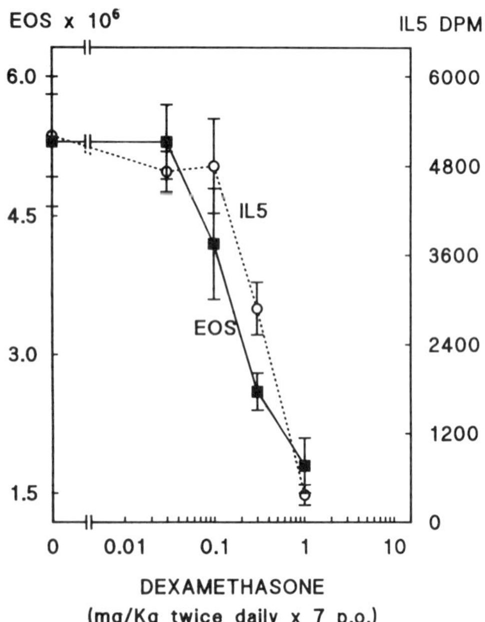

Fig. 11.4 The effect of dexamethasone on marrow eosinophilia and serum IL-5. Mice infected with *M. corti* larvae 7 days earlier were dosed orally twice daily (morning and afternoon) for 7 days with dexamethasone suspended in carboxymethyl cellulose. Eosinophil counts were determined in marrow of pair femurs using Discombes fluid and serum IL-5 by bioassay on Ly.H7.B13 cells. Each result represents the mean ± S.E.M. of six mice.

of IL-5 from T-lymphocytes and inhibition of its actions on eosinophils occur in the same concentration range.

Conclusion

Dramatic progress has been made in recent years in the unravelling of cytokine involvement in eosinophil myelopoiesis and function. *In vitro* studies have suggested that GM–CSF, IL-3 and IL-5 promote eosinophil proliferation and differentiation, with IL-5 being critical for maturation. Studies in parasite-infected mice and sensitized guinea-pigs, on the other hand, have demonstrated an almost complete inhibition of the eosinophilia by administration of an antibody to IL-5 (but not to GM–CSF and IL-3), indicating a central role for this cytokine *in vivo*. Supporting this view, IL-5 transgenic mice have high levels of circulating, mature eosinophils. Hypereosinophilic patients reportedly have increased levels of IL-5 and in patients with onchocerciasis the eosinophilia is preceded by a transient increase in serum IL-5. Antigen-challenge also increases levels of IL-5 mRNA in biopsy specimens from skin, nose and the tracheobronchial tree of allergic subjects.

Glucocorticoids are the most potent drugs available for the treatment of hypereosinophilia in experimental studies as well as in patients. These drugs act at several levels to suppress eosinophil development, survival and function. Glucocorticoids appear to have little effect on the eosinophil itself but may rather act to inhibit IL-5 and other cytokines involved in eosinophil myelopoiesis and allergy which are produced by a subpopulation of T helper lymphocytes, mast cells and possibly other structural cells in the airways (e.g. fibroblasts, endothelial cells, epithelial cells). The most important source of these cytokines in allergic disease remains to be established, together with the extent to which the anti-inflammatory actions of glucocorticoids can be explained by modification of cytokine networks. A further understanding of these processes and their regulation in health and disease may help to further our knowledge of allergic airways disease and provide new opportunities for discovery of novel anti-allergic therapies.

References

Ädelroth, E., Rosenhall, L., Johannson, S.-Å., Linden, M. and Venge, P. (1990). Inflammatory cells and eosinophil activity in asthmatics investigated by bronchoalveolar lavage. The effects of antiasthmatic treatments with budesonide or terbutaline. *Am. Rev. Respir. Dis.* **142**, 91–99.

Altman, L.C., Hill, J.S., Hairfield, W.M. and Mullarkey, M.F. (1981). Effects of corticosteroids on eosinophil chemotaxis and adherence. *J. Clin. Invest.* **67**, 28–36.

Anderson, V. (1969). Autoradiographic studies of eosinophil kinetics: Effects cortisol. *Cell Tissue Kinet.* **2**, 139–146.

Arya, S.K., Wong-Stall, F. and Gallo, R.C. (1984). Dexamethasone-mediated inhibition of human T cell growth factor and γ-interferon messenger RNA. *J. Immunol.* **133**, 273–276.

Bainton, D.F. and Farquhar, M.G. (1970). Segregation and packaging of granule enzymes in eosinophilic leukocytes. *J. Cell. Biol.* **5**, 54–73.

Beeson, P.B. and Bass, D.A. (1977). Mechanisms of accelerated eosinophil production. *In* "The Eosinophil, Major Problems in Internal Medicine Series". (P.B. Beeson and D.A. Bass, eds), vol. xiv, pp. 79–89. W.B. Saunders, Philadelphia.

Begley, C.G., Lopenz, A.F., Nicola, N.A. *et al.* (1986). Purified colony-stimulating factors enhance the survival of human neutrophils and eosinophils in vitro: a rapid and sensitive micro-assay for colony stimulating factors. *Blood* **68**, 162–166.

Bjornson, B.H., Havey, J.M. and Rose, L. (1985). Differential effect of hydrocortisone on eosinophil and neutrophil proliferation. *J. Clin. Invest.* **76**, 924–929.

British Thoracic Society (1990). Guidelines for management of asthma in adults: I-chronic persistent asthma. *Brit. Med. J.* **301**, 651–653.

Burke, L.A., Hallsworth, M.P., Lichtfield, T.M., Davidson, R. and Lee, T.H. (1991). Identification of the major activity derived from cultured human peripheral blood mononuclear cells, which enhances eosinophil viability, as granulocyte macrophage colony stimulating factor (GM–CSF). *J. Allergy Clin. Immunol.* **88**, 226–235.

Butterfield, J.H. and Gleich, G.J. (1989). *In* "Anti-inflammatory Steroid Action: Basic and Clinical Aspects" (R.P. Schleimer, H.W. Claman and A. Oronsky, eds), pp. 151-–197. Academic Press, London.

Butterfield, J.H., Leiferman, K.M., Abrams, J., Silver, J.E., Bower, J., Gonchoroff, N. and Gleich, G.J. (1992). Elevated serum levels of interleukin-5 in patients with the syndrome of episodic angio-edema and eosinophilia. *Blood* **79**, 688–692.

Butterfield, M.D., Ackerman, S.J., Weiler, M.S., Eisenbrey, A.B. and Gleich, G.J. (1986). Effects of glucocorticoids on eosinophil colony growth. *J. Allergy Clin. Immunol.* **78**, 450–457.

Butterworth, A.E. (1984). Cell mediated damage to helminths. *Adv. Parasitol.* **23**, 143–235.

Chand, N., Harrison, J.E., Rooney, S., Pillar, J., Jakubicki, R., Nolan, K., Diamantis, W. and Sofia, R.D. (1992). Anti-IL-5 monoclonal antibody inhibits allergic late phase bronchial eosinophilia in guinea pigs: a therapeutic approach. *Eur. J. Pharmacol.* **211**, 121–123.

Cheever, A.W., Xu, Y.H., Sher, A. and Macedonia, J.G. (1991). Analysis of egg granuloma formation in *Schistosoma japonicum*- infected mice treated with antibodies to Interleukin-5 and gamma interferon. *Infect. Immun.* **59**, 4071–4074.

Chihara, J., Plumas, J., Gruart, V., Tavernier, J., Prin, L., Capron, A. and

Capron, M. (1990). Characterization of a receptor for interleukin 5 on human eosinophils. Variable expression and induction of granulocyte/macrophage colony-stimulating factor. *J. Exp. Med.* **172**, 1347–1351.

Churchill, L., Friedman, B., Schleimer, R.P. and Proud, D. (1992). Production of granulocyte macrophage colony stimulating factor by cultured human tracheal epithelial cells. *Immunology* **75**, 189–195.

Clutterbuck, E.J., Hirst, E.M.A. and Sanderson, C.J. (1989). Human interleukin-5 (IL-5) regulates the production of eosinophils in human bone marrow cultures: Comparison and interaction with IL-1, IL-3, IL-6 and GM–CSF. *Blood* **73**, 1504–1512.

Coëffier, E., Joseph, D. and Vargaftig, B.B. (1991). Activation of guinea pig eosinophils by human recombinant IL-5. *J. Immunol.* **147**, 2595–2602.

Coffman, R.L., Seymour, B.W.P., Hudak, S., Jackson, J. and Rennick, D. (1989). Antibody to interleukin-5 inhibits helminth-induced eosinophilia in mice. *Science* **245**, 308–310.

Cohen, J.J. (1989). *In* "Anti-inflammatory Steroid Action. Basic and Clinical Aspects" (R.P. Schleimer, H.N. Claman and A. Oronsky, eds), pp. 110–131. Academic Press, San Diego.

Culpepper, J. and Lee, F. (1985). Regulation of IL-3 expression by glucocorticoids in cloned murine T lymphocytes. *J. Immunol.* **135**, 3191–3197.

Denburg, J.A., Dolovich, J. and Harnish, D. (1989). Basophil, mast cell and eosinophil growth and differentiation factors in human allergic disease. *Clin. Exp. Allergy* **19**, 249–254.

Dent, L.A., Strath, M., Mellor, A.L. and Sanderson, C.J. (1990). Eosinophilia in transgenic mice expressing interleukin-5. *J. Exp. Med.* **172**, 1425–1431.

Desreumaux, P., Janin, A., Colombel, J.F., Prin, L., Plumas, J., Emilie, D., Tarpier, G., Capron, A. and Capron, M. (1992). Interleukin 5 messenger RNA expression by eosinophils in the intestinal mucosal of patients with coeliac disease. *J. Exp. Med.* **175**, 293–296.

Dunsky, E.H., Zweiman, B., Fishchler, E. and Levy, D.A. (1979). Early effects of corticosteroids on basophils, leukocyte histamine and tissue histamine. *J. Allergy Clin. Immunol.* **64**, 426–432.

Durham, S.R., Ying, S., Varney, V.A., Jacobson, M.R., Sudderick, R.M., Mackay, I.S., Kay, A.B. and Hamid, Q.A. (1992). Cytokine messenger RNA expression for IL-3, IL-4, IL-5, and granulocyte/macrophage colony-stimulating factor in the nasal mucosa after local allergen provocation: relationship to tissue eosinophilia. *J. Immunol.* **148**, 2390–2394.

Ebsworth, K.J., Lawrence, C.E. and DeBrito, F.B. (1991). Glucocorticoids inhibit interleukin-5 induced maturation of eosinophils. *Clin. Exp. Allergy 22*, 125.

Ema, H., Suda, T., Nagayoshi, K., Miura, Y., Civin, C.I. and Nakauchi, H. (1990). Target cells for granulocyte colony-stimulating factor, interleukin-3, and Interleukin-5 in differentiation pathways of neutrophils and eosinophils. *Blood* **76**, 1956–1961.

Enokihara, H., Nagashima, S., Noma, T., Kajitani, H., Hamaguchi, H., Saito, K., Furusawa, S., Shishido, H. and Honjo, T. (1988). Effect of human recombinant interleukin-5 and G–CSF on eosinophil colony formation. *Immunol. Letts* **18**, 73–76.

Enokihara, H., Furusawa, S., Nakakubo, H., Kajitani, H., Nagashima, S., Satio-

K., Shishido, H., Hitoshi, Y., Takatsu, K. and Noma, T. (1989). T cells from eosinophilic patients produce interleukin-5 with interleukin-2 stimulation. *Blood* **73**, 1809–1813.

Enokihara, H., Kajitani, H., Nagashima, S., Tsunogake, S., Takano, N., Saito, K., Furusawa, S., Shishido, H., Hitoshi, Y. and Takatsu, K. (1990). Interleukin 5 activity in sera from patients with eosinophilia. *Brit. J. Haematol.* **75**, 458–462.

Estes, D.M. and Teale, J.M. (1991). *In vivo* effects of anticytokine antibodies on isotype restriction in *mesocestoides corti*-infected BALB/c mice. *Infect. Immun.* **59**, 836–842.

Fabian, I., Lass, M., Kletter, Y. and Golde, D.W. (1992). Differentiation and functional activity of human eosinophilic cells from an eosinophil HL-60 subline: response to recombinant hematopoietic growth factors. *Blood* **80**, 788–794.

Fattah, D., Quint, D.J., Proudfoot, A., O'Malley, R., Zanders, E.D. and Champion, B.R. (1990). *In vitro* and *in vivo* studies with purified recombinant human interleukin-5. *Cytokine* **2**, 112–121.

Fauci, A.S. (1982). The Idiopathic hypereosinophilic syndrome. *Ann. Intern. Med.* **97**, 78–92.

Frendl, G. (1992) Interleukin-3: from colony-stimulating factor to pluripotent immunoregulatory cytokine. *Int. J. Immunopharmacol.* **14**, 421–430.

Gibson, P.G., Dolovich, J., Girgis-Gabardo, A., Morris, M.M., Anderson, M., Hargreave, F.E. and Denburg, J.A. (1990). The inflammatory response in asthma exacerbation: changes in circulating eosinophils, basophils and their progenitors. *Clin. Exp. Allergy* **20**, 661–668.

Gibson, P.G., Manning, P.J., O'Byrne, P.M., Girgis-Gabardo, A., Dolovich, J., Denburg, J.A. and Hargreave, F.E. (1991). Allergen-induced asthmatic responses. Relationship between increases in airway responsiveness and increases in circulating eosinophils, basophils, and their progenitors. *Am. Rev. Respir. Dis.* **143**, 331–335.

Gillis, S., Grabtree, G.R. and Smith, K.A. (1979). Glucocorticoid-induced inhibition of T cell growth factor production. I. The effect on mitogen-induced lymphocyte proliferation. *J. Immunol.* **123**, 1624–1631.

Griffin, E., Håkansson, Formgren, H., Jörgensen, K., Peterson, C. and Venge, P. (1991). Blood eosinophil number and activity in relation to lung function in patients with asthma and with eosinophilia. *J. Allergy Clin. Immunol.* **87**, 548–557.

Gulbenkian, A.R., Egan, R.W., Fernandez, X., Jones, H., Kreutner, W., Kung, T., Payvandi, F., Sullivan, L., Zurcher, J.A. and Watnick, A.S. (1992). Interleukin-5 modulates eosinophil accumulation in allergic guinea pig lung. *Am. Rev. Respir. Dis.* **146**, 263–265.

Hallsworth, M.P., Litchfield, T.M. and Lee, T.H. (1992). Glucocorticoids inhibit granulocyte-macrophage colony-stimulating factor- and interleukin-5 enhanced *in vitro* survival of human eosinophils. *Immunology* **75**, 382–385.

Hamid, Q., Azzawi, M., Ying, S., Moqbel, R., Wardlaw, A.J., Corrigan, C.J., Bradley, B., Durham, S.R., Collins, J.V., Jeffery, P.K., Quint, D.J. and Kay, A.B. (1991). Expression of mRNA for interleukin-5 in mucosal bronchial biopsies from asthma. *J. Clin. Invest.* **87**, 1541–1546.

Her, E., Frazer, J., Austen, K.F. and Owen, Jr. W.F. (1991). Eosinophil hematopoietins antagonize the programmed cell death of eosinophils. *J. Clin. Invest.* **188**, 1982–1987.

Howell, C.J., Pujol, J.-L., Crea, A.E.G., Davidson, R., Gearing, A.J.H., Godard, P.H. and Lee, T.H. (1989). Identification of an alveolar macrophage-derived activity in bronchial asthma that enhances leukotriene C_4 generation by human eosinophils stimulated by ionophore A23187 as a granulocyte-macrophage colony-stimulating factor. *Am. Rev. Respir. Dis.* **140**, 1340–1347.

Hughes, J.M., Rolfe, F.G., Sewell, W.A., Black, J.L. and Armour, C.L. (1992). Corticosteroid inhibition of interleukin-5 expression in human peripheral blood mononuclear cells. *Am. Rev. Respir. Dis.* **145**, A264.

Inoue, C., Ichikawa, A., Hotta, T. and Saito, H. (1990). Constructive gene expression of interleukin-5 in Kimura's disease. *Brit. J. Haematol.* **76**, 554–559.

Kaneko, M., Hitoshi, Y., Takatsu, K. and Matsumoto, S. (1991). Role of interleukin-5 in local accumulation of eosinophils in mouse allergic peritonitis. *Int. Arch. Allergy Appl. Immunol.* **96**, 41–45.

Kawabori, S., Soda, K., Perdue, M.H. and Bienenstock, J. (1991). The dynamics of intestinal eosinophil depletion in rats treated with dexamethasone. *Lab. Invest.* **64**, 224–233.

Kay, A.B., Ying, S., Varney, V., Gaga, M., Durham, S.R., Moqbel, R., Wardlaw, A.J. and Hamid, Q. (1991). Messenger RNA expression of the cytokine gene cluster, interleukin-3 (IL-3), IL-4, IL-5 and granulocyte/macrophage colony-stimulating factor, in allergen-induced late-phase cutaneous reactions in atopic subjects. *J. Exp. Med.* **173**, 775–778.

Kellgren, J.H. and Janus, O. (1951). The eosinopenic response to cortisone and ACTH in normal subjects. *Br. Med. J.* **2**, 1183.

Kita, H., Abu-Ghazaheh, R., Sanderson, C.J. and Gleich, C.J. (1991a). Effect of steroids on immunoglobulin-induced eosinophil degranulation. *J. Allergy Clin. Immunol.* **87**, 70–77.

Kita, H., Ohnishi, T., Okubo, Y., Weiler, D., Abrams, J.S. and Gleich, G.J. (1991b). Granulocyte/macrophage colony-stimulating factor and interleukin-3 release from human peripheral blood eosinophils and neutrophils. *J. Exp. Med.* **174**, 745–748.

Korenaga, M., Hitoshi, Y., Yamaguchi, N., Sato, Y., Takatsu, K. and Tada, I. (1991). The role of interleukin-5 in protective immunity to strongyloides venezuelensis infection in mice. *Immunology* **72**, 502–508.

Lamas, A.M., Leon, O.G. and Schleimer, R.P. (1991). Glucocorticoids inhibit eosinophil responses to granulocyte-macrophage colony-stimulating factor. *J. Immunol.* **147**, 254–259.

Liesveld, J.L. and Abboud, C.N. (1991). State of the Art: The Hypereosinophilic Syndromes. *Blood Rev.* **5**, 29–37.

Liesveld, J.L., Abboud, C.N., Slovick, F.T., Rowe, J.M. and Brennan, J.K. (1988). Effect of hydrocortisone and interleukins-1 and -2 on eosinophil progenitors in hypereosinophilic states. *Int. J. Cell Cloning* **6**, 404–416.

Limaye, A., Abrams, J.S., Silver, J.E., Ottesen, E.A. and Nutman, T.B. (1990). Regulation of parasite-induced eosinophilia: Selectively increased interleukin 5 production in helminth-infected patients. *J. Exp. Med.* **172**, 399–402.

Limaye, A.P., Abrams, J.S., Silver, J.E., Awadzi, K., Francis, H.F., Ottesen, E.A. and Nutman, T.B. (1991). Interleukin-5 and the posttreatment eosinophilia in patients and onchocerciasis. *J. Clin. Invest.* **88**, 1418–1421.

Lopez, A.F., Sanderson, C.J., Gamble, J.R. *et al.* (1988). Recombinant human interleukin-5 is a selective activator of human eosinophil function. *J. Exp. Med.* **167**, 219–224.

Lopez, A.F., Eglington, J.M., Lyons, A.B., Tapley, P.M., To, L.B., Park, L.S., Clark, S.C. and Vadas, M.A. (1990). Human interleukin-3 inhibits the binding of granulocyte-macrophage colony-stimulating factor and interleukin-5 to basophils and strongly enhances their functional activity. *J. Cell Phys.* **145**, 66–77.

Lu, L., Lin, Z.-H., Shen, R.-N., Warren, D.J., Leemhuis, T. and Broxmeyer, H.E. (1990). Influence of interleukins 3, 5, and 6 on the growth of eosinophil progenitors in highly enriched human bone marrow in the absence of serum. *Exp. Haematol.* **18**, 1180–1186.

Lübbert, M., Jonas, D. and Herrmann, F. (1990). Animal models for the biological effects of continuous high cytokine levels. *Blut* **61**, 253–257.

Macdonald, D., Gordon, A.A., Kajitani, H., Enokihara, H. and Barrett, A.J. (1990). Interleukin-2 treatment-associated eosinophilia is mediated by interleukin-5 production. *Brit. J. Haematol.* **76**, 168–173.

Madden, K.B., Urban, J.F. Jr., Ziltener, H.J., Schrader, J.W., Finkelman, F.D. and Katona, I.M. (1991). Antibodies to IL-3 suppress helminth-induced intestinal mastocytosis. *J. Immunol.* **147**, 1387–1391.

Mirza, S. and DeBrito, F.B. (1992). Cyclosporin A and FK-506 inhibit cytokine secretion from T-helper-2 lymphocytes. *Clin. Exp. Allergy* **22**, 125.

Murata, Y., Yamaguchi, N., Hitoshi, Y., Tominaga, A. and Takatsu, K. (1990). Interleukin-5 and interleukin-3 induce serine and tyrosine phosphorylations of several cellular proteins in an interleukin-5-dependent cell line. *Biochem. Biophys. Res. Commun.* **73**, 1102–1108.

Ohno, I., Lea, R., Finotto, S., Marshall, J., Denburg, J., Dolovich, J., Gauldie, J. and Jordana, M. (1991). Granulocyte/macrophage colony-stimulating factor (GM–CSF) gene expression by eosinophils in nasal polyposis. *Am. J. Respir. Cell Molec. Biol.* **5**, 505–510.

Otsuka, H., Dolovich, J., Richardson, M., Bienenstock, J. and Denburg, J.A. (1987). Metachromatic cell progenitors and specific growth and differentiation factors in human nasal mucosa and polyps. *Am. Rev. Respir. Dis.* **136**, 710–717.

Owen, W.F. Jr., Rothenberg, M.E., Silberstein, D.S., Gasson, J.C., Stevens, R.L., Austen, K.F. and Soberman, R.J. (1987). Regulation of human eosinophil viability, density, and function by granulocyte/macrophage colony-stimulating factor in the presence of 3T3 fibroblasts. *J. Exp. Med.* **166**, 129.

Owen, W.F., Rothenberg, M.E., Petersen, J., Weller, P.F., Silberstein, D., Sheffer, A.L., Stevens, R.L., Soberman, R.J. and Austen, K.F. (1989). Interleukin-5 and phenotypically altered eosinophils in the blood of patients with the idiopathic hypereosinophilic syndrome. *J. Exp. Med.* **170**, 343–348.

Owen, W.F., Petersen, J., Sheff, D.M., Folkerth, R.D., Anderson, R.J., Corson, J.M., Sheffer, A.L. and Austen, F.K. (1990). Hypodense eosinophils and interleukin-5 activity in the blood of patients with the eosinophilia-myalgia syndrome. *Proc. Natl. Acad. Sci. U.S.A.* **87**, 8647–8651.

Parronchi, P., Manetti, R., Simonelli, C., Rugiu, F.S., Piccinni, M.-P., Maggi, E. and Romagnani, S. (1991). Cytokine production by allergen (Der pI)-specific $CD4^+$ T cell clones derived from a patient with severe atopic disease. *Int. J. Clin. Lab. Res.* **21**, 186–189.

Pin, I., Freitag, A.P., O'Byrne, P.M., Girgis-Gabardo, A., Watson, R.M., Dolovich, J., Denburg, J.A. and Hargreave, F.E. (1992). Changes in the cellular profile of induced sputum after allergen-induced asthmatic responses. *Am. Rev. Respir. Dis.* **145**, 1265–1269.

Plaut, M., Pierce, J.H., Watson, C.J., Hanley-Hyde, J., Nordan, R.P. and Paul, W.E. (1989). Mast cell lines produce lymphokines in response to cross-linkage of FcεRI or to calcium ionophores. *Nature* **339**, 64–71.

Pretolani, M., Lefort, J., Leduc, D. and Vargaftig, B.B. (1992). Effect of human recombinant interleukin-5 on *in vitro* responsiveness of PAF of lung from actively sensitized guinea-pigs. *Brit. J. Pharmacol.* **106**, 677–684.

Robinson, D.S., Hamid, Q., Ying, S., Tsicopoulos, A., Barkans, J., Bentley, A.M., Corrigan, C., Durham, S. and Kay, B. (1992). Predominant T_{H2}-like bronchoalveolar T-lymphocyte population in atopic asthma. *New Engl. J. Med.* **326**, 298–304.

Rothenberg, M.E., Owen, W.F. Jr., Silberstein, D.S., Soberman, R.J., Austen, K.F. and Stevens, R.L. (1987). Eosinophils cocultured with endothelial cells have increased survival and functional properties. *Science* **237**, 645–647.

Rothenberg, M.E., Owen, W.F. Jr., Silberstein, D.S., Wood, J., Soberman, R.J., Austen, K.F. and Stevens, R.L. (1988). Human eosinophils have prolonged survival, enhanced functional properties, and become hypodense when exposed to human interleukin-3. *J. Clin. Invest.* **81**, 1986–1992.

Rothenberg, M.E.J., Peterson, R.L., Stevens, D.S., Silberstein, D.T., McKenzie, K.F., Austen, K.F. and Owen, W.F. (1989). IL5-dependent conversion of normodense human eosinophils to the hypodense phenotype uses 3T3 fibroblasts for enhanced viability, accelerated hypodensity, and sustained antibody-dependent cytotoxicity. *J. Immunol.* **143**, 2311–2316.

Samoszuk, M. and Nansen, L. (1990). Detection of interleukin-5 messenger RNA in deed stevnberg cells of Hodgkin's disease with eosinophilia. *Blood* **75**, 13–16.

Sanderson, C.J. (1990). The biological role of interleukin-5. *Int. J. Cell Cloning* **8** (Suppl. 1), 147–154.

Sanderson, C.J., Warren, D.J. and Strath, M. (1985). Identification of a lymphokine that stimulates eosinophil differentiation in vitro. Its relationship to IL3 and functional properties of eosinophils produced in cultures. *J. Exp. Med.* **162**, 60–74.

Sanjar, S., McCabe, P.J., Fattah, D., Humbles, A.A. and Pole, S.M. (1992). TRFK5, an antibody to interleukin-5, selectively inhibits antigen-induced eosinophil accumulation in the guinea pig lung. *Am. Rev. Respir. Dis.* **145**, A40.

Schleimer, R.P. (1990). Effects of glucocorticosteroids on inflammatory cells relevant to their therapeutic applications in asthma. *Am. Rev. Respir. Dis.* **141**, S59–S69.

Schleimer, R.P., Claman, H.N. and Oronsky, A. (1989). "Anti-inflammatory Steroid Action. Basic and Clinical Aspects". Academic Press, London.

Sedgwick, J.B., Calhoun, W.J., Gleich, G.J., Kita, H., Abrams, J.S., Schwartz, L.B., Volovitz, B., Ben-Yaakov, M. and Busse, W.W. (1991). Immediate and late airway response of allergic rhinitis patients to segmental antigen challenge. *Am. Rev. Respir. Dis.* **144**, 1274–1281.

Sher, A., Coffman, R.L., Hieny, S., Scott, P. and Cheever, A.W. (1990). Interleukin-5 is required for the blood and tissue eosinophilia but not granuloma formation induced by infection with *Schistosoma mansoni*. *Proc. Natl. Acad. Sci. U.S.A.* **87**, 61–65.

Silberstein, D.S., Austen, K.F. and Owen, W.F. (1989). Glycoprotein hormones that regulate the development of inflammation in eosinophilia-associated disease. *Haematol. Oncol. Clin. North Am.* **3**, 511–533.

Slovick, F.T., Abboud, C.N., Brennan, J.K. and Lichtman, M.A. (1985). Modulation of *in vitro* eosinophil progenitors by hydrocortisone: role of accessory cells and interleukins. *Blood* **66**, 1072–1079.

Sonoda, Y., Arai, N. and Ogawa, M. (1989). Humoral regulation of eosinophilopoiesis in vitro: analysis of the targets of interleukin-3, granulocyte/macrophage colony-stimulating factor (GM–CSF), and interleukin-5. *Leukaemia* **3**, 14–18.

Spry, C.J.F. (1988). *In* "Eosinophils, A Comprehensive Review, and Guide to the Scientific and Medical Literature" (C.J.F. Spry, ed.), pp. 10–28. Oxford University Press, Oxford.

Street, N.E. and Mosmann, T.R. (1991). Functional diversity of T lymphocytes due to secretion of different cytokine patterns. *FASEB J.* **5**, 171–177.

Suda, T., Miura, Y., Ijima, H., Ozawa, K., Motoyoshi, K. and Takaku, F. (1983). The effect of hydrocortisone on human granulopoiesis in vitro with cytochemical analysis of colonies. *Exp. Haematol.* **11**, 114–121.

Tavernier, J., Devos, R., Cornelis, S., Tuypens, T., Heyden, der V., Fiers, W. and Plaetinck, G. (1991). A human high affinity interleukin-5 receptor (IL5R) is composed of an IL-5-specific alpha chain and a beta chain shared with the receptor for GM–CSF. *Cell* **66**, 1175–1184.

Terada, N., Konno, A., Tada, H., Shirotori, K., Ishikawa, K. and Togawa, Kiyoshi. (1992). The effect of recombinant human interleukin-5 on eosinophil accumulation and degranulation in human nasal mucosa. *J. Allergy Clin. Immunol.* **90**, 160–168.

Thorens, B., Mermod, J.-J. and Vassalli, P. (1987). Phagocytosis and inflammatory stimuli induce GM–CSF mRNA in macrophages through posttranscriptional regulation. *Cell* **48**, 671–679.

Urban, J.F. Jr., Katona, I.M., Paul, W.E. and Finkelman, F.D. (1991). Interleukin-4 is important in protective immunity to a gastrointestinal nematode infection in mice. *Proc. Natl. Acad. Sci. U.S.A.* **88**, 5513–5517.

Van Leeuwen, B.H., Martinson, M.E., Webb, G.C. and Young, I.G. (1989). Molecular organization of the cytokine gene cluster, involving the human IL-3, IL-4, IL-5, and GM-CSF genes, on human chromosome 5. *Blood* **73**, 1142–1148.

Varney, V.A., Jacobson, M.R., Sudderick, R.M., Robinson, D.S., Irani, A.-M. A., Schwartz, L.B., Mackey, I.S., Kay, A.B. and Durham, S.R. (1992). Immunohistology of the nasal mucosa following allergen-induced rhinitis. *Am. Rev. Respir. Dis.* **146**, 170–176.

Venge, P., Henriksen, J. and Dahl, R. (1991). Eosinophils in exercise-induced asthma. *J. Allergy Clin. Immunol.* **88**, 699–704.

Walker, C., Bode, E., Boer, L., Hansel, T.T., Blaser, K. and Virchow, J.-C. Jr. (1992). Allergic and non-allergic asthmatics have distinct patterns of T-cell activation and cytokine production in peripheral blood and bronchoalveolar lavage. *Am. Rev. Respir. Dis.* **146**, 109–115.

Wallen, N., Kita, H., Weiler, D. and Gleich, G.J. (1991). Glucocorticoids inhibit cytokine-mediated eosinophil survival. *J. Immunol.* **147**, 3490–3495.

Wang, J.M., Rambaldi, A., Biondi, A., Chen, Z.G., Sanderson, C.J. and

Mantovani, A. (1989). Recombinant human interleukin-5 is a selective eosinophil chemoattractant. *Eur. J. Immunol.* **19**, 701–705.

Warren, D.J. and Moore, M.A.S. (1988). Synergism among interleukin 1, interleukin-3, and interleukin-5 in the production of eosinophils from primitive hemopoietic stem cells. *J. Immunol.* **140**, 94–99.

Whetton, A.D. and Dexter, T.M. (1989). Myeloid haemopoietic growth factors. *Biochim. Biophys. Acta* **989**, 111–132.

Wierenga, E.A., Snoek, M., Jansen, H.M., Bos, J.D., Lier, R.A.W. and Kapsenberg, M.L. (1991). Human atopen-specific types 1 and 2 T-helper cell clones. *J. Immunol.* **147**, 2942–2949.

Wu, C.Y., Fargeas, C., Nakajima, T. and Delespesse, G. (1991). Glucocorticoids suppress the production of interleukin-4 by human lymphocytes. *Eur. J. Immunol.* **21**, 2645–2647.

Yamaguchi, Y., Suda, T., Suda, J., Eguchi, M., Miura, Y., Harada, N., Tominaga, A. and Takatsu, K. (1988). Purified interleukin-5 supports the terminal differentiation and proliferation of murine eosinophilic precursors. *J. Exp. Med.* **167**, 43–48.

Yamaguchi, Y., Matsui, T., Kasahara, T., Etoy, S., Tominaga, A., Takatsu, K., Miura, Y. and Suda, T. (1990a). In vivo changes of hemopoietic progenitors and the expression of the interleukin-5 gene in eosinophilic mice infected with *Toxocara canis*. *Exp. Hematol.* **18**, 1152–1157.

Yamaguchi, Y., Suda, T., Shiozaki, H., Miura, Y., Hitoshi, Y., Tominaga, A., Takatsu, K. and Kasahara, T. (1990b). Role of IL-5 in IL-2 induced eosinophilia. *J. Immunol.* **145**, 873–877.

Yamaguchi, Y., Suda, T., Ohta, S., Tominaga, K., Miura, Y. and Kasahara, T. (1991). Analysis of the survival of mature human eosinophils: interleukin-5 prevents apoptosis in mature human eosinophils. *Blood* **78**, 2542–2547.

12

Immunopharmacology of the Eosinophil in Asthma

A.R. LEFF

Department of Medicine MC6076, Section of Pulmonary and Critical Care Medicine, The University of Chicago, 5841 S. Maryland Ave., Chicago, IL 60637, USA

Until recently, the eosinophil was regarded largely as a benign participant in asthmatic inflammation, and substantially more attention was paid to the role of mast cell secretion for which the pharmacological regulation has been well defined (Kaliner *et al.*, 1972; Garrity *et al.*, 1983; Leff *et al.*, 1983). With the advent of bronchoalveolar lavage (BAL) techniques and studies, a broader recognition arose that chronic, severe asthma in humans was more closely approximated by models of the late phase reaction to antigen challenge. This resulted in a direction of focus toward granulocytic inflammation in asthma and to the role of cells and specific mediators of these responses. Early investigations first implicated the neutrophil as the responsible granulocyte (Marsh *et al.*, 1985; Murphy *et al.*, 1986); however, more recently, it has been suggested that eosinophils are at least equally responsible for the airway hyperresponsiveness. While virtually all investigators now believe that inflammation is a *sine qua non* for the hyperreactivity of human asthma, many also now believe that eosinophilic infiltration of the conducting airways may also be a requisite event (Leff *et al.*, 1991).

Eosinophils are difficult to isolate in the inactive state. To do so requires isolation of the cells from the peripheral blood since eosinophils in BAL fluid are largely hypodense and highly activated. This isolation with high purification is a cumbersome process. Recent investigations

T-Lymphocyte and Inflammatory Cell Research in Asthma
ISBN 0-12-388170-6

have demonstrated that eosinophils cultured from umbilical cord blood share characteristic adhesion molecules and other receptors (Walsh *et al.*, 1990); however, these cells must be derived under stimulated conditions and their immaturity and/or influence of cytokines in culture results in certain differences in phenotypic properties.

The difficulty of isolating eosinophils in large numbers in natively inactive states poses some distinct difficulties in pharmacological and pathophysiological assessment. Because of these difficulties, the vast majority of studies have implicated the pathogenetic role of the eosinophil by association rather than by direct experimental intervention. The inability to obtain large numbers of highly purified cells also has limited substantially studies of the molecular biology of the cell and prospective studies assessing the role of the physiological effect of these eosinophils activated *ex vivo*.

This chapter examines first the evidence for a pathogenetic role of the eosinophil in human asthma. The potential role of T cell and cytokine regulation will be considered briefly. Recent experimental evidence has linked the role of molecular adhesion molecules on the eosinophil to airway hyperresponsiveness, and these data also are considered. It has also been suggested that eosinophils may induce airway hyperresponsiveness indirectly through modulation of epithelial function. Finally, the potential for pharmacological manipulation of eosinophil function as a potential therapeutic modality is considered. It should be recognized that these are somewhat premature attempts to link diverse data into a somewhat more unified view. Other interpretations certainly may apply and ultimately prevail.

Which is the Responsible Granulocyte?

Prior investigations have made a reasonable case for the role of the polymorphonuclear leukocyte in experimental airway hyperresponsiveness. Ozone inhalation causes airway hyperresponsiveness in a number of species, including normal humans, and is associated with neutrophilic infiltration into the airways (Holtzman *et al.*, 1983). However, Murlas and Roum (1985) have shown that airway hyperresponsiveness in guinea-pigs exposed to ozone precedes tissue infiltration with neutrophils. Hyperresponsiveness in sensitized rabbits (Marsh *et al.*, 1985; Murphy *et al.*, 1986) is attenuated by granulocyte depletion and restored by repletion. In these studies, it was assumed that neutrophils, the majority constituents of the granulocytic population, were the responsible cell type. However, this was not specifically evaluated. It seems that the classification of both eosinophils and polymorphonuclear leukocytes as "granulocytes", a morphological description, was, for some time, taken as an implication of functional association. Indeed, the function and morphology of eosinophils and neutrophils differ entirely, as summarized in Table 12.1.

Other investigations have demonstrated that neutrophils from asthmatic patients have diminished responsiveness to adenosine and that stimulation of asthmatic neutrophils with formyl-Met-Leu-Phe (fMLP) caused greater superoxide production than in neutrophils from non-asthmatic subjects (Sustiel *et al.*, 1989); however, eosinophils also were not evaluated in these studies. Where it has been studied specifically in fatal asthma, it has been suggested that the neutrophil usually does not infiltrate tissues in allergic inflammation (Fujisawa *et al.*, 1990). On the other hand, there has been a large number of studies implicating specifically the eosinophil in airway hyperresponsiveness, and some studies have indicated that eosinophils or their ghost proteins (such as major basic protein, see below) always are present in asthmatic patients in states of airway hyperresponsiveness.

Bascom and co-workers (1988) demonstrated an influx of inflammatory cells, which included both eosinophils and neutrophils, into the nasal washings during the late response to antigen challenge. Corticosteroid treatment prevented the influx only of eosinophils. Cookson *et al.* (1989) demonstrated a decrease in the peripheral eosinophil count paralleling the time-course and severity of the late asthmatic response. Dunn and co-workers (1988) demonstrated a prolonged "eosinophil-rich" infiltrate bronchoconstriction in guinea-pigs after ovalbumin-sensitization. It may be that eosinophil activation occurs, at least in part, before tissue infiltration occurs. Frick *et al.* (1989) found an increase in hypodense eosinophils (presumed to be more active than normodense) in patients manifesting late phase asthmatic responses to antigen challenge, an effect

Table 12.1
Eosinophils are not red neutrophils

How they differ from neutrophils:

1. Eosinophils have no phagocytic function
2. Eosinophils contain core and granular proteins not found in neutrophils
3. Eosinophils disintegrate to release granular and core proteins after initial degranulation
4. Eosinophils combat parasitic infections by release of granular proteins after immune activation
5. Eosinophils augment airway smooth muscle contractility in animal models

that was absent in patients not having a late phase response. They speculated that hypodense eosinophils may be important in the cascade of events causing late asthmatic responses, as well as being a determinant of asthmatic severity. Bousquet and co-workers (1990) also found that eosinophilic inflammation in humans, measured in peripheral blood and biopsy specimens as cellular constituency and by characteristic proteins, was correlated to the severity of the asthma. Other studies have correlated the late phase reaction in humans specifically to eosinophilic infiltration. Diaz and co-workers (1989) further suggested that eosinophils also may be associated with macrophage activation (Rossi *et al.*, 1991). Preliminary studies suggest that activated macrophages may augment substantially airway responsiveness by inducing oedema formation in the conducting airways (Padrid *et al.*, 1993).

It is important to note that relationship between inflammatory cells and airway hyperresponsiveness is not unequivocal. Djukanovic *et al.* (1990) found no correlation between either mast cells or eosinophils and indices of disease activity or methacholine responsiveness in atopic asthmatics. While some preliminary studies (Strek *et al.*, 1991) indicate that activated eosinophils but not neutrophils can upregulate contractile responses in guinea-pig airways, the mechanism by which this occurs, the specificity of a particular inflammatory cell, and the prodromal and antedromal events of granulocytic activation in airways requires further exploration. At the present time, it none the less seems that the case for the eosinophil being the responsible granulocyte in human asthma is considerably stronger than that for the neutrophil. However, without definitive knowledge of how eosinophils actually may cause airway hyperresponsiveness, it is premature (however tempting) to attribute a primal role to the eosinophil in human asthma.

Eosinophils and Airway Epithelium

An impressive histological picture is painted by the infiltrating eosinophil as it homes in on the lamina propria of the airway, eventually causing epithelial denudation (Laitinen *et al.*, 1985) (Fig. 12.1). This, in turn, leads to several events that theoretically could exacerbate asthma. Oedema and swelling of the epithelium cause lumenal narrowing. By the principle of Laplace, this amplifies the translation of tensile constrictor forces in the wall of the airway to decreased cross-sectional area of the conducting airways of the lung and causes augmented bronchoconstriction. Taken alone, epithelial "damage" may be a misleading concept. The time-course of this response is uncertain; based upon *in vitro* studies,

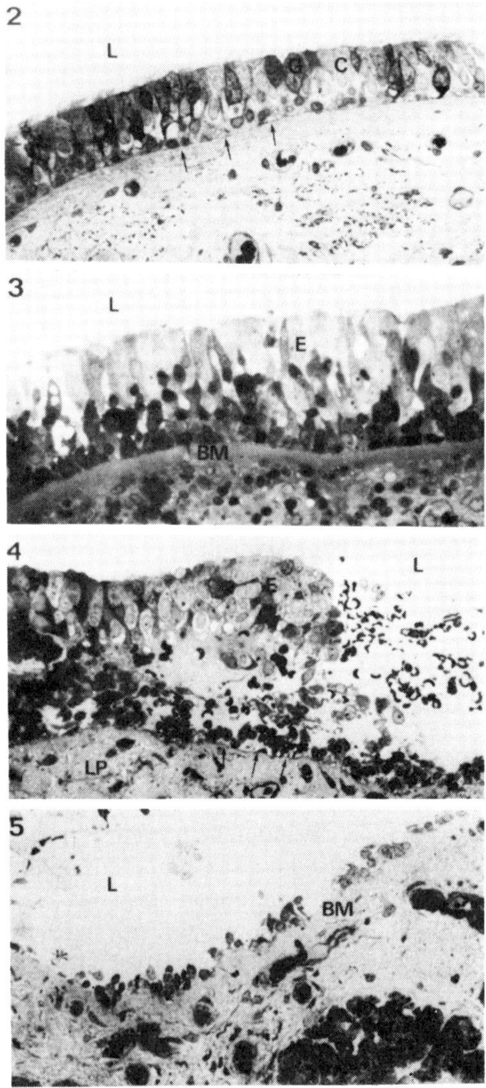

Fig. 12.1 Stages of epithelium denudation in asthma. (2) Control subject with normal basement membrane (arrows) and epithelium with ciliated (C) and goblet cells (G). (3) Asthma patient. Note vacuolation and early thickening of the basement membrane (BM). (4) More advanced pathology in asthma patient. Upper part of the epithelium is shedding off and being separated from the basal layer of cells and, possibly, oedema fluid. There is pronounced oedema in the lamina propria. (5) Extreme damage to epithelium in patient with asthma. The epithelium is virtually entirely shed. (From Laitinen *et al.*, 1985; reproduced with permission from the publisher.)

cytotoxic effects caused by eosinophil products on the epithelium do not occur immediately (Frigas *et al.*, 1980), yet activated eosinophils cause augmented airway contraction *in vivo* almost immediately (White *et al.*, 1990). Non-specific hyperresponsiveness has been induced in the airways of two non-human species almost immediately after application (Flavahan *et al.*, 1988; Barnes *et al.*, 1985). *In vitro*, epithelial cell removal appears to cause slight augmentation of airway contractility (Barnes *et al.*, 1985; Flavahan *et al.*, 1985; Stuart-Smith and Vanhoutte, 1987), although the degree of augmentation is small and the magnitude of the contractile response is not increased. It has been suggested that this effect could, at least in part, result from a diffusion phenomenon. In canine (Brofman *et al.*, 1989) and guinea-pig airways (White *et al.*, 1990) *in situ*, there is no effect of epithelial removal *per se* on either the contractile or relaxation response (Fig. 12.2). However, application of the highly cationic major basic protein of eosinophils (MBP) causes direct and sustained contraction of the guinea-pig trachea that is abolished by epithelial removal (Fig. 12.3). In both canine and guinea-pig airways *in vivo* (Brofman *et al.*, 1989; White *et al.*, 1990) and *in vitro* (Flavahan *et al.*, 1988), the response to contractile agonists is augmented after pretreatment with MBP (Fig. 12.4). This non-specific hyperresponsiveness is also abolished by epithelial cell ablation. It remains unclear whether epithelially mediated hyperresponsiveness caused by MBP is receptor-mediated. There has been no demonstration to date of a specific MBP receptor, and it is possible that epithelial activation caused by MBP may be a result of the high charge density of the molecule.

MBP is a core protein that is unique to the eosinophil (Fig. 12.5). There are three other unique eosinophilic proteins – eosinophil peroxidase (EPO), eosinophil cationic protein (ECP), and eosinophil-derived neurotoxin (EDN). These non-core, granular proteins appear to have a more important function in combating parasitic infestation than in the pathogenesis of experimental airway hyperresponsiveness. Although a preliminary report suggested that ECP might cause profound bronchoconstriction, albeit of short duration (Strek *et al.*, 1991), more recent evidence indicates that ECP may co-elute in the purification process with eosinophil phospholipase A_2 (PLA_2) (Fig. 12.6), which has the identical physiological fingerprint presumed previously for ECP (Strek *et al.*, 1993a). These studies are based upon PLA_2 from *Naja naja* venom, which contains many isoforms of the enzyme. Topical application of this PLA_2 causes augmentation of airway responsiveness as well as direct contraction, and this response does not depend upon the presence of an intact epithelium.

It is interesting to note that EPO secretion is often used as an index

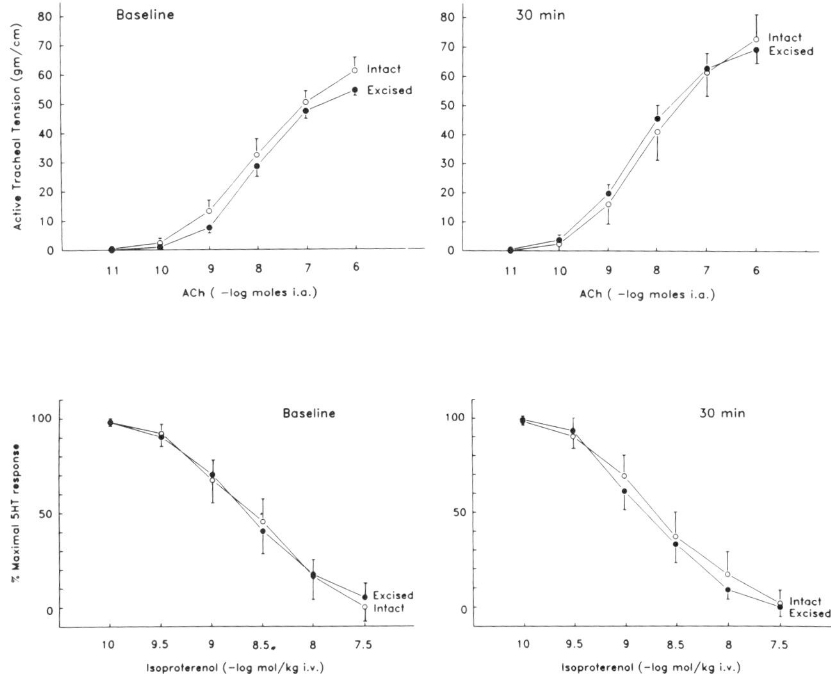

Fig. 12.2 Effect of epithelial removal on airway contraction to muscarinic stimulation (above) and relaxation of tone caused by serotonin (below) caused by isoproterenol *in vivo* in guinea-pig trachealis. Unlike results obtained *in vitro*, there is no effect of epithelium removal when agonists are administered intravenously. Active tension (AT) is measured isometrically *in situ* in a segment of guinea-pig trachealis. Baseline: initial responses before epithelial excision (left); 30 min: response 30 min after epithelial removal. (From White *et al.*, 1990 and Brofman *et al.*, 1989; reproduced with permission from the publishers.)

of eosinophil activation. However, this protein is not biologically active in guinea-pig airways, and secretion of EPO *in vitro* does not correlate directly with the ability of stimulated eosinophils to induce experimental airway hyperresponsiveness (Strek *et al.*, 1993b). The secretion of EPO also varies substantially according to the mode of activation but not as a function of the bioactivity of the activated eosinophil *in vivo*.

While MBP appears to be the fundamental bioactive bronchoconstricting protein of eosinophils, the mechanism by which it acts is undefined and is still the subject of some controversy. Some investigators have presumed that the cytotoxic effect of MBP inhibits the function of putative epithelial-derived relaxing factor (EpDRF) (Stuart-Smith and Vanhoutte, 1988, 1990) and that this is translated into augmented contraction of the

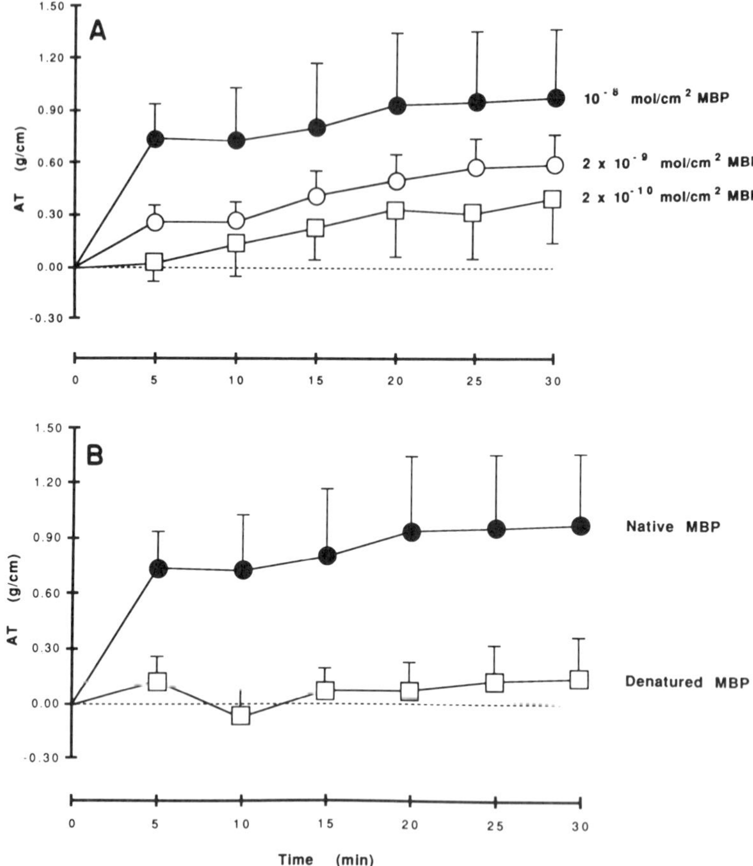

Fig. 12.3 Effect of major basic protein (MBP) of human eosinophils on guinea-pig trachea with topical application. There is sustained, dose-related contraction (A) that is dependent upon an intact epithelium (not shown). Heat denaturation also abolishes the contractile activity of MBP (B). AT: Active tension in guinea-pig trachealis *in situ* (see Fig. 12.2). (From White *et al.*, 1990; reproduced with permission from the American Physiological Society.)

underlying airway smooth muscle. While there are several candidates for EpDRF, including prostaglandin E_2 and nitric oxide, there are no definitive data that identify the EpDRF. The observation that airway contraction begins immediately after application of MBP to the lumenal surface of guinea-pig airways *in situ* (White *et al.*, 1990) suggests that the early effects of MBP may be *stimulatory* rather than inhibitory and that MBP causes airway hyperresponsiveness by induction of epithelial secretion of a bronchoconstricting agent. This putative bronchoconstricting

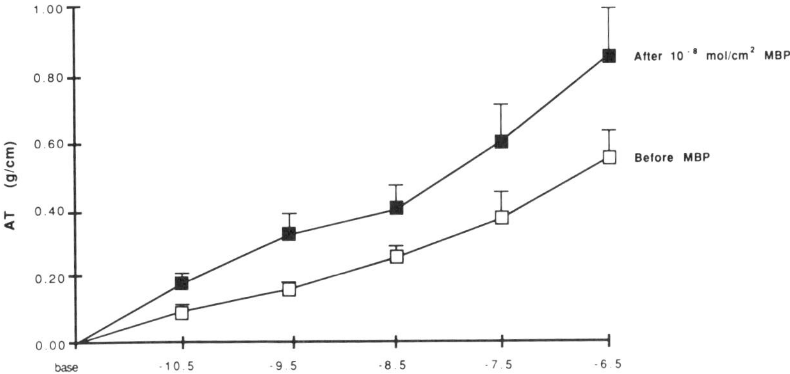

Fig. 12.4 Augmented muscarinic contraction of guinea-pig trachealis after treatment with major basic protein (MBP). Abbreviations are as above. (From White *et al.*, 1990; reproduced with permission from the American Physiological Society.)

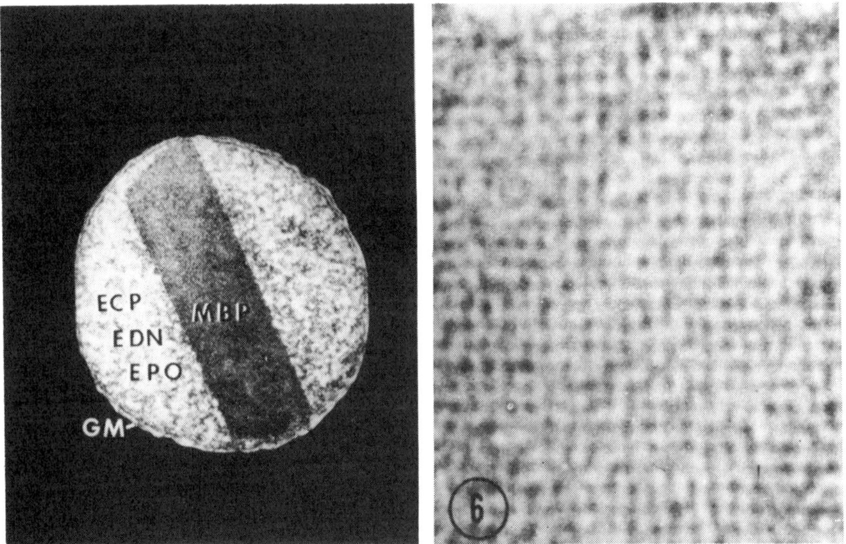

Fig. 12.5 Electron photomicrographs demonstrating the granular matrix of the eosinophil. The central matrix is the core protein, MBP. The protein has an extremely orderly architecture within the core (right). The other three proteins, ECP, EDN and EPO are stored separately from the core within the granule.

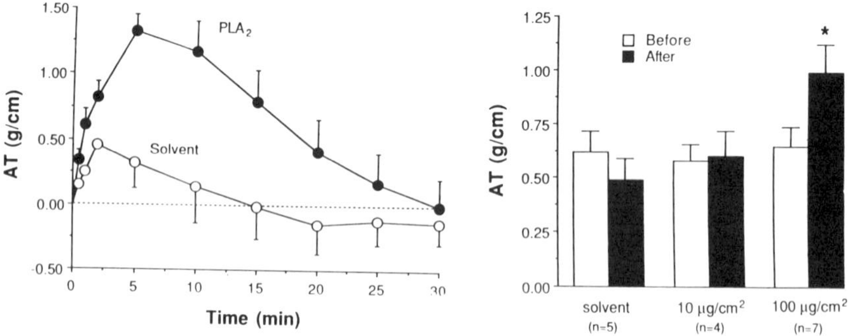

Fig. 12.6 Effect of *Naja naja* phospholipase A_2 (PLA_2) on isometric contraction of guinea-pig trachealis. Topical application of PLA_2 caused immediately forceful contraction of short duration (left). This is identical to the effect previously attributed to ECP. Right: PLA_2 also causes augmentation of muscarinic contraction. Unlike the response elicited by MBP, PLA_2 does not require an intact epithelial to induce contraction or augment muscarinic responsiveness. (From Strek *et al.*, 1993a; reproduced with permission from the publisher.)

substance also has not been identified. It is noteworthy that differences in epithelial–smooth muscle interactions occur when the identical tissues are studied *in vitro* (Stuart-Smith and Vanhoutte, 1988, 1990) or *in vivo* (Brofman *et al.*, 1989; White *et al.*, 1990). It is not surprising that results vary not only among species, but also as a consequence of the preparation that is employed. Based upon a scenario synthesized from *in vivo* and *in vitro* observations within the same species, the following seems likely.

Eosinophils infiltrate airways by mechanisms still only partially defined (see below) and initiate a hyperresponsive state by stimulating secretion of a bronchoactive constricting agent(s) from the epithelium/lamina propria through secretion of MBP. In time (24–48 h), cytotoxic effects of epithelial proteins, including MBP, cause epithelial damage and eventual cell death (Frigas *et al.*, 1980). Assuming the presence of an as yet unidentified EpDRF, it is at this stage that augmentation of airway responsiveness occurs by inhibition of the synthesis of this factor. The process is exacerbated by the sloughing of the epithelium and oedema formation (Rowan *et al.*, 1990) and airway occlusion from secretion and cellular debris. It should be noted that the epithelium is capable of extremely rapid regrowth, and the process of epithelial migration, epithelial activation/cytotoxic damage, and sloughing may be in flux at any particular site in the bronchopulmonary tree and in any particular stage at a given site. The elucidation of this process and the final determination of the mechanism of action of eosinophil core protein promises to be an exciting area of future investigation.

Role of Granulocyte Adhesion Molecules in Airway Hyperresponsiveness

In a previous section, the interaction of eosinophils with airway lamina propria and eosinophils was suggested to play an important role in the induction of airway hyperresponsiveness. Adhesion molecules play an important role in cell–cell attachments in numerous biological processes including viral infection. The mechanism(s) by which granulocytes are localized to the interstices of the conducting airways in human asthma still remain largely undefined. Chemotaxis may certainly play an important initiating role. However, it is not well understood how eosinophils, a minority constituent of the peripheral blood, become so highly and selectively concentrated in the airway. Recent thought has implicated the role of specific molecular adhesion molecules both on the surface of the eosinophils and upon the endothelium. By far the greatest amount of data related to these adhesion molecules have been derived from studies of neutrophils, which share some of the identical adhesion molecules of eosinophils. Thus, it is presumed that cellular migration of eosinophils and neutrophils may proceed similarly, at least with respect to their shared adhesion molecules.

The accumulation of granulocytes within the airway interstices requires slowing and trapping of the cells from the circulating blood, adherence to the endothelium, diapedesis through the epithelium, and migration to the more superficial layers of the airway. The importance of leukocyte adhesion molecules on neutrophils has been demonstrated in patients who genetically lack the integrin (CD18) family of leukocyte adhesion receptors (Anderson *et al.*, 1985; Anderson and Springer, 1987). Leukocyte adhesion deficiency (LAD) results in progressive soft tissue infections, impaired pus formation and a marked leukocytosis. These findings indicate the inability of neutrophils to migrate along chemotactic gradients to sites where inflammatory healing is necessary. There is no known complication of eosinophil deficiency, but it is interesting to consider whether the ability to induce impaired eosinophil adhesion would substantially ameliorate asthma. A detailed review of these molecules and their properties has recently been published by Leff *et al.* (1991). The following discussion is derived in large part from that review.

Granulocyte Adhesion Receptors

β_2-Integrin (CD18) family

This group consists of three adhesion receptors that are found only on leukocytes. Because they cause adhesion to other cells, these receptors also are termed LeuCAM (leukocyte-cell adhesion molecules) and are members of the integrin supergene family. They are comprised of two chains (α and β). There is a common β-chain and three separate α-chains for the members of this family: LFA-1 (CD11a), Mac-1 (macrophage antigen-1 or CD11b), and p150,95 or CD11c) (Table 12.2).

VLA (CD29) family

The term VLA refers to the very late activation family. When first identified, these receptors were found to appear > 2 weeks after antigenic activation on lymphocytes *in vitro*. There are six VLA designations: there is a common β-chain (CD29) and CD49 α-chains (a–f). These VLA receptors bind to extracellular matrix and collagen.

MEL-14/LAM-1

MEL-14/LAM-1 (leukocyte adhesion molecule-1) is a member of the selectin class of molecules. This molecule is proteolysed *in vivo* from the cellular membrane of neutrophils, and this process may also aid in the detachment process after initial adhesion, which is necessary for further migration.

Endothelial Adhesion Molecules

ICAM-1 (CD54)

The intercellular adhesion molecule-1 (ICAM-1) first was discovered as the ligand for LFA-1α in lymphocyte aggregation (Rothlein *et al.*, 1986). The molecule is a member of the immunoglobulin supergene family and has five immunoglobulin-like domains and a cytoplasmic tail upon which adhesion function apparently does not depend. This is the adhesion receptor utilized by rhinoviruses in the common cold, which is a major factor in exacerbating all forms of asthma.

ICAM is the endothelial cell adhesion molecule that attaches to LFA-1α and Mac-1 (Staunton *et al.*, 1990). Induction of this molecule requires protein synthesis *de novo* which occurs within 2–4 h and is maximal at 8–24 h post-stimulation. This induction is an important mechanism in regulating leukocyte infiltration (Dustin *et al.*, 1986; Prober *et al.*, 1986; Wegner *et al.*, 1990).

(ELAM-1), PADGEM/GMP-140 (CD62)

The endothelial leukocyte adhesion molecule (ELAM-1) is a glycoprotein of the selectin family (Table 12.2) that is induced after cytokine activation. Like ICAM, this molecule is involved in adhesion of leukocytes to the endothelium. The PADGEM (platelet activation-dependent granule-external membrane protein or granule membrane protein M) is also a glycoprotein of the selectin family. This molecule is mobilized quickly on activation to the surface where it promotes leukocyte adhesion. Like ICAM and ELAM, PADGEM is thus an inducible regulator of leukocyte adhesion.

VCAM

Vascular cell adhesion molecule (VCAM) is expressed maximally on cultured human endothelial cells 24 h after stimulation with interleukin-1 (IL-1), tumour-necrosis factor (TNF) or lipopolysaccharide (LPS). VCAM is the endothelial ligand for VLA-4, the β_1-integrin expressed on eosinophils, but not neutrophils. Interestingly, IL-4 has recently been found to induce selectively VCAM expression, but not that of ICAM-1 or ELAM, on cultured endothelial cells.

Granulocyte Migration and Adhesion

Much of the adhesion process has been deduced from studies of the various steps of the process *in vitro*. These involve studies of neutrophil adhesion to cultured monolayers of human umbilical vein endothelial cells (HUVECs). In non-activated neutrophils, adhesion is inhibited by monoclonal antibodies to ICAM-1, LFA-1α, MEL-14, and ELAM-1 (Barker *et al.*, 1989; Lusinskas *et al.*, 1989) but not Mac-1 (Smith *et al.*, 1989). Adhesion by these receptors is additive, suggesting the concept of an obligate receptor-ligand relationship of LFA-1α and ICAM-1 (Marlin and Springer, 1987). For activated neutrophils, adhesion is not inhibited by monoclonal antibodies to MEL-14 and ELAM-1 (Smith *et al.*, 1990), but partial inhibition results from monoclonal antibodies to LFA-1α and Mac-1 and near complete inhibition results from monoclonal antibodies to ICAM-1 and LFA-1α. The data suggest that adhesion occurs by a series of steps as outlined in Fig. 12.7. Again, it is noted that this sequence of events is defined for neutrophils, and the extent to which this pertains to eosinophils is unclear. Of particular note is the fact that eosinophils, unlike neutrophils, do not marginate in blood vessels.

Table 12.2
Adhesion receptors of the integrin superfamily

Family name	α-subunits	Molecular mass (α/β) (kDa)	Distribution	Ligands
β_1-VLA (CD29), platelet gpIIa, receptor b, chicken integrin band 3	α_1-VLA (CD49a)	210/130	Lymphocytes, fibroblasts, basement membrane	Laminin, collagen
	α_2-LA-2 platelet, qpla, ECMRII (CD49b)	165/130	T-lymphocytes, platelets, fibroblasts, endothelium, epithelium	Collagen, laminin
	α_3-VLA-3, ECMRI (CD49c)	130/130	Epithelium, fibroblasts	Fibronectin, laminin (collagen?)
	α_4-VLA-4, LPAM-1 (CD49d)	150/130	Most leukocytes, neural crest, fibroblasts	Fibronectin, VCAM-1
	α_5-VLA-6, fibronectin receptor,	135/130	Thymocytes, T-lymphocytes,	Fibronectin

	ECMRV1, platelet gplc (CD49e)		fibroblasts, epithelium, endothelium, platelets	
	α_6-VLA-6, platelet gp1C+ (CD49f)	120/130	T-lymphocytes, platelets	Laminin
β_2-LFA-1 (CD18), LeuCAM, leukocytes Integrins	α_L-LFA-1 (CD11a)	180/95	Most leukocytes	ICAM-1, ICAM-2
	α_m-Mac-1, Mo-1, CR3, OKM-1, OKM-10, Leu 15 (CD11b)	170/95	Macrophages/monocytes, granulocytes	ICAM-1, C3bi, gen, Factor X, LPS
	α_1-p150,95, LeuK5, CR4 (CD11c)	150/95	Macrophages/monocytes granulocytes	(C3bi?)
β_3-Platelet gpIIIa, Vitronectin receptor β (CD61)	α_{11b}-gpIIb (CD41)	120/105	Platelets	Fibronectin, fibrinogen, von Willebrand factor
	α_v-vitronectin receptor (CD51)	135/105	B-lymphocytes, macrophages/ monocytes, endothelium	Vitronectin, fibrinogen, von Willebrand factor, thrombospondin

VLA, very late antigen, LFA-1, lymphocyte function-associated antigen-1; LeuCAM, leukocyte cell adhesion molecules.

Reprinted from Leff *et al.*, 1991 with permission from the American Physiological Society.

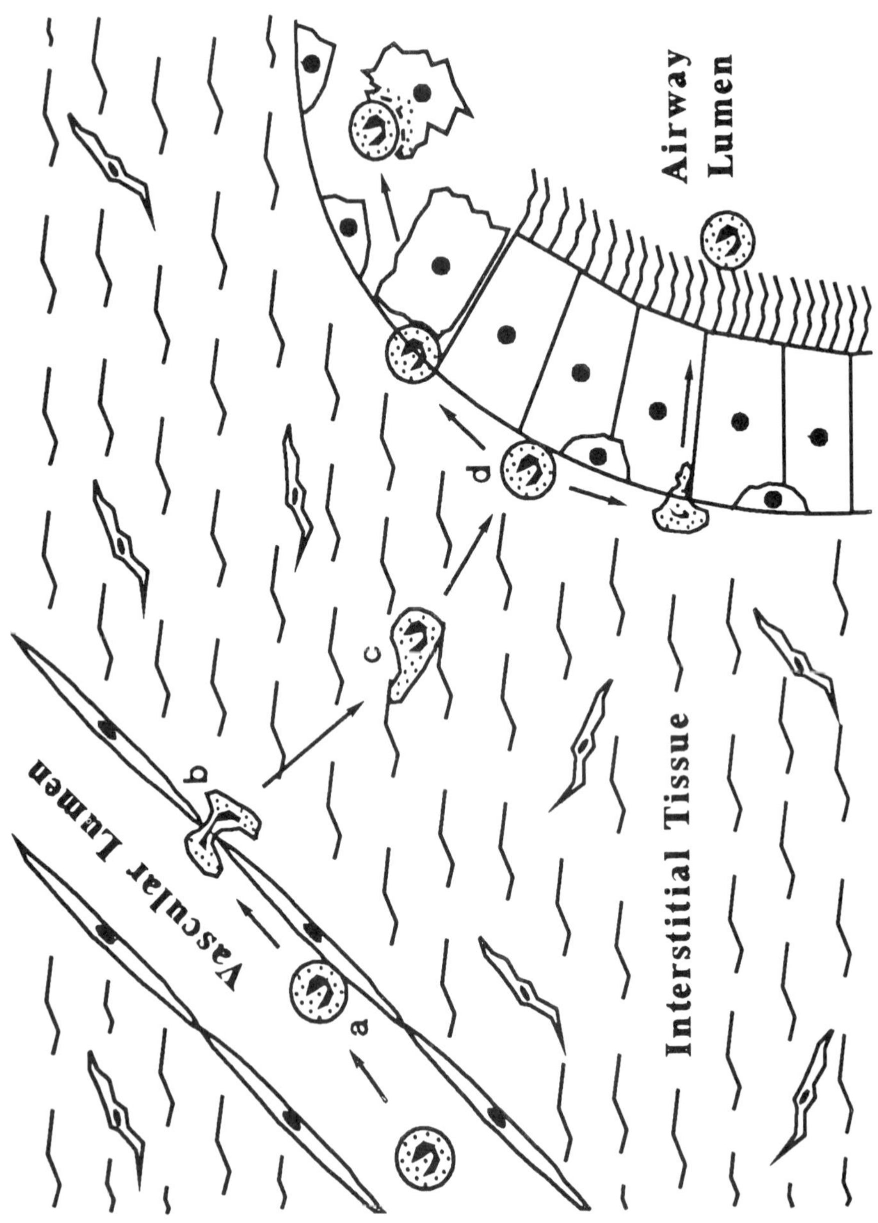

Airway Lumen
Interstitial Tissue
Vascular Lumen
a
b
c
d

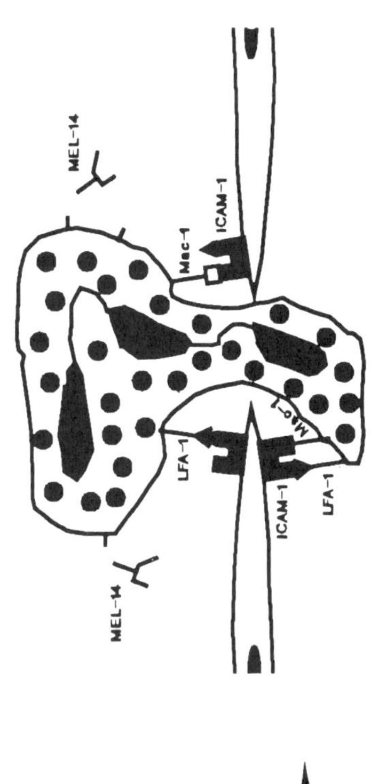
A Margination
Neutrophil
MEL-14
LFA-1
ICAM-1
ELAM-1
PADGEM/
GMP-140
Endothelium

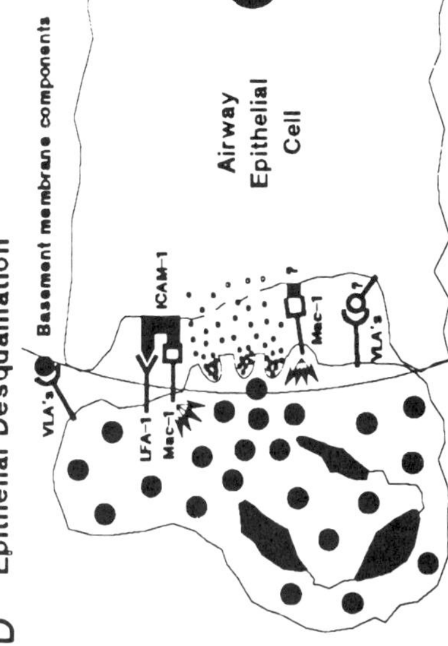
B Transendothelial Migration
MEL-14
Mac-1
ICAM-1
LFA-1

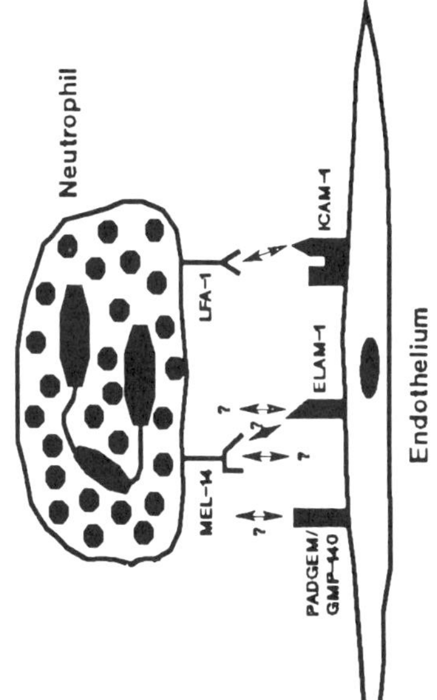
C Interstitial Migration
Extravascular
Matrix Proteins
VLA's
Mac-1 ?

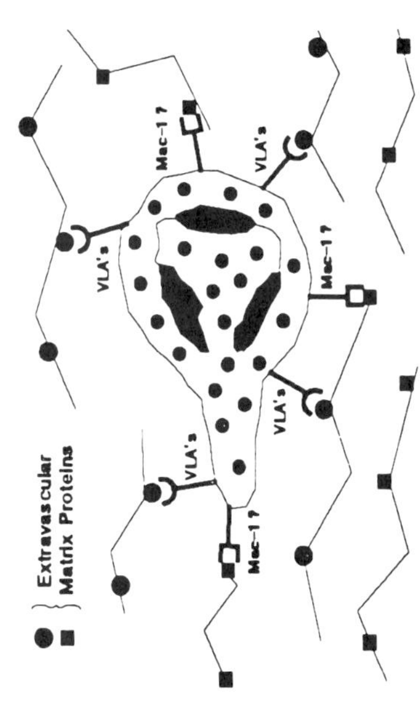
D Epithelial Desquamation
Basement membrane components
Airway
Epithelial
Cell
ICAM-1
LFA-1
Mac-1
VLA's

Step 1 is the adhesion of the granulocyte to the endothelium, and this is mediated by MEL-14, ELAM-1 and LFA-1α/ICAM-1 (Fig. 12.7A). MEL-14 then is shed and Mac-1 is activated, thus regulating transendothelial migration (Fig. 12.7B); this occurs through binding to ICAM-1 by Mac-1. The role of other adhesion molecules in this process is still incompletely defined. This completes diapedesis, and granulocyte migration now proceeds through the submucosal layers of the airway (Fig. 12.7C). It is presumed that a chemoattractant gradient (?leukotriene B_4) is involved here. It is probably at this point that VLA receptor activation plays a role in the movement through the airway matrix. The final step requires leukocyte retention and activation (Fig. 12.7D). This activation results in the inflammatory burst activity of neutrophils (e.g., H_2O_2 production) and/or eosinophils (EPO?).

Relationship between Eosinophilia and Adhesion

The complex process of adhesion and migration suggests that the absence of any essential step will prevent selective migration of inflammatory cells to the site of inflammation. This offers some encouragement from a pharmacological perspective, since the opportunity to intervene in the process of molecular adhesion could variously be applied to both antiviral and anti-inflammatory therapy, including that which causes human asthma (see below). The caveat, of course, is that inhibition of granulocyte adhesion also may prevent the essential components of the inflammatory

Fig. 12.7 Stages of eosinophil migration. Adhesion molecules believed to contribute during each of four steps of granulocyte migration from vascular lumen to airway lumen. Evidence suggests (see text) that LFA-1 to ICAM-1, MEL-14, ELAM-1, and PADGEM/GMP-140 mediate the initial adhesion (margination) of neutrophils to endothelium (A). MEL-14 is then shed and adhesion via ELAM-1 (and possibly PADGEM/GMP-140) released as the granulocyte becomes activated, with Mac-1 and LFA-1 binding to endothelial ICAM-1 controlling transendothelial migration (B). Migration through the interstitium (C) is then presumably managed via Mac-1 and the VLA family of receptors binding to extravascular matrix proteins (i.e. fibronectin, laminin and collagen). Finally, at the epithelium, adhesion and migration are regulated via VLA receptors to basement membrane components, Mac-1 and LFA-1 to epithelial ICAM-1, and VLA receptors and Mac-1 to yet undetermined epithelial cell adhesion ligands. Epithelial desquamation (D) would be aided by this adhesion, promoting and sustaining a high local cytotoxin concentrations in an enclosed pocket between the granulocyte and epithelial cell, as well as Mac-1 adhesion-dependent enhancement of granulocyte activation. (From Leff *et al.*, 1991; reproduced with permission from the American Physiological Society.)

process that combats infection, as in leukocyte adhesion deficiency (LAD) disease.

It also seems apparent that there is no essential linkage between processes causing granulocyte demargination or peripheral blood eosinophilia and the necessary complex cascade of events that promote tissue eosinophilia, such as that seen in the conducting airways in human asthma. This likely accounts for the failure of hypereosinophilic animal models to demonstrate airway hyperresponsiveness. Similarly, while patients suffering from eosinophilia-myalgia syndrome have numerous ills, these apparently do not include invasion of the conducting airways or concomitant airway hyperresponsiveness (Hertzman *et al.*, 1990; Culpepper *et al.*, 1991). It appears that the process that promotes eosinophil proliferation and survival and may largely be dependent upon cytokines, such as IL-5, is both selective for this granulocyte and independent of other stages of its biological activation.

Evidence for Involvement of Eosinophil Adhesion Molecules in Airway Hyperresponsiveness

There has been much less study of the adhesion molecules on eosinophils, but some limited data indicate relevant similarities to studies of neutrophil adhesion (Jutila *et al.*, 1989; Wegner *et al.*, 1989). Possible differences exist in the degree to which the various receptors are utilized between eosinophils and neutrophils and in the cytokines that may activate and upregulate these receptors. The VLA-4 adhesion molecule exists only on the eosinophil, but its mode of activation and adhesion in airway hyperresponsiveness remains unknown. Relative to neutrophil adhesion, Mac-1 and P150,95 (Te Velde *et al.*, 1987) may contribute more than MEL-14 and ELAM-1 in eosinophil adhesion in studies utilizing *in vitro* studies of HUVECs (Fig. 12.8).

A few investigations have examined the events of eosinophil adhesion *in vivo*. Antigen inhalation has been shown to induce ICAM-1 expression in sensitized airways (Wegner *et al.*, 1990). Both the vascular endothelium and airway epithelium stains heavily for ICAM-1 after repeated antigen inhalation. Staining for LFA-1α demonstrates intense leukocyte infiltration immediately below the basement membrane (adjacent to the site of ICAM-1 expression) in chronically inflamed airways of monkeys. This is not observed in acutely inflamed airways.

In monkeys treated with mouse anti-human ICAM-1 monoclonal antibody R6.5 for 8 days, infiltration of eosinophils is substantially inhibited and airway responsiveness is attenuated (Fig. 12.9). Intravenous infusion of monoclonal antibody to ICAM-1 reduced the number

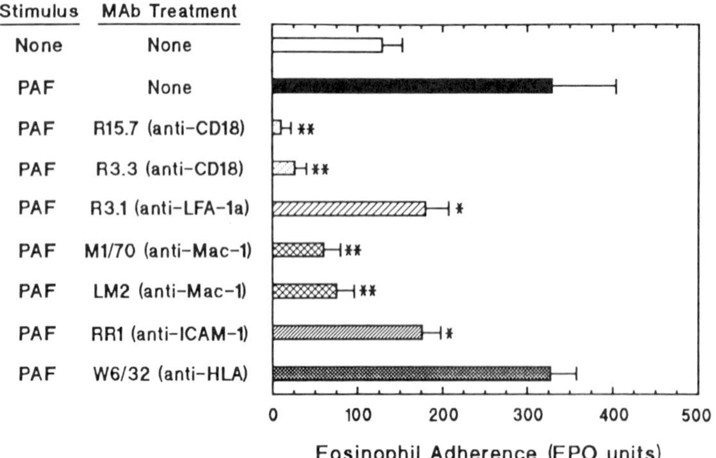

Fig. 12.8 Effects of various monoclonal antibodies (1:4 dilution of supernatants) to adhesion molecules on platelet-activating factor (PAF, 10^{-7} M)-induced primate lung eosinophil adhesion to cultured monolayers of human umbilical vein endothelial cells. Adhered eosinophils were quantitated by a colorimetric assay for eosinophil peroxidase (EPO units, mean ± S.D.). *Significant (Dunnett's multiple comparison test, $P < 0.05$) attenuation of PAF-induced adherence. (From Young *et al.*, 1986; reproduced with permission from the American Physiological Society.)

of eosinophils present in the bronchoalveolar fluid measured during methacholine challenge in immune-sensitized monkeys. This decrease in eosinophils was associated with a comparable decrease in airway response to inhaled methacholine.

Role of Cytokines and Arachidonate Metabolites in Chemotaxis and Activation

Products of the arachidonate pathway (LTB_4, 5-HETE and 5-HPETE) cause chemotaxis of eosinophils (Nagy *et al.*, 1982). Prostaglandin D_2 causes selective accumulation of eosinophils in canine isolated trachea. Administration of platelet-activating factor (PAF) to guinea-pigs causes eosinophil infiltration that is inhibited by PAF antagonists (Lellouch-Tubiana *et al.*, 1988). However, PAF also causes infiltration of neutrophils as well.

The cytokines IL-3 and IL-5 have multiple and varied effects on eosinophils. IL-5 is essential for the maturation of eosinophils from immature precursor cells (Clutterbuck *et al.*, 1989; Warren and Moore,

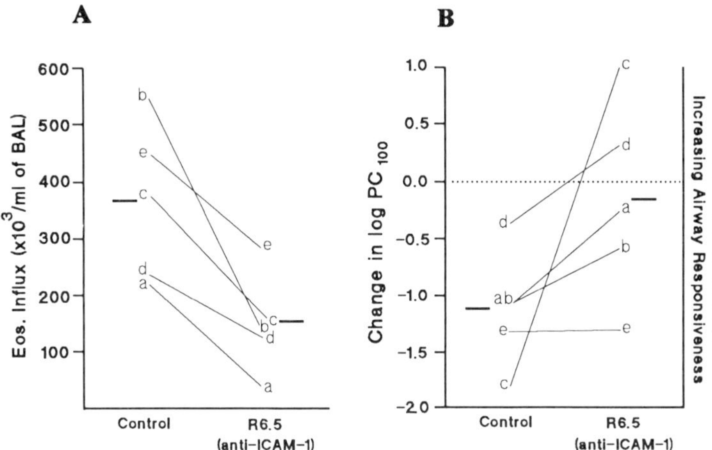

Fig. 12.9 Effects of monoclonal antibody R6.5 to ICAM-1 (1.76 mg/kg per day, intravenous) on airway eosinophilia (assessed by bronchoalveolar lavage, BAL) and increase in airway responsiveness (inhaled methacholine PC_{100}) induced by 3 alternate-day antigen inhalations in monkeys. Studies with R6.5 treatment are compared with mean of bracketing control studies on each animal. Bars, mean of five animals individually identified by letters a–e. R6.5 treatment significantly attenuated eosinophil influx when tested versus bracketing control values by 2-way analysis of variance (P = 0.0133) and versus post-R6.5 control study by Friedman's test (P = 0.0212); Friedman's for R6.5 versus pre-R6.5 control was P + 0.0755. R6.5 treatment significantly inhibited decrease in log PC_{100} versus pre-R6.5 control Friedman's test (P = 0.0002); Friedman's for R6.5 versus post-R6.5 control was P = 0.667. (From Wegner *et al.*, 1990; reproduced with permission from the American Physiological Society.)

1988) and is a selective chemoattractant for eosinophils (Yamaguchi *et al.*, 1988; Wang *et al.*, 1989). IL-5 also augments the magnitude of eosinophil degranulation stimulated by secretory immunoglobulin A (IgA) on Sepharose beads. IL-3 also prolongs eosinophil survival, and it has been suggested that these cytokines may play an important role in the selective accumulation of eosinophils in conducting airways in asthma (Lamas *et al.*, 1989). Granulocyte–macrophage colony-stimulating factor (GM–CSF) also enhances eosinophil survival in culture. This cytokine is produced by airway epithelial cells and suggests another potential role of the epithelium in the inflammatory events of asthma. GM–CSF also primes eosinophils by inducing enhanced surface receptor expression and increased leukotriene C_4 production (Howell *et al.*, 1989).

HUVECs stimulated with tumour necrosis factor demonstrate increased expression of vascular cell adhesion molecule-1 (VCAM-1) (Kyan-Aung *et al.*, 1991); treatment with monoclonal antibody directed against VCAM-1 preferentially inhibited eosinophil- versus neutrophil-adhesion, but only when eosinophils were pretreated with a monoclonal antibody directed against the common β-chain of the CD11/CD18 complex. Although eosinophils bind to VCAM-1, this effect is probably minor compared with the activity of CD11/CD18 adhesion molecules. Rand and co-workers (Rand *et al.*, 1991) demonstrated that the T cell-derived cytokine IL-2 was a potent chemoattractant for eosinophils from normal and eosinophilic donors. The role of IL-1 receptor inhibition on the eosinophil in mediating airway hyperresponsiveness in humans is currently being examined.

Formulating a Therapeutic Strategy

Because eosinophils appear to play no vital role in the human immune response except for parasitic infestation, therapeutic approaches directed toward inhibition of eosinophil function seem particularly appealing. This, of course, presumes that eosinophil is either an essential or fundamental component of the human asthmatic response. Despite correlative evidence that suggests that eosinophils induce airway hyperresponsiveness *in vivo*, the role of the eosinophil as an effector cell in asthma has not been verified. Other cellular components of immune hyperresponsiveness have been implicated, namely the mast cell and the T-lymphocyte (Azzawi *et al.*, 1990; Frew *et al.*, 1990; Garssen *et al.*, 1991; Rochester and Rankin, 1991). Over the years, therapies directed against the mast cell have been only minimally successful in treating human asthma. There is one report suggesting an effect in the treatment of steroid-dependent human asthmatics with cyclosporin, which inhibits specifically T cell function (Alexander *et al.*, 1992). However, this radical and potentially toxic suppression of the immune system hardly seems the basis upon which to launch a therapeutic strategy. Indeed, these studies probably serve more to implicate the role of T cell mediation of eosinophil (and other cell) functions in human asthma. Thus, the advantages of devising specific therapeutic inhibition of eosinophil function are clear, but perhaps still a bit premature.

These concerns aside, there are several obvious approaches. Corticosteroids substantially inhibit eosinophilia and the inflammation of human asthma, and they remain the predominant mode of "anti-eosinophil" treatment today. While effective, the side-effects from long-term use are prodigious. Although it is likely that more potent topically administered corticosteroids (e.g. aerosols) will be even more effective than currently available agents, there is ample reason to consider more specific anti-eosinophil therapies.

Eosinophils and mast cells possess β-adrenergic receptors of the β_2-subtype that are coupled to adenylyl cyclase. However, unlike mast cells, in eosinophils these receptors do not appear to modulate oxidative metabolism or eosinophil degranulation (Yukawa *et al.*, 1990), and so the utility of this approach seems rather limited. Eosinophils produce substantial quantities of leukotriene C_4 when activated. Antagonists directed at the leukotriene C_4 receptor or, more globally, at 5-lipoxygenase inhibition have been shown in preliminary studies (White *et al.*, 1993) to inhibit the effects of eosinophil activation on guinea-pig airways. These compounds currently are undergoing clinical trials in humans. While somewhat effective, they do not, at present, reverse completely the bronchoconstriction of even moderate human asthma.

The notion that certain cytokines induce what may be essential components of eosinophil survival, adhesion and activation suggests that a specific intervention in eosinophil function having no other effects on immune function is possible. There is a naturally circulating IL-1 receptor antagonist, but its utility as a pharmacological agent in treating inflammatory states remains to be tested. To date, there are no IL-5 receptor antagonists that are approved for human use. Since IL-5 appears to be essential for eosinophil survival beyond the marrow precursor stage, development of a selective IL-5 antagonist has particular appeal. The difficulty will be to produce an IL-5 (or other cytokine) antagonist that also is not immunogenic in humans. Because such antagonists likely will be proteins, parenteral administration will be required, and this further constrains enthusiasm.

The blockade of molecular adhesion is an approach for which there is some experimental verification in primates (Wegner *et al.*, 1990). This is a highly complicated approach, because the responsible and eosinophil-specific adhesion molecules remain to be defined more fully. Once this is done, other concerns apply. Blockade of adhesion must be specific for eosinophils, as neutrophil function must remain intact for combating infection. There is also the reasonable concern that anti-adhesion molecule, even if highly specific, also may be immunogenic.

These concerns should not be taken as cause for discouragement but rather as reason for enthusiasm and excitement. The elucidation of the role of the eosinophil in asthma may provide one of the first novel approaches to the treatment of asthma in more than 20 years. There are ample data already to suggest that this will be a productive approach to the development of better therapies for human asthma.

References

Alexander, A.G., Barnes, N.C. and Kay, A. (1992). Trial of cyclosporin in corticosteroid-dependent severe asthma. *Lancet* **339**, 324–328.

Anderson, D.C. and Springer, T.A. (1987). Leukocyte adhesion deficiency: an inherited defect in the Mac-1, LFA-1 and p150, 95 glycoproteins. *Annu. Rev. Med.* **38**, 175–194.

Anderson, D.C., Schmalsteig, F.C., Finegold, M.J., Hughes, R., Rothlein, L.J., Miller, S., Kohl, M.F., Tosi, R., Jacobs, L., Waldrop, T.C., Goldman, A.S., Shearer, W.T. and Springer, T.A. (1985). The severe and moderate phenotypes of heritable Mac-1, LFA-1 deficiency: their quantitative definition and relation to leukocyte dysfunction and clinical features. *J. Infect. Dis.* **152**, 668–689.

Azzawi, M., Bradley, B., Jeffery, P.K., Frew, A.J., Wardlaw, A.J., Knowles, G., Assoufi, B., Collins, J.V., Durham, S. and Kay, A.B. (1990). Identification of activated T lymphocytes and eosinophils in bronchial biopsies in stable atopic asthma. *Am. Rev. Respir. Dis.* **142**, 1407–1413.

Barker, R.L., Loegering, D.A., Ten, R.M., Hamann, K.J., Pease, L.R. and Gleich, G.J. (1989). Eosinophil cationic protein cDNA. Comparison with other toxic cationic proteins and ribonucleases. *J. Immunol.* **143**, 952–955.

Barnes, P.J., Cuss, F.H. and Palmer, J.B. (1985). The effect of airway epithelium on smooth muscle contractility in bovine trachea. *Brit. J. Pharmacol.* **86**, 685–692.

Bascom, R., Pipkorn, U., Lichtenstein, L.M. and Naclerio, R.M. (1988). The influx of inflammatory cells into nasal washings during the late response to antigen challenge. Effect of systemic steroid pretreatment. *Am. Rev. Respir. Dis.* **138**, 406–412.

Bousquet, J., Chanez, P., Lacoste, J.Y., Barneon, G., Ghavanian, N., Enander, I., Venge, P., Ahlstedt, S., Simony-Lafontaine, J., Godard, P. and Michel, F.-B. (1990). Eosinophilic inflammation in asthma. *New Engl. J. Med.* **323**, 1033–1039.

Brofman, J.D., White, S.R., Blake, J.S., Munoz, N.M., Gleich, G.J. and Leff, A.R. (1989). Epithelial augmentation of trachealis contraction caused by MBP of eosinophils. *J. Appl. Physiol.* **66**, 1867–1873.

Clutterbuck, E.J., Hirst, E.M.A. and Sanderson, C.J. (1989). Human interleukin-5 (IL-5) regulates the production of eosinophils in human bone marrow cultures: comparison and interaction with IL-1, IL-3, IL-6 and GM–CSF. *Blood* **73**, 1504–1512.

Cookson, W.O.C.M., Craddock, C.F., Benson, M.K. and Durham, S.R. (1989). Falls in peripheral eosinophil counts parallel the late asthmatic response. *Am. Rev. Respir. Dis.* **139**, 458–462.

Culpepper, R.C., Williams, R.G., Mease, P.J., Koepsell, T.D. and Kobayashi, J.M. (1991). Natural history of the eosinophilia-myalgia syndrome. *Ann. Intern. Med.* **115**, 437–442.

Diaz, P., Gonzalez, M.G., Galleguillos, F.R., Ancic, P., Cromwell, O., Shepherd, D., Durham, S.R., Gleich, G.J. and Kay, A.B. (1989). Leukocytes and mediators in bronchoalveolar lavage during allergen-induced late-phase asthmatic reactions. *Am. Rev. Respir. Dis.* **139**, 1383–1389.

Djukanovic, R., Wilson, J.W., Britten, K.M., Wilson, S.J., Walls, A.F., Roche, W.R., Howarth, P.H. and Holgate, S.T. (1990). Quantitation of mast cells and eosinophils in the bronchial mucosa of symptomatic atopic asthmatics and in healthy control subjects using immunohistochemistry. *Am. Rev. Respir. Dis.* **142**, 863–871.

Dunn, C.J., Elliott, G.A., Oostveen, J.A. and Richards, I.M. (1988). Development of a prolonged eosinophil-rich inflammatory leukocyte infiltration in the guinea-pig asthmatic response to ovalbumin inhalation. *Am. Rev. Respir. Dis.* **137**, 541–547.

Dustin, M.L., Rothlein, R., Bhan, A.K., Dinarello, C.A. and Springer, T.A. (1986). Induction by IL1 and interferon: tissue and distribution, biochemistry, and function of a natural adherence molecule (ICAM-1). *J. Immunol.* **137**, 245–252.

Flavahan, N.A., Aarhus, L.L., Rimele, T.J. and Vanhoutte, P.M. (1985). Respiratory epithelium inhibits bronchial smooth muscle tone. *J. Appl. Physiol.* **58**, 834–838.

Flavahan, N.A., Slifman, N.R., Gleich, G.J. and Vanhoutte, P.M. (1988). Human eosinophil major basic protein causes hyperreactivity of respiratory smooth muscle. Role of the epithelium. *Am. Rev. Respir. Dis.* **138**, 685–688.

Frew, A.J., Moqbel, R., Azzawi, M., Hartnell, A., Barkans, J., Jeffery, P.K., Kay, A.B., Scheper, R.J., Varley, J., Church, M.K. and Holgate, S.T. (1990). T lymphocytes and eosinophils in allergen-induced late-phase asthmatic reactions in the guinea-pig. *Am. Rev. Respir. Dis.* **141**, 407–413.

Frick, W.E., Sedgwick, J.B. and Busse, W.W. (1989). The appearance of hypodense eosinophils in antigen-dependent late phase asthma. *Am. Rev. Respir. Dis.* **139**, 1401–1406.

Frigas, E., Loegering, D.A. and Gleich, G.J. (1980). Cytotoxic effects of guinea pig eosinophil major basic protein on tracheal epithelium. *Lab. Invest.* **42**, 35–43.

Fujisawa, T., Kephart, G.M., Gray, B.H. and Gleich, G.J. (1990). The neutrophil and chronic allergic inflammation. *Am. Rev. Respir. Dis.* **141**, 689–697.

Garrity, E.R., Stimler, N., Munoz, N.M., Fried, R. and Leff, A.R. (1983). Response of bronchial smooth muscle to mast cell degranulation *in situ*. *J. Appl. Physiol.* **55**, 1803–1810.

Garssen, J., Nijkamp, F.P., Van Der Vliet, H. and Van Loveren, H. (1991). T-cell-mediated induction of airway hyperreactivity in mice. *Am. Rev. Respir. Dis.* **144**, 931–938.

Hertzman, P.A., Blevens, W.L., Mayer, J., Greenfield, B., Ting, M. and Gleich, G.J. (1990). Association of the eosinophilia-myalgia syndrome with the ingestion of tryptophan. *New Engl. J. Med.* **322**, 869–873.

Holtzman, M.J., Fabri, L.M., O'Byrne, P.M., Gold, B.D., Aizawa, H., Walters, E.H., Alpert, S.E. and Nadel, J.A. (1983). Importance of airway inflammation for hyperresponsiveness induced by ozone. *Am. Rev. Respir. Dis.* **127**, 686–690.

Howell, C.J., Pujol, J.L., Crea, A.E.G., Davidson, R., Gearing, A.J.H., Godard, P.H. and Lee, T.H. (1989). Identification of an alveolar macrophage-derived activity in bronchial asthma that enhances leukotriene C4 generation by human eosinophils stimulated by ionophore A23187 as a granulocyte-macrophage colony-stimulating factor. *Am. Rev. Respir. Dis.* **140**, 1340–1347.

Jutila, M.A., Rott, L., Berg, E.L. and Butcher, E.C. (1989). Function and regulation of the neutrophil MEL-14 antigen in vivo: comparison with LFA-1 and Mac-1. *J. Immunol.* **143**, 3318–3324.

Kaliner, M.A., Orange, R.P. and Austen, K.F. (1972). Immunological release of histamine and slow reacting substances of anaphylaxis from human lung.

IV. Enhancement by cholinergic and alpha-adrenergic stimulation. *J. Exp. Med.* **136**, 556–557.

Kyan-Aung, U., Haskard, D.O. and Lee, T.H. (1991). Vascular cell adhesion molecule-1 and eosinophil adhesion to cultured human umbilical vein endothelial cells *in vitro*. *Am. J. Respir. Cell Molec. Biol.* **5**, 445–450.

Laitinen, L.A., Heino, M., Laitinen, A., Kava, T and Haahtela, T. (1985). Damage of the airway epithelium and bronchial reactivity in patients with asthma. *Am. Rev. Respir. Dis.* **131**, 599–606.

Lamas, A.M., Marcotte, C.V. and Schleimer, R.P. (1989). Human endothelial cells prolong eosinophil survival. Regulation by cytokines and glucocorticoids. *J. Immunol.* **142**, 3978–3984.

Leff, A., Brown, J.K., Frey, M., Reed, B.R. and Gold, W.M. (1983). Biochemical and physiological effects of compound 48/80 on canine trachea *in vivo*. *J. Appl. Physiol.* **54**, 720–729.

Leff, A.R., Hamann, K.J. and Wegner, C.D. (1991). Inflammation and cell–cell interactions in airway hyperresponsiveness. *Am. J. Physiol.; Lung Cell. Molec. Physiol.* **260** (4), L189–L206.

Lellouch-Tubiana, A., Lefort, J., Simon, M.T., Pfister, A. and Vargaftig, B.B. (1988). Eosinophil recruitment into guinea pig lungs after PAF-acether and allergen administration. Modulation by prostacyclin, platelet depletion, and selective antagonists. *Am. Rev. Respir. Dis.* **137**, 948–954.

Lusinskas, F.W., Brock, A.F., Arnaout, M.A. and Gimbrone, M.A. Jr., (1989). Endothelial-leukocyte adhesion molecule-1-dependent and leukocyte (CD11/CD18)-dependent mechanisms contribute to polymorphonuclear leukocyte adhesion to cytokine-activated human vascular endothelium. *J. Immunol.* **142**, 2257–2263.

Marlin, S.D. and Springer, T.A. (1987). Purified intercellular adhesion molecule-1 (ICAM-1) is a ligand for lymphocyte function-associated antigen (LFA-1). *Cell* **51**, 813–819.

Marsh, W.R., Irvin, C.G., Murphy, K.R., Behrens, B.L. and Larsen, G.L. (1985). Increases in airway reactivity to histamine and inflammatory cells in bronchoalveolar lavage after the late asthmatic response in an animal model. *Am. Rev. Respir. Dis.* **131**, 875–879.

Murlas, C. and Roum, J.H. (1985). Bronchial hyperreactivity occurs in steroid-treated guinea pigs depleted of leukocytes by cyclophosamide. *J. Appl. Physiol.* **58**, 1630–1637.

Murphy, K.R., Wilson, M.C. and Irvin, C.G. (1986). The requirement for polymorphonuclear leukocytes in the late asthmatic response and heightened airway reactivity in an animal model. *Am. Rev. Respir. Dis.* **134**, 62–68.

Nagy, L., Lee, T.H., Goetzi, E.J., Picket, W.C. and Kay, A.B. (1982). Complement receptor enhancement and chemotaxis of human neutrophils and eosinophils by leukotrienes and other lipoxygenase products. *Clin. Exp. Immunol.* **47**, 541–547.

Padrid, P.A., Wolf, R., Spaethe, S., Munoz, N., Kalk, A., Finucane, T. and Leff, A.R. (1993). Selective attenuation by 5-lipoxygenase blockade of peripheral airway hyperresponsiveness and edema caused by activated alveolar macrophage. *Am. Rev. Respir. Dis.* (in press).

Prober J.S., Gimbrone, M.A. Jr., Lapierre, L.A., Mendrick, D.L., Fiers, W., Rothlein, R. and Springer, T.A. (1986). Overlapping patterns of activation of human endothelial cells by interleukin-1, tumor necrosis factor, and immune interferon. *J. Immunol.* **137**, 1893–1896.

Rand, T.H., Silberstein, D.S., Kornfeld and Weller, P.F. (1991). Human eosinophils express functional interleukin 2 receptors. *J. Clin Invest.* **88**, 825–832.

Rochester, C.L. and Rankin, J.A. (1991). Is asthma T-cell mediated? *Am. Rev. Respir. Dis.* **144**, 1005–1007.

Rossi, G.A., Crimi, E., Lantero, S., Gianiorio, P., Oddera, S., Crimi, P. and Brusasco, V. (1991). Late-phase asthmatic reaction to inhaled allergen is associated with early recruitment of eosinophils in the airways. *Am. Rev. Respir. Dis.* **144**, 379–383.

Rothlein, R., Dustin, M.L., Marlin, S.D. and Springer, T.A. (1986). A human intercellular adhesion molecule (ICAM-1) distinct from LFA-1. *J. Immunol.* **137**, 1270–1274.

Rowan, J.L., Mithyde, D. and McDonald, R.J. (1990). Eosinophils cause acute edematous injury in isolated perfused rat lung. *Am. Rev. Respir. Dis.* **42**, 215–220.

Smith, C.W., Marlin, S.D., Rothlein, R., Lawrence, M.B., McIntire, L.V. and Anderson, D.C. (1989). Role of ICAM-1 in the adherence of human neutrophils to human endothelial cells *in vitro*. *In* "Leukocyte Adhesion Molecules: Structure, Function and Regulation" (T.A. Springer, D.C. Anderson, A.S. Rosenthal and R. Rothlein, eds), pp. 170–189. Springer-Verlag, New York.

Smith, C.W., Kishimoto, T.K., Abbassi, O., McIntire, L.V. and Anderson, D.C. (1990). Human MEL-14 antigen contributes to the CD11/CD18-independent adhesion of neutrophils to endothelial cells. *FASEB J.* (abst.).

Staunton, D.W., Dustin, M.L., Erickson, H.P. and Springer, T.A. (1990). The arrangement of the immunoglobulin-like domains of ICAM-1 and the binding sites for LFA-1 and rhinovirus. *Cell* **61**, 243–254.

Strek, M.E., Morgan, D.W., Bak, C.E.T., Gleich, G.J., Abrahams, C., Leff, A.R. and White, S.R. (1991). Phospholipase A_2 copurifying with eosinophil cationic protein causes tracheal smooth muscle contraction and augments muscarinic responsiveness. *Am. Rev. Respir. Dis.* **143**, A558.

Strek, M.E., Garland, A., Abrahams, C., Leff, A.R. and White, S.R. (1993a). Direct effects and augmentation of airway smooth muscle contraction caused by phospholipase A_2. *Am. Rev. Respir. Dis.* (in press).

Strek, M.E., White, S.R., Hsieu, T.R., Kulp, G.V.P. and Leff, A.R. (1993b). Effect of mode of activation on tracheal smooth muscle contraction caused by isolated human eosinophils. *Am. Rev. Respir. Dis.* (abst.) (in press).

Stuart-Smith, K. and Vanhoutte, P.M. (1987). Heterogeneity in the effects of epithelial removal in the canine bronchial tree. *J. Appl. Physiol.* **63**, 2510–2515.

Stuart-Smith, K. and Vanhoutte, P.M. (1988). Airway epithelium modulates the responsiveness of porcine bronchial smooth muscle. *J. Appl. Physiol.* **65**, 721–727.

Stuart-Smith, K. and Vanhoutte, P.M. (1990). Epithelium, contractile tone, and responses to relaxing agonists in canine bronchi. *J. Appl. Physiol.* **69**, 678–685.

Sustiel, A.M., Joseph, B., Rocklin, R.E. and Borish, L. (1989). Asthmatic patients have neutrophils that exhibit diminished responsiveness to adenosine. *Am. Rev. Respir. Dis.* **140**, 1556–1561.

Te Velde, A.A., Keizier, G.D. and Figdor, C.G. (1987). Differential function of LFA-1 family molecules (CD11 and CD18) in adhesion of human monocytes to melanoma and endothelial cells. *Immunology* **61**, 261–267.

Walsh, G.M., Hartnell, A., Moqbel, R., Cromwell, O., Nagy, L., Bradley, B., Furitsu, T., Ishizaka, T. and Kay, A.B. (1990). Receptor expression and functional status of cultured human eosinophils derived from umbilical cord blood mononuclear cells. *Blood* **76**, 105–111.

Wang, J.M., Rambaldi, A., Biondi, A., Chen, Z.G., Sanderson, C.J. and Mantovani, A. (1989). Recombinant human interleukin-5 is a selective eosinophil chemoattractant. *Eur. J. Immunol.* **19**, 701–705.

Warren, D.J. and Moore, M.A.S. (1988). Synergism among interleukin 1, interleukin-3, and interleukin-5 in the production of eosinophils from primitive hemopoietic stem cells. *J. Immunol.* **140**, 94–99.

Wegner, C.D., Smith, C.W. and Rothlein, R. (1989). CD18 dependence of primate eosinophil adherence *in vitro*. *In* "Leukocyte Adhesion Molecules: Structure, Function and Regulation" (T.A. Springer, D.C. Anderson, A.S. Rosenthal and R. Rothlein, eds), pp. 208–214. Springer-Verlag, New York.

Wegner, C.D., Gundel, R.H., Reilly, P., Haynes, N., Letts, L.G. and Rothlelin, R. (1990). *Science* **247** 456–459.

White, S.R., Ohno, S., Munoz, N.M., Gleich, G.J., Abrahams, C., Solway, J. and Leff, A.R. (1990). Epithelium-dependent contraction of airway smooth muscle caused by eosinophil MBP. *Am. J. Physiol.; Lung Cell Molec. Physiol.* **259** (3), L294–L303.

White, S.R., Strek, M.E., Kulp, G.V., Burch, R.A. and Leff, A.R. (1993). Down-regulation of human eosinophil activation and degranulation by inhibition of phospholipase A_2. *Am. Rev. Respir. Dis.* (abst.) (in press).

Yamaguchi, Y., Hayashi, Y., Sugama, Y., Miura, Y., Kasahara, T., Kitamura, S., Torisu, M., Mita, S., Toiminaga, A., Takatsu, K. and Suda, T. (1988). Highly purified murine interleukin-5 (IL-5) stimulates eosinophil function and prolongs *in vitro* survival. IL-5 as an eosinophil chemotactic factor. *J. Exp. Med.* **167**, 1737–1742.

Young, J.D., Peterson, C.G.B., Venge, P. and Cohn, Z.A. (1986). Mechanism of membrane damage by humane cationic protein. *Nature* **321**, 613–616.

Yukawa, T., Ukena, D., Kroegel, C., Chanez, P., Dent, G., Chung, K.F. and Barnes, P.J. (1990). $Beta_2$-adrenergic receptors on eosinophils. Binding and functional studies. *Am. Rev. Respir. Dis.* **141**, 1446–1452.

13

Regulation of Matrix Production in the Airways

J.S. CAMPA, N.K. HARRISON and G.J. LAURENT

Biochemistry Unit, Department of Thoracic Medicine, National Heart and Lung Institute, University of London, Manresa Road, London SW3 6LR, UK

Introduction

Deposition of scar tissue, comprised of collagen, elastin and other less abundant extracellular matrix materials, is a fundamental feature of host defence. When this occurs in structures of internal organs requiring a high compliance or fine structure for transport and exchange of molecules, there are often life-threatening consequences.

In the lung there are several diseases in which excessive or disordered matrix deposition leads to impaired respiratory function (see Shock and Laurent, 1990 for review). These include bronchopulmonary dysplasia, chronic bronchitis, cryptogenic fibrosing alveolitis (or idiopathic pulmonary fibrosis), acute respiratory distress syndrome, sarcoidosis and asthma. In these conditions the location of the disease is variable but in every case a common pattern has emerged, with an ongoing inflammation, oedema and movement of white cells from the circulation. These events are inevitably associated with damage to existing structures and deposition of matrix molecules. If this deposition is such that histologically the scar tissue is deemed excessive compared with normal, the term fibrosis is often used. In the airways of patients with asthma there is evidence for such changes and the term subepithelial fibrosis has been applied to

T-Lymphocyte and Inflammatory Cell Research in Asthma
ISBN 0-12-388170-6

describe them. In this chapter we will describe the matrix components of the normal airway, evidence for their deposition in asthma and current theories as to the mechanisms leading to their deposition.

Matrix Components of the Normal Airway

The lung extracellular matrix is a complex and dynamic meshwork with a large number of components each contributing to the microenvironment of the cells. Some of the components of the normal human airway are shown in Fig. 13.1. Collagens, of at least eight different types, account for at least 60% of the extracellular matrix proteins and 15–20% of the dry weight of the normal adult lung. Figure 13.1 shows diagrammatically the structure of interstitial fibrillar collagens types I, II and III and

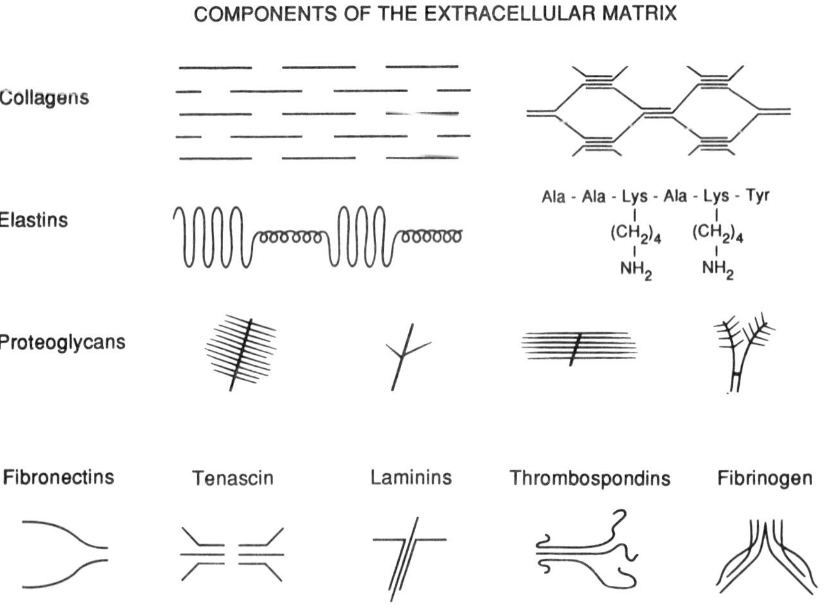

Fig. 13.1 Components of the extracellular matrix. A diagrammatic presentation of the structures of the major components of the extracellular matrix of the lung. Structures in the top panel are typical of interstitial (left) and basement membrane (right) collagens. The panel for proteoglycans structures demonstrates the diversity in size and relative composition of the carbohydrate side-chains and protein cores.

contrasts the parallel array and overlap observed for adjacent molecules of these types with the basement membrane collagens type IV. The latter has a so-called "chicken-wire" structure providing a 3-dimensional network within which cells and other matrix proteins are embedded.

Elastin is the next most abundant matrix protein, conveying upon its structures an ability to stretch and undergo elastic recoil. Elastin is synthesized as a single polypeptide chain, 65–70 kDa, termed tropoelastin. Insolubility and tertiary structure is achieved by the cross-linking of lysyl residues (Fig. 13.1) in reactions catalysed by lysyl oxidase. This ultimately forms the covalent cross-links desmosine and isodesmosine, structures which are unique biochemical markers for elastin. Proteoglycans and glycosaminoglycans play important roles in matrix hydration, fibre formation, cell–matrix and cell–cell interactions. They consist of a protein core with one or more glycosaminoglycan side-chains (Fig. 13.1), attached covalently to the core by *O*-glycosidic linkages. The most abundant lung glycosaminoglycans are hyaluronic acid (non-sulphated) and the sulphated chondroitin sulphate, heparan sulphate and dermatan sulphate (Kjellen and Lindahl, 1991).

Also found in the alveolar matrix are several structural glycoproteins, some of which are illustrated in Fig. 13.1. Fibronectin is a disulphide-linked dimer comprising subunits of approximate M_r230 000–250 000. It is present in extracellular matrices, basal lamina, cell surfaces and blood. Fibronectin has been implicated in a variety of cell contact processes, including cell attachment and migration, opsonization and wound healing. Two major forms of the molecule have been distinguished: a plasma form, which is a soluble heterodimer, and a cell surface, cellular associated form, which consists of dimers and multimers. The latter have a fibrillar structure and are highly insoluble. Each subunit of fibronectin contains specific sites for binding to cells and a range of molecules, including collagen, fibrin and heparin (Hynes, 1990; Ingber *et al.*, 1990; Sottiile *et al.*, 1991).

Tenascin, also known as cytotactin, is a large disulphide-linked glycoprotein of six identical subunits of reported M_r of 190 000–320 000. It inhibits cell adhesion, migration and alterations in cell shape and these functions are mediated by binding to fibronectin, proteoglycans and heparin (Chiquet-Ehrismann, 1990). A view is emerging that proteins such as tenascin, which disrupt cell adhesion and consequently lead to a breakdown of the cytoskeleton, could greatly affect cellular function, possibly via the release of cytoskeletal-associated factors acting within secondary messenger pathways (Ben-Ze'v, 1991).

The major glycoprotein in basement membranes is laminin (M_r 800 000), a cross-shaped molecule composed of three polypeptides, A, B1 and B2 chains. These chains are *N*-glycosylated and disulphide bound. The current models suggest a "bunch of three flowers" structure, where each chain forms a short arm and the rest of the chains project down to form the triple-chained long arm. Laminins bind collagen and heparan sulphate proteoglycans and are reported to play important roles in cell adhesion, migration, growth and differentiation (Timpl *et al.*, 1983).

The thrombospondins are a family of proteins generated by alternative splicing and gene duplication, which contain binding sites for many soluble proteins and up to five cellular receptors. A typical family member is the human platelet thrombospondin. TS1p180, a homotrimer with three identical chains. Thrombospondin can regulate cellular migration and proliferation and roles have been proposed in developmental growth, angiogenesis, tumorigenesis and wound healing (Lawler, 1986; Lawler and Hynes, 1986).

Fibrinogen, a 340-kDa blood protein composed of six polypeptide chains (two Aα, two Bβ and two γ), is not typically found in the normal extracellular matrix. Its presumed major function is in blood haemostasis, where it forms fibrin, the final product of the clotting cascade. However, fibrinogen and fibrinogen-derived peptides have been implicated in other cell functions including cell migration (Senior *et al.*, 1986) and proliferation (Gray *et al.*, 1990). It seemed appropriate to include fibrinogen here as it is a key matrix component in the setting of injury and inflammation and is present in asthma where plasma exudation and oedema are common features (Rogers and Evans, 1992).

Shown in a stylized way in Fig. 13.2 are the interactions between components of the matrix, as well as their interactions with adjacent cells. The diagram also shows interaction between cytoskeletal elements within a cell and their external environment. These elements, including microtubules (α- and β-tubulin), intermediate filaments (cytokeratins, vimentin, desmin and lamin proteins), α-actinin and actin, interact via cell-surface molecules with the extracellular matrix. One group of cell-surface molecules is the superfamily of the α-and β-integrins, transmembrane receptors which link actin-associated proteins to the extracellular matrix and to adhesion receptors on cell surfaces. Integrins are likely to play pivotal roles in the transmission of forces to and from the cytoskeleton (Ingber, 1991).

Matrix components may also have more specific receptors (Buck and Hoewitz, 1987). Fibroblasts and other migratory cells possess a 67-kDa membrane-associated receptor protein which binds laminin, collagen and a specific amino acid sequence in elastin (Mecham *et al.*, 1989; Senior *et al.*, 1989). The precise role of these receptors is still uncertain, but clearly their role in matrix–cell signalling needs to be assessed.

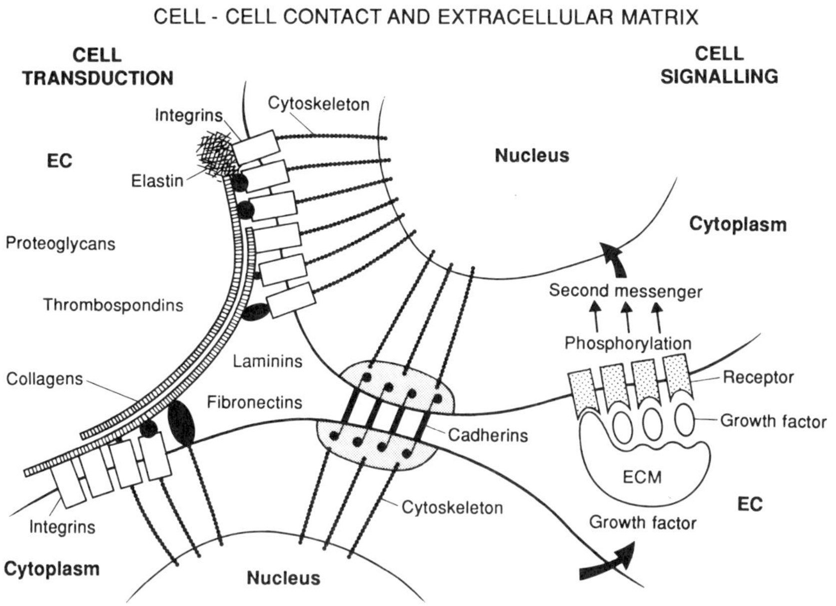

Fig. 13.2 Cell–cell contact and extracellular matrix. Stylized representation of the components involved in cell-to-cell contacts and cell-to-extracellular matrix interactions.

Figure 13.3 shows the localization of some of the airway structures defined above. In normal lung, there is a basement membrane underneath airway-lining cells, comprised largely of type IV collagen, proteoglycans, laminin and fibronectin (Roche *et al.*, 1989). These components have several critical functions: as substrates interacting with and regulating functions of adherent cells, and in the regulation of ion transport and flux of small and large molecules. In this way the basement membrane partly regulates both the nutrition of adjoining airway cells and the composition of the fluids in which they are bathed. Beneath the basement membrane of the normal respiratory bronchiole is stromal tissue comprised of predominantly two types of mesenchymal cells – fibroblasts and smooth muscle cells embedded in a matrix which likely contains all the structures shown in Fig. 13.1. The major components, collagens (types I and III) and elastin, are the primary determinants of the mechanical properties of airways. In the upper airway there is the additional support of the cartilaginous structures, themselves comprised predominantly of type II collagen although other minor collagens (types IX, X and XI) are also found in such cartilage.

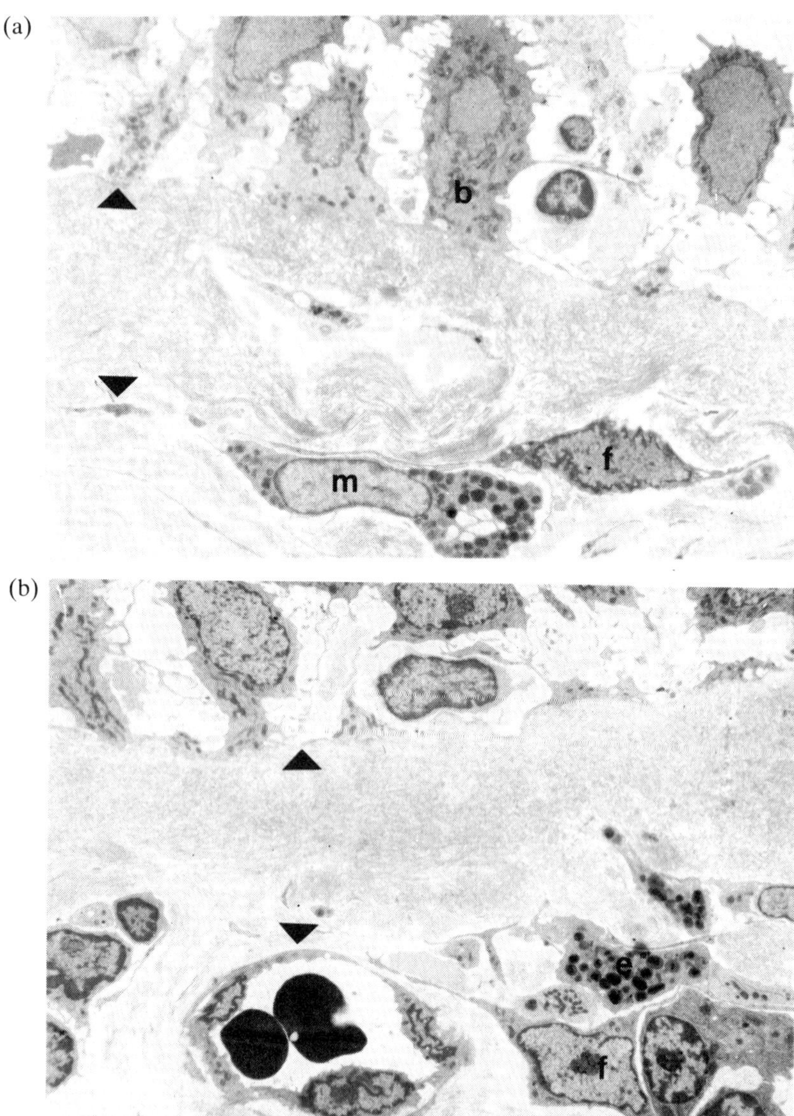

Fig. 13.3 Lung architecture in asthma. (a) Electron micrograph of subepithelial tissues from a fibreoptic bronchial biopsy taken from a subject with mild atopic asthma. Beneath the basal cells (b) of the surface epithelium there is a thin basal lamina associated with a thickened zone of reticular collagen (arrows). Fibroblast-like cells (f) and mast cells (m) may contribute either alone or by their interaction to increase the resultant deposition of a collagenous matrix. Glutaraldehyde and osmium tetroxide: uranyl acetate and lead citrate staining. × 3750. (b) A further subject with mild atopic asthma whose subepithelial tissue shows the marked thickening of reticular collagen and nearby eosinophils (e) and fibroblast (f) in close association. A bronchial vessel is also shown. × 3000. (Prepared and reproduced by permission of Dr Peter K. Jeffery.)

In lung, the key matrix-producing cells are believed to be mesenchymal cells, particularly fibroblasts, although chondrocytes will be responsible for type II collagen production in the bronchi and upper airways. It is also important to consider changes in both synthetic and degradative pathways as determinants of collagen deposition, since these cells are actively synthesizing and degrading matrix components throughout development and into old age (Laurent, 1987; Mays *et al.*, 1991).

Collagen Deposition in the Airways

The histological abnormalities which characterize asthma are variable (Jeffery, 1992), but most descriptions include a degree of epithelial injury with an oedematous submucosa, thickening of the epithelial basement membrane, mucus gland hyperplasia, the presence of leukocytes, degranulated mast cells and smooth muscle hypertrophy. The thickening of the basement membrane has not been extensively studied, although this observation, originally made over 30 years ago (Dunnill, 1960), has recently been reaffirmed. Several groups have used morphometric techniques to quantitate basement membrane thickness in patients with mild atopic asthma and reported a thickening of this structure (Jeffery *et al.*, 1989; Brewster *et al.*, 1990). Figure 13.3a shows a section from such a patient and identifies the basement membrane. It has also been demonstrated that this membrane was comprised predominantly of interstitial collagen types I, III and V, rather than type IV (Roche *et al.*, 1989), suggesting that excess collagen was laid down by interstitial fibroblasts rather than epithelial cells.

The clinical implications of the findings with respect to collagen deposition in asthma are uncertain. However, it has been suggested that this event may explain, at least in part, why many asthmatics develop a degree of irreversible airflow obstruction which is not responsive to drugs affecting airway smooth muscle tone. This clearly requires further investigation, particularly in those patients with advanced and apparently intractable disease.

The cells responsible for the so-called subepithelial fibrosis are uncertain. One obvious candidate is the fibroblast-like cell seen in Fig. 13.3a,b. It has been suggested that these cells are myofibroblast in lineage and a correlation between the number of such cells and the degree of subepithelial fibrosis has been shown (Brewster *et al.*, 1990; Roche, 1990). Other cell types should also be considered; smooth muscle cells are capable of elaborating matrix molecules and non-mesenchymal cell types may also play a role. Mast cells have recently been shown to express collagen genes in cell culture (see Fig. 13.3a) and epithelial cells have also been reported to produce extracellular matrix components (Crouch *et al.*, 1987; Federspiel *et al.*, 1991).

Regulation of Matrix Production

A variety of mechanisms have been proposed for the regulation of collagen production. The agents which affect collagen production *in vitro* are diverse (Table 13.1), however, in broad terms their likely mechanisms fall into four categories:

1) *Substrate regulation in which, for example, amino acids might regulate production.* An example of this would be the suggested regulation by glutamine (Bellon *et al.*, 1987). Another is oxygen, required for the hydroxylation of

Table 13.1
Agents which affect collage production *in vitro*

Agent	Effect	References
TGF-β	↑	Raghu *et al.* (1989)
IL-1	↑	Goldring and Krane (1987)
Insulin-like growth factor 1	↑	Goldstein *et al.* (1989)
Insulin	↑	Goldstein *et al.* (1989)
Ascorbate	↑	Pinnell (1985)
Oestradiol	↑	Frankel *et al.* (1988)
Bleomycin	↑	Sterling *et al.* (1986)
Glutamine	↑	Bellon *et al.* (1987)
Retinoic Acid	↑	Federspiel *et al.* (1991)
Leukotriene C_4	↑	Phan *et al.* (1988)
	↑	
Carboxy-propeptides (collagen)	↑	Katayama *et al.* (1991)
Collagen peptides (mature)	↑	Pacini *et al.* (1990)
Mechanical stress	↑	Sumpio *et al.* (1988)
Hypoxia (oxygen tension)	↑	Chvapil and Hurych (1968)
PGE_2	↓	Varga *et al.* (1987)
Corticosteroids	↓	Cockayne *et al.* (1986)
Interferon-γ	↓	Czaja *et al.* (1987)
Retinoic acid	↓	Nelson and Balian (1984)
Vitamin D_3	↓	Rowe and Kream (1982)
Carboxy-propeptides (collagen)	↓	Katayama *et al.* (1991)
Amino-propeptides (collagen)	↓	Wu *et al.* (1986)
Parathyroid hormone	↓	Kream *et al.* (1980)
TNF-α	↓	Solis-Herruzo *et al.* (1988)

proline and lysine residues, which has profound effects on collagen synthesis both directly (Crouch *et al.*, 1989) and indirectly via stimulation of other cellular factors (Peacock *et al.*, 1991; Falanga *et al.*, 1991).
2) *Feedback by procollagen or its products*. The products of collagen metabolism have feedback effects which have been shown for collagen (Pacini *et al.*, 1990) and procollagen peptides (Wiestner *et al.*, 1979; Katayama *et al.*, 1991).
3) *Mechanical processes*. The mechanical environment of the cells also affects collagen production as has been shown *in vitro* for both fibroblasts (Banes *et al.*, 1985; Carver *et al.*, 1991) and smooth muscle cells (Sumpio *et al.*, 1988).
4) *Hormonal*. Finally, hormone regulation by endocrine, autocrine or paracrine agents has also been proposed and this is the most intensively investigated area.

Another possible mechanism for increasing collagen production at a specific location is the action of agents which induce proliferation and/or migration of collagen-producing cells. Again, there are a variety of candidate molecules and a challenge for the future will be to resolve which of these molecules (or others still to be discovered) are playing roles in the fibroproliferative response in airways of patients with respiratory disorders where fibrosis is a feature.

One of the most promising candidates is the recently discovered polypeptide endothelin-1. This compound is produced by a variety of cells including epithelial (Mattoli *et al.*, 1990, 1991) and endothelial (Yanagisawa *et al.*, 1988) cells, and is known from immunohistochemical studies to be synthesized in the airways of patients with asthma (Springall *et al.*, 1991; Mattoli *et al.*, 1991). Endothelin-1 is known to promote fibroblast replication and chemotaxis (Peacock *et al.*, 1992), and there is a report of enhanced collagen production in scleroderma (Kahaleh, 1991). Thus it is possible that endothelin is exerting effects both on airway tone and the composition of the matrix and contributing to several features of the asthmatic process.

There is undoubtedly a network of mediators which have both positive and negative effects on collagen synthesis and degradation, fibroblast replication and chemotaxis. The balance between the events stimulated by these agents dictates the amount of collagen produced. Listed in Table 13.1 are some of these, but this list is incomplete and additions will emerge through discovery of new agents and examination of the effects of known mediators, as they are tested in cell culture. One of the current challenges in research is to apply imaging techniques with antibody and oligonucleotide probes to visualize which of these mediators are playing the key roles in asthma.

Eosinophils as Mediators of Collagen Deposition

There are several observations suggesting that eosinophils may play a role in the stimulation of collagen production. Asthmatic subjects frequently have an eosinophilia in blood and sputum, and increased numbers of eosinophils can be demonstrated beneath the epithelial basement membrane of asthmatic airways. The presence of one such cell apparently in close proximity with collagen underlying the surface epithelial cells is shown in Fig. 13.3b. There are other pathological conditions in which excess eosinophils are associated with collagen deposition and tissue fibrosis. These include the hypereosinophilic syndrome, in which endomyocardial fibrosis is a complication (Spry *et al.*, 1983), and cryptogenic fibrosing alveolitis, in which an elevated eosinophil count in bronchoalveolar lavage is often associated with a more rapid progression to lung fibrosis (Turner-Warwick and Haslam, 1987). There is increasing recognition that tissue-dwelling eosinophils and fibroblasts may interact. It has been demonstrated that eosinophil lysates can stimulate fibroblast DNA synthesis (Pincus *et al.*, 1987). Furthermore, it has been reported that eosinophil cationic protein (a highly basic protein secreted from eosinophil granules) can stimulate fibroblasts in culture to synthesize hyaluronon and proteoglycans (Sarnstrand *et al.*, 1989). Finally, we have preliminary evidence that eosinophil-conditioned media can stimulate human lung fibroblasts to proliferate and that this function is mediated via sequence-specific cell receptors (Shock *et al.*, 1991). Results of these studies are shown in Fig. 13.4.

The discovery that eosinophils can release polypeptide cytokines is likely to be crucial to the regulation of lung collagen in disease states. Recently it has been shown that human blood eosinophils produce the mRNA for transforming growth factor-β (TGF-β) and the protein product (Wong *et al.*, 1991). TGF-β is a 25-kDA polypeptide and in our experience the most potent stimulator of collagen production (McAnulty *et al.*, 1991). In addition, it has been shown to be active on human lung fibroblasts *in vitro* (Harrison *et al.*, 1990). It occurs in high concentrations in macrophages and platelets, and is present in the epithelial lining fluid of the normal human respiratory tract (Yamauchi *et al.*, 1988). Furthermore, an important role for TGF-β in interstitial pulmonary fibrosis has been proposed based on studies using immunohistochemical and *in situ* hybridization techniques (Broekelman *et al.*, 1991; Khalil *et al.*, 1991).

Recent research has drawn our attention to the fibrosis occurring in asthma. Future studies should aim to define more precisely the nature

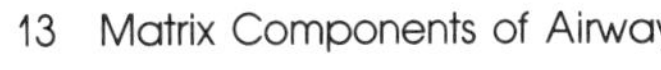

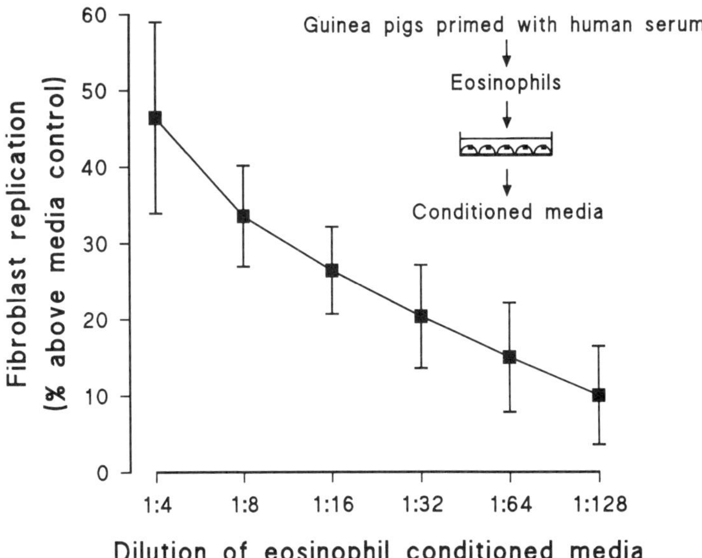

Fig. 13.4 Effect of eosinophil-derived conditioned media on fibroblast replication. Data taken from Shock *et al.* (1991) shows stimulation of fibroblast replication in the presence of serially diluted media from eosinophils cultured for 3 h. Each point represents the mean (± S.D.) from experiments performed on six eosinophil preparations.

of the mediators which induce this fibrosis. If the structure of these molecules and their receptors can be delineated this would provide the first step in a programme to develop specific inhibitors aimed at preventing collagen deposition in the lung.

References

Banes, A.J., Gilbert, J., Taylor, D. and Monbureau, O. (1985). A new vacuum-operated stress-providing instrument that applies static or variable duration cyclic tension or compression to cell in vitro. *J. Cell Sci.* **75**, 35–42.

Bellon, G., Monboisse, J.C., Randoux, A. and Borel, J.P. (1987). Effects of preformed proline and proline amino acid precursors including glutamine on collagen synthesis in human fibroblast cultures. *Biochim. Biophys. Acta* **930**, 39–47.

Ben-Ze'v, A. (1991). Animal cell shape changes and gene expression. *BioEssays* **13**, 207–211.

Brewster, C.E.P., Howarth, P.H., Djukanovic, R., Wilson, J., Holgate, S.T. and Roche, W.R. (1990). Myofibroblasts and subepithelial fibrosis in bronchial asthma. *Am. J. Respir. Cell Molec. Biol.* **3**, 507–511.

Broekelman, T.J., Limper, A.H., Colby, T.V. and McDonald, J.A. (1991). Transforming growth factor β_1 is present at sites of extracellular matrix gene expression in human pulmonary fibrosis. *Proc. Natl. Acad. Sci. U.S.A.* **88**, 6642–6646.

Buck, C.A. and Hoewitz, A.F. (1987). Cell surface receptors for extracellular matrix molecules. *Annu. Rev. Cell Biol.* **3**, 179–205.

Carver, W., Nagpal, M.L., Nachtigal, M., Borg, T.K. and Terracio, L. (1991). Collagen expression in mechanically stimulated cardiac fibroblasts. *Circ. Res.* **69**, 116–122.

Chiquet-Ehrismann, R. (1990). What distinguishes tenascin from fibronectin? *FASEB J.* **4**, 2598–2604.

Chvapil, M. and Hurych, J. (1968). Control of collagen biosynthesis. *Int. Rev. Connective Tissue Res.* **4**, 166–177.

Cockayne, D., Sterling, K.M., Shull, S., Mintz, K.P., Illeyne, S. and Cutroneo, K.R. (1986). Glucocorticoids decrease the synthesis of type 1 procollagen mRNAs. *Biochemistry* **25**, 3202–3209.

Crouch, E.C., Moxley, M.A. and Longmore, W. (1987). Synthesis of collagenous proteins by pulmonary type II epithelial cells. *Am. Rev. Respir. Dis.* **135**, 1118–1123.

Crouch, E.C., Parks, W.C., Rosenbaum, J.L., Chang, D., Whitehouse, L., Wu, L., Stenmark, K.R., Orton, E.C. and Mecham, R.P. (1989). Regulation of collagen production by medial smooth muscle cells in hypoxic pulmonary hypertension. *Am. Rev. Respir. Dis.* **140**, 1045–1051.

Czaja, M.J., Weiner, F.R., Eghbali, M., Giambrone, M.A. and Zern, M.A. (1987). Differential effects of gamma interferon on collagen and fibronectin gene expression. *J. Biol. Chem.* **262**, 3348–3351.

Dunnill, M.S. (1960). The pathology of asthma, with special reference to changes in the bronchial mucosa. *J. Clin. Pathol.* **13**, 27–33.

Falanga, V., Qian, S.W., Danielpour, D., Katz, M.H., Roberts, A.B. and Sporn, M.B. (1991). Hypoxia upregulates the synthesis of TGF-β_1 by human dermal fibroblasts, *J. Invest. Dermatol.* **97**, 634–637.

Federspiel, S.J., DiMari, S.J., Howe, A.M., Guerry-Force, M.L. and Haralson, M.A. (1991). Extracellular matrix biosynthesis by cultured fetal rat lung epithelial cells. IV. Effects of chronic exposure to retinoic acid on growth, differentiation, and collagen biosynthesis. *Lab. Invest.* **65**, 441–450.

Frankel, F.R., Hsu, C.-Y.J. and Myers, J.C. (1988). Regulation of α_2(I), α_1(III) and α_2(V) collagen mRNAs by estradiol in the immature rat uterus. *DNA* **7**, 347–354.

Goldring, M.B. and Krane, S.M. (1987). Modulation by recombinant interleukin-1 of synthesis of types I and III collagens and associated procollagen mRNA levels in cultured human cells. *J. Biol. Chem.* **262**, 16724–16729.

Goldstein, R.H., Polkis, C.F., Pilch, P.F., Smith, B.D. and Fine, A. (1989). Stimulation of collagen formation by insulin and insulin-like growth factor I in cultures of human lung fibroblasts. *Endocrinology* **124**, 964–970.

Gray, A.J., Reeves, J.T., Harrison, N.K., Winlove, P. and Laurent, G.J. (1990). Growth factors for human fibroblasts in the solute remaining after clot formation. *J. Cell Sci.* **96**, 271–274.

Harrison, N.K., Argent, A.C., McAnulty, R.J., Cambrey, A.D., Campa, J.S., Black, C.M. and Laurent, G.J. (1990). Collagen synthesis and degradation by lung fibroblasts from patients with systemic sclerosis. *Am. Rev. Respir. Dis.* **141**, A704 (abst.).

Hynes, R.O. (1990). "Fibronectins". Springer-Verlag, New York.

Ingber, D. (1991). Integrins as mechanochemical transducers. *Curr. Opinion Cell Biol.* **3**, 841–848.

Ingber, D.E., Prusty, D., Frangioni, J.V., Gragoe, E.J.J.R., Lechene, C. and Schwartz, M.A. (1990). Control of intracellular pH and growth by fibronectin in capillary endothelial cells. *J. Cell Biol.* **110**, 1803–1811.

Jeffery, P.K. (1992). Pathology of asthma. *Brit. Med. Bull.* **48** (1), 23–39.

Jeffery, P.K., Wardlaw, A.J., Nelson, F.C., Collins, J.V. and Kay, A.B. (1989). Bronchial biopsies in asthma. *Am. Rev. Respir. Dis.* **140**, 1745–1753.

Kahaleh, M.B. (1991). Endothelin, an endothelial-dependent vasoconstrictor in scleroderma. Enhanced production and profibrotic action. *Arth. Rheum.* **34** (8), 978–983.

Katayama, K., Seyer, J.M., Raghow, R. and Kang, A.H. (1991). Regulation of extracellular matrix production by chemically synthesized subfragments of type I collagen carboxy propeptide. *Biochemistry* **30**, 7097–7104.

Khalil, N., O'Connor, R.N., Unruh, H.W., Warren, P.W., Flanders, K.C., Kemp, A., Bereznay, O.H. and Greenberg, A.H. (1991). Increased production and immunohistochemical localization of transforming growth factor-β in idiopathic pulmonary fibrosis. *Am. J. Respir. Cell. Molec. Biol.* **5**, 155–162.

Kjellen, L. and Lindahl, U. (1991) Proteoglycans: structure and interactions. *Annu. Rev. Biochem.* **60**, 443–475.

Kream, B.E., Rowe, D.W., Gworek, S.C. and Raisz, L.G. (1980). Parathyroid hormone alters collagen synthesis and procollagen mRNA levels in fetal rat calvaria. *Proc. Natl. Acad. Sci. U.S.A.* **77**, 5641–5658.

Laurent, G.J. (1987). Dynamic state of Collagen: pathways of collagen degradation *in vivo* and their possible role in regulation of collagen mass. *Am. J. Physiol.* **251**, C1–C9.

Lawler, J. (1986). The structural and functional properties of thrombospondin. *Blood* **67**, 1197–1209.

Lawler, J. and Hynes, R. (1986). The structure of human thrombospondin and adhesive glycoproteins with multiple calcium-binding sites and homologies with different proteins. *J. Cell Biol.* **103**, 1635–1648.

Mattoli, S., Mezzetti, M., Riva, G., Allegra, L. and Fasoli, A. (1990). Specific binding of endothelin on human bronchial smooth muscle cells in culture and secretion of endothelin-like material from bronchial epithelial cells. *Am. J. Respir. Cell. Molec. Biol.* **3**, 145–151.

Mattoli, S., Soloperto, M., Marini, M. and Fasoli, A. (1991). Levels of endothelin in the bronchoalveolar lavage fluid of patients with symptomatic asthma and reversible airflow obstruction. *J. Allergy Clin. Immunol.* **88**, 376–384.

Mays, P.K., McAnulty, R.J., Campa, J.S. and Laurent, G.J. (1991). Age related changes in collagen synthesis and degradation in rat tissue: importance of degradation of newly synthesised collagen in regulating collagen production. *Biochem. J.* **276**, 307–313.

McAnulty, R.J., Campa, J.S., Cambrey, A.D. and Laurent, G.J. (1991). The effect of transforming growth factor β on rates of procollagen synthesis and degradation in vitro. *Biochim. Biophys. Acta* **1091**, 231–235.

Mecham, R.P., Hinek, A., Griffin, G.L., Senior, R.M. and Liotta, L.A. (1989).

The elastin receptor shows structural and functional similarities to the 67-kDa tumor cell laminin receptor. *J. Biol. Chem.* **264**, 16652–16657.

Nelson, D.L. and Balian, G. (1984). The effect of retinoic acid on collagen synthesis by human dermal fibroblasts. *Collagen Rel. Res.* **4**, 119–128.

Pacini, A., Gardi, G., Corradeschi, F., Viti, A., Belli, C., Calzoni, P. and Lungarella, G. (1990). *In vivo* stimulation of lung collagen synthesis by collaged derived peptides. *Res. Commun. Chem. Pathol. Pharmacol.* **68**, 89–101.

Peacock, A., Dawes, K.E., Shock, A., Gray, A.J., Reeves, J.T. and Laurent, G.J. (1992). Endothelin 1 and Endothelin 3 induce chemotaxis and replication of pulmonary artery fibroblasts. *Am. J. Respir. Cell Mol. Biol.* **7**, 492–499.

Peacock, A.J., Dawes, K.E. and Laurent, G.J. (1991). Hypoxia stimulates endothelial cells (EC) to produce a growth factor and chemoattractant for fibroblasts. *Am. Rev. Respir. Dis.* **143**, A378 (abst.).

Phan, S.H., McGarry, B.M., Loeffler, K.M. and Kunkel, S.L. (1988). Binding of Leukotriene C4 to rat lung fibroblasts and stimulation of collagen synthesis *in vitro*. *Biochemistry (USA)* **27**, 2846–2853.

Pincus, S.J., Ramesch, K.S. and Wyner, D.J. (1987). Eosinophils stimulate fibroblast DNA synthesis. *Blood* **70**, 572–574.

Pinnell, S.R. (1985). Regulation of collagen biosynthesis by ascorbic acid: a review. *Yale J. Biol. Med.* **58**, 553–559.

Raghu, G., Mastra, S., Meyers, D. and Narayanan, A.S. (1989). Collagen synthesis by normal and fibrotic lung fibroblasts and the effect of transforming growth factor-β. *Am. Rev. Respir. Dis.* **140**, 95–100.

Roche, W.R. (1990). Myofibroblasts. *J. Pathol.* **161**, 281–282.

Roche, W.R., Beasley, R., Williams, J.H. and Holgate, S.T. (1989). Subepithelial fibrosis in the bronchi of asthmatics. *Lancet* **i**, 520–523.

Rogers, D.F. and Evans, T.W. (1992). Plasma exudation and oedema in asthma. *Brit. Med. Bull.* **48** (1), 120–134.

Rowe, D.W. and Kream, B.E. (1982). Regulation of collagen synthesis in fetal rat calvaria by 1,25-dihydroxyvitamin D_2. *J. Biol. Chem.* **262**, 6955–6958.

Sarnstrand, B., Hernnas, J., Peterson, C., Venge, P. and Malmstrom, A. (1989). Eosinophil cationic protein stimulates synthesis of hyaluron and proteoglycan in fibroblast cultures. *Am. Rev. Respir. Dis.* **139**, A209.

Senior, R.M., Skogen, W.F., Griffin, G.L. and Wilner, G.D. (1986). Effects of fibrinogen derivatives upon the inflammatory response: studies with human fibrinopeptide B. *J. Clin. Invest.* **77**, 1014–1019.

Senior, R.M., Hinek, A., Griffin, G.L., Pipoly, D.J., Crouch, E.C. and Mecham, R.P. (1989). Neutrophils show chemotaxis to type IV collagen and its 7S domain and contain a 67 kD type IV collagen binding protein with lectin properties. *Am. J. Respir. Cell. Molec. Biol.* **1**, 479–487.

Shock, A. and Laurent, G.J. (1990). Leucocytes and pulmonary disorders: mobilization, activation and role in pathology. *Molec. Aspects Med.* **11**, 425–526.

Shock, A., Rabe, K.F., Dent, G., Chambers, R.C., Gray, A.J., Chung, K.F., Barnes, P.J. and Laurent, G.J. (1991). Eosinophils adhere to and stimulate replication of lung fibroblasts *in vitro*. *Clin. Exp. Immunol.* **86**, 185–190.

Solis-Herruzo, J.A., Brenner, D.A. and Chojkier, M. (1988). Tumor necrosis factor α inhibits collagen gene transcription and collagen synthesis in cultured human fibroblasts. *J. Biol. Chem.* **263**, 5841–5845.

Sottiile, J., Schwarzbauer, J.E., Selegue, J. and Mosher, D.F. (1991). Five type I modules of fibronectin from a functional unit that bind to fibroblasts and Staphylococcus aureus. *J. Biol. Chem.* **266**, 12840–12843.
Springall, D.R., Howarth, P.H., Counihan, H., Djukanovic, R., Holgate, S.T. and Polak, J.M. (1991). Endothelin immunoreactivity of airway epithelium in asthmatic patients. *Lancet* **337**, 697–701.
Spry, C.J.F., Davies, J., Tai, P.C., Olsen, E.J.G., Oakley, C.M. and Goodwin, J.F. (1983). Clinical features of fifteen patients with hypereosinophilic syndrome. *Q. J. Med.* **205**, 1–22.
Sterling, K.M., Harris, M.J., Mitchell, J.J. and Cutroneo, K.R. (1986). Bleomycin treatment of chick fibroblasts causes an increase of polysomal type I procollagen mRNAs. *J. Biol. Chem.* **258**, 14438–14444.
Sumpio, B.E., Banes, A.J., Link, W.G. and Johnson, G. (1988). Enhanced collagen production by smooth muscle cells during repetitive mechanical stretching. *Arch. Surg.* **123**, 1233–1236.
Timpl, R., Engel, J. and Martin, G.R. (1983). Laminin, a multifunctional protein of basement membranes. *Trends Biochem. Sci.* **8**, 207–209.
Turner-Warwick, M. and Haslam, P.L. (1987). The value of serial bronchoalveolar lavages in assessing the clinical progress of patients with cryptogenic fibrosing alveolitis. *Am. Rev. Respir. Dis.* **135**, 26–34.
Varga, J., Diaz-Perez, A., Rosenbloom, J. and Jimenez, S.A. (1987). PGE_2 causes a coordinate decrease in the steady state levels of fibronectin and types I and III procollagen mRNAs in normal human dermal fibroblasts. *Biochem. Biophys. Res. Commun.* **147**, 1282–1288.
Wiestner, M., Kreig, T., Horlein, D., Glanville, R.W., Fietzek, P. and Muller, P.K. (1979). Inhibiting effect of procollagen peptides on collagen biosynthesis in fibroblast cultures. *J. Biol. Chem.* **254**, 7016–7023.
Wong, D.T.W., Elovic, A., Matossian, K., Nagura, N., McBride, J., Chou, M.Y., Gordon, J.R., Rand, T.H., Galli, S.J. and Weller, P.F. (1991). Eosinophils from patients with blood eosinophilia express transforming growth factor β_1. *Blood* **10**, 2702–2707.
Wu, C.H., Donovan, C.B. and Wu, G.Y. (1986). Evidence for pretranslational regulation of collagen synthesis by procollagen propeptides. *J. Biol. Chem.* **261**, 10482–10484.
Yamauchi, K., Martinet, Y., Basset, P., Fells, G.A. and Crystal, R.G. (1988). High levels of transforming growth factor-β are present in the epithelial lining fluid of the normal human lower respiratory tract. *Am. Rev. Respir. Dis.* **137**, 1360–1363.
Yanagisawa, M., Kurihara, H., Kimura, S., Tomobe, M., Kobayashi, M., Mitsui, Y., Yazaki, Y., Goto, K. and Masaki, T. (1988). A novel potent vasoconstrictor peptide produced by vascular endothelial cells. *Nature* **332**, 411–415.

Discussion

S.T. Holgate
This is a very much underworked area, which I think we all appreciate. One aspect of this which Dr Laurent touched on is the possible factors that may be chemoattractant for fibroblasts or this particular cell, which

we believe is a myofibroblast, and whether there are any local elements that could be involved in this. Recently, we have described the presence of marked upregulation of endothelin in the bronchial epithelium of asthmatics. Could you comment on your work with Andrew Peacock which has shown that this is a fibroblast chemoattractant and also increases collagen synthesis?

G.J. Laurent
In this lecture I focussed on enhanced collagen syntheses and fibroblast proliferation as two possible ways leading to excessive collagen deposition. The third possibility you are mentioning is that fibroblasts might be attracted into specific areas. There are indeed a variety of chemoattractants for fibroblasts. Platelet-derived growth factor (PDGF) is the one most commonly studied – an agent which is both a chemoattractant and a growth factor for fibroblasts. It can abstract fibroblasts along a concentration gradient from the source of PDGF. The fibroblasts are thought to move along the gradient, and when they reach the higher PDGF concentrations replication occurs.

We were surprised that endothelin was also a potent mitogen for fibroblasts. In fact, it also stimulates collagen production by individual fibroblasts, and is a fibroblast mitogen. If endothelin is present, it has to be a key candidate for mediating the sorts of changes we are seeing. If you are showing it is present based on immunohistochemical studies, this is very interesting.

S.T. Holgate
A recent paper published in the *Journal of Allergy and Clinical Immunology* showed quite marked elevation of endothelin levels in lavage fluid from asthmatics, which is reduced when patients are treated with steroids. Furthermore, work at St Bartholomew's Hospital, London, has shown that myofibroblasts (which we think these are) are remarkably responsive in terms of contraction to endothelin. There now becomes a real possibility that the endothelin generated by the epithelium by mechanisms so far unknown might, in addition to producing myofibroblast migration, also be responsible for the contraction of the mucosa, a second level of muscular contraction which is much more superficial, and would therefore have profound effects in folding the epithelium into the characteristic way that it folds in patients with asthma. There are some dynamic aspects of this cell about which we need to think in addition to the matrix protein and possibly more static aspects.

G.J. Laurent
There are endothelin antibodies which we know can block the activities about which I am talking – growth and chemotaxis – with which progress could be made. I think Andrew Peacock and Keith Dawes examined lavage fluids from Professor Holgate's laboratory in terms of these assays. Chemotaxis occurred in response to lavage fluids from asthmatics, but the precise construction of endothelin was not assesssed.

P. Venge
Do you think this physical contact between the eosinophil and the fibroblast is a necessary interaction in order for the eosinophil to promote a response?

G.J. Laurent
I do not believe contact between the oesinophil and the fibroblast is necessary. In our studies the growth factor activity comes from the oesinophil supernatants. It has not been possible to get fibroblast to divide in co-culture with oesinophils. If the eosinophils are playing a role, we would probably need to argue that it is from a distance rather than first having first to come in contact.

A.B. Kay
This is a very difficult area, and a lot more information is needed before we can come to any conclusions. Dr Laurent has posed the problems very nicely: that we have this complex mixture beneath a true basement membrane, and that this is probably likely to be far more complex than we realize – not only collagen deposition of various types, but also various macroglobulins and proteoglycans. We are assuming – and it is not a proven assumption – a direct relationship between that deposition, that heterogeneous mess, and the symptoms of the disease.

I am unconvinced that this connection actually exists. I am more struck by the fact that even in the very mildest asthmatics – so mild that they *just* make the diagnosis – there are quite marked changes. In some of the earliest biopsies we did in 1986 and 1987, we saw these gross changes in people only occasionally using bronchodilators.

Now that we have more experience, we can probe the airways of people with more severe disease. I am not convinced that those changes are any different as the disease increases in severity. I am far more impressed with the inflammatory cell infiltrate, and possibly the amount of mucus hypersecretion. The changes at the basement membrane level seem to me very similar in the moderately severe asthma. Would Professor Holgate feel that these changes relate to the severity of the disease?

S.T. Holgate

We have measured the thickness of that subepithelial band, and in fact it does not reflect either duration or severity. Recently we have gone into deep biopsies using a monoclonal antibody against the myofibroblasts, and have found that these cells spread out much deeper into the airway and into the smooth muscle itself. The question now is whether the hypertrophy of the smooth muscle which is so frequently quoted to occur in asthma is not actually an increase in the presence of myofibroblast cells, and that we have a mixture of muscle and fibrosis occurring in the smooth muscle component, which of course would have profound effects on long-term airway function.

Furthermore, we have just completed a study in the over-65-year-old age group (a very neglected group of patients), and have found an extremely strong association between the presence of serum IgE in the lung – allergen-specific IgE – and the basal level of airways obstruction, which frequently drops down to 30% of predicted. There is nothing to tell us that in the long term, that is over 40 or 50 years, an atopic with a very low level of inflammatory response might not actually get into quite serious problems in a way that we often find in patients with chronic obstructive pulmonary disease.

We have to be very open-minded about this. I endorse everything Dr Kay has said in terms of gathering more information.

C. Page

A number of people have said today that asthma is a reversible disease. It has been shown that the inflammatory cells can be removed with chronic steroids, but the thickness of this basement membrane, at least, is possibly difficult to reverse. Bearing in mind, as you say, that we are usually not looking deeper at the muscle, we have no idea whether that smooth muscle, whether it be myofibroblasts and muscle or just muscle, is reversible. Do you also feel, Professor Holgate, that we have to start thinking of this disease much more like atherosclerosis where long-term anatomical changes are looked at?

S.T. Holgate

Yes, I agree – we have to keep our imagination open.

N.C. Barnes

I would like to address the same issue as Dr Kay and Professor Holgate from a slightly different angle. In patients with bad asthma in later life there are several patterns which do not really fit with irreversible and chronic asthma being due to some structural change. Some patients who are lifelong non-smokers will say that they had no problem with breathing until they had a particular viral infection – and they then developed sudden devastating asthma which is never fully reversible with all forms of treatment.

The reverse picture is also seen: people who have had long-term, poorly controlled asthma, which has never been properly treated, are given one course of steroids, their lung function returns to normal, and they can then be kept completely well with small doses of inhaled steroids.

This strikes me as not being a permanent fibrotic problem, but some sort of biochemical or cellular switch. Evidence for this is accumulating, for example, from Dr Lee, that people whose asthma is not fully reversible with conventional treatment and with steroids, have a cellular defect in that they cannot respond normally to steroids.

G.J. Laurent
It is clear we must keep an open mind regarding the role of connective tissue deposition in chronic asthma. What is clear is that changes in matrix metabolism and composition will have marked effects on tissue function. It is crucial to keep compiling information on this under-researched area.

Part III

Monocytes, Macrophages and Mast Cells in Asthma

14

Monocyte and Macrophage Function in Asthma

T.H. LEE, M. HALLSWORTH, L. BURKE,
C. HOWELL, S.J. LANE, C. SOH and V. GANT

*Department of Allergy and Allied Respiratory Disorders, UMDS,
Guy's Hospital, London SE1 9RT, UK*

Introduction

The macrophage is a very versatile cell and is able to participate in immune responses by the generation of potent biological mediators as well as playing a critical role in antigen presentation. It is present in large numbers in the lungs, and in bronchoalveolar lavage (BAL) it comprises over 85% of the recovered cell population. Using bronchoalveolar lavage with balloon catheters, it has been shown that the macrophage is a predominant cell in the airways of patients with asthma as well as in normal subjects. From its location, it would be expected to be readily exposed to inhaled allergens and particles.

Evidence for Monocyte and Macrophage Activation in Asthma

In the early 1970s Capron and co-workers discovered evidence for immunoglobulin G (IgE) receptors ($Fc_{\epsilon}R$) on macrophages (Capron *et al.*, 1975). It is now known that the $Fc_{\epsilon}R$ which is expressed on the surface of macrophages is linked to secretory responses. This receptor is referred to as $Fc_{\epsilon}RII$ and differs both structurally and functionally from

T-Lymphocyte and Inflammatory Cell Research in Asthma
ISBN 0-12-388170-6

the $Fc_{\epsilon}RI$ on mast cells and basophils. The $FC_{\epsilon}RII$ is a low-affinity receptor with an estimated affinity constant for monomeric IgE binding to macrophages and to U937 cells of approximately 10^7 mol/litre. This is approximately 200-fold lower than that of IgE binding to the high-affinity $Fc_{\epsilon}RI$.

Approximately 10% of peripheral blood mononuclear cells and lung macrophages from normal non-atopic humans bear $Fc_{\epsilon}R$ receptors (Melewicz *et al.*, 1982). The numbers of IgE-bearing macrophages and monocytes increase in atopic subjects. Patients with severe asthma and atopic dermatitis who have been treated with corticosteroids have the lowest percentage of IgE-positive peripheral blood monocytes (Melewicz *et al.*, 1981). Spiegelberg (1984) noted that monocytes from severely atopic subjects induce more chromium release from IgE-coated red blood cells than monocytes from non-atopic or mildly atopic subjects (Joseph *et al.*, 1983). Lung macrophages from subjects with mild atopic asthma demonstrate that approximately 20% of these cells are $Fc_{\epsilon}RII$-positive (Spiegelberg *et al.*, 1984).

Thus, monocytes and macrophages isolated from patients with asthma have enhanced expression of $Fc_{\epsilon}RII$, which can be modulated by corticosteroid treatment. Monocytes from patients with asthma also show increased complement receptor expression and greater enhancement of receptor expression following stimulation with casein than those of non-asthmatic individuals (Kay *et al.*, 1981).

Furthermore, a defect of monocyte responsiveness to corticosteroids has been identified in asthmatic subjects who do not respond clinically to corticosteroid treatment (Poznansky *et al.*, 1984). Metzger and colleagues (1987) have found that the total number of monocytes in bronchoalveolar lavage fluid increases at 40–96 h after allergen challenge. This suggests that following allergen challenge there is active recruitment of monocytes into the airway compartment.

Mediator Generation by Monocytes and Macrophages

Dessaint *et al.* (1979) demonstrated that rat peritoneal macrophages were able to release granule-associated enzymes and superoxide anion when stimulated with IgE–antigen complexes. Bach and colleagues (1980) observed that rat peritoneal macrophages released leukotriene C_4 (LTC_4) following antigen stimulation and Rankin and colleagues (1982, 1986) demonstrated that rat alveolar macrophages could be activated by monoclonal IgE and specific antigen to release both LTB_4 and LTC_4. Ferreri *et al.* (1986) challenged peripheral blood monocytes *in vitro* with chemically aggregated IgE and found that they released small quantities of eicosanoid mediators. Fuller *et al.* (1986) also observed the release of LTB_4, prostaglandin $F_{2\alpha}$, thromboxane B_2 and β-glucuronidase from macrophages, obtained from patients with a variety of lung diseases, when these cells were challenged with anti-IgE. The respiratory burst of *in vitro* cultured macrophages from subjects with asthma is increased compared with that of macrophages from normal subjects (Cluzel *et al.*, 1987). Furthermore, the number of monocytes which demonstrate expression of complement receptors is enhanced in patients after allergen bronchial provocation (Carroll *et al.*, 1985).

In vivo studies also support the view that macrophages may play a role in mechanisms of asthma. The amount of β-glucuronidase measured in the bronchoalveolar fluid of patients with asthma increased following antigen challenge, with simultaneous depletion of macrophage intracellular levels. This suggests that macrophage secretory processes were activated by allergen (Tonnel *et al.*, 1983).

Monocyte and Granulocyte Interactions in Asthma

Macrophages may participate in airway inflammation in patients with asthma not only through the release of inflammatory products, but also by the release of factors which can modulate the function of other cells. These include chemotactic factors and cytokines. We have recently demonstrated enhanced generation of a granulocyte-activating factor from monocytes derived from asthmatic subjects (Wilkinson *et al.*, 1989). Characterization of the enhancing activity revealed that the predominant factor had an isoelectric point of 7.1 and a molecular weight of 3000 Da. Activity was heat-sensitive and was sensitive to pronase but not to neuraminidase treatment. The secretion of the activity by monocytes was inhibited by steroids *in vitro* in subjects who were sensitive to prednisolone, with major improvements in FEV_1 following the administration of this drug. However, in subjects who are corticosteroid-resistant, monocyte secretion of the 3-kDa molecule was not inhibited by corticosteroid *in vitro*. These experiments suggest that the monocyte may be a target for drug action in asthma.

Alveolar Macrophages in Asthma

The incubation of eosinophils with culture supernatants of alveolar macrophages from asthmatic patients, followed by stimulation with calcium ionophore, resulted in enhancement of their capacity to secrete LTC_4. Macrophage supernatants from normal individuals had no enhancing effect when compared to culture media. There was an inverse correlation between the percentage enhancement and the baseline LTC_4 production. Partial purification of the enhancing activity and subsequent neutralization with specific antibody indicated that the major activity responsible for the eosinophil-priming effect was granulocyte–macrophage colony-stimulating factor (GM–CSF) (Howell *et al.*, 1989).

Measurement of GM–CSF by ELISA techniques in macrophage-derived supernatants demonstrated that asthmatic macrophages produce two- to threefold more GM-CSF than normal macrophages. The secretion of GM-CSF could be enhanced by stimulation with lipopolysaccharide and, in allergic asthmatic patients, by specific allergen. Incubation of macrophages from allergic asthmatic patients with an allergen to which the subject was not sensitive did not lead to the release of this cytokine. These results increase the context in which IgE-dependent stimuli may lead to cytokine release and suggest a further mechanism for the amplification of antigen-specific chronic inflammation (Hallsworth and Lee, in preparation). Immunohistochemical analysis of the airways in moderately severe asthma demonstrated a profound infiltration with macrophages of an immature phenotype, with characteristics of blood monocytes (Poston *et al.*, 1992). Furthermore, there was a significant increase in the numbers of T cells and eosinophils. There was no significant difference in the neutrophil numbers between asthmatic and non-asthmatic subjects. The cells which infiltrated the airway mucosa exhibited increased HLA-DR expression as did the basoepithelial cell layer in the asthmatic biopsies. These experiments indicate that macrophage activation and infiltration can be prominent features of biopsies obtained from patients with asthma.

In view of the association in biopsies of macrophages of an immature phenotype and eosinophilia, we have recently looked at interactions of blood monocytes with eosinophils (Burke *et al.*, 1991). Specifically, we have looked at the capacity of blood monocytes from asthmatic individuals to secrete molecules which could enhance the survival of the eosinophil. Our results show that asthmatic monocytes secrete increased quantities of GM–CSF at concentrations which are capable of promoting the survival of eosinophils in culture. The upregulation of cytokine release by asthmatic monocytes is not restricted to GM–CSF, since similar patterns of enhanced cytokine secretion are also seen for interleukin-1β, tumour necrosis factor (TNF-α) and interleukin-8. Thus, upregulation of cytokine generation by monocytes is a feature of the asthmatic diathesis and the major cytokine which contributes to eosinophil survival is GM–CSF.

Antigen Presentation by Lung Macrophages and Monocytes in Asthma

Because bronchial biopsies from asthmatic patients contain both immature macrophages and activated T-lymphocytes, we investigated whether alveolar macrophages recovered from asthmatics are able to present two recall antigens to autologous peripheral blood T-lymphocytes as effectively as peripheral blood monocytes. Alveolar macrophages from some asthmatic patients presented antigens as effectively as blood monocytes; when the asthmatic group was taken as a whole, a correlation was found between alveolar macrophage antigen presenting ability and the number of lymphocytes recovered in the BAL fluid (unpublished data). This provides evidence for a local interaction between these two cell types and suggests a possible mechanism whereby alveolar macrophages promote lymphocyte infiltration and activation within the lung, thus contributing to persisting inflammation in asthma.

References

Bach, M.K., Brashler, J.R., Hammarström, S. and Samuelsson, B. (1980). Identification of leukotriene C_1 as a major component of slow reacting substance from rat mononuclear cells. *J. Immunol.* **125** (1), 115–117.

Burke, L.A., Hallsworth, M.P., Litchfield, T.M., Davidson, R. and Lee, T.H. (1991). Identification of the major activity derived from cultured human peripheral blood mononuclear cells, which enhances eosinophil viability, as granulocyte macrophage colony stimulating factor (GM–CSF). *J. Allergy Clin. Immunol.* **88**, 226–235.

Capron, A., Dessaint, J.P., Capron, M. and Bazin, H. (1975). Specific IgE antibodies in immune adherence of normal macrophages to *Schistosoma mansoni* schistosomules. *Nature* **253** (5491), 474–475.

Carroll, M.P., Durham, S.R., Walsh, G. and Kay, A.B. (1985). Activation of neutrophils and monocytes after allergen and histamine-induced bronchoconstriction. *J. Allergy Clin. Immunol.* **75** (2), 290–296.

Cluzel, M., Damon, M., Chanez, P., Bousquet, J., Crastes de Paulet, A., Michel, F.B. and Godard, P. (1987). Enhanced alveolar cell lumonil-dependent chemiluminescence in asthma. *J. Allergy Clin. Immunol.* **80** (2), 195–201.

Dessaint, J.P., Capron, A., Joseph, M. and Bazin, H. (1979). Cytophilic binding of IgE to the macrophage. II. Immunologic release of lysosomal enzyme from macrophages by IgE and anti-IgE in the rat. *Cell Immunol.* **46** (1), 24–34.

Ferreri, N.R., Howland, W.C. and Spiegelberg, H. (1986). Release of leukotrienes C_4 and B_4 and prostaglandin E_2 from human monocytes stimulated with aggregated IgG, IgA and IgE. *J. Immunol.* **135**, 4188–4193.

Fuller, R.W., Morris, P.K., Sykes, D., Varndell, I.M., Kemeny, D.M., Cole, P.J.Y., Dollery, C.T. and MacDermot, J. (1986). Immunoglobulin E-dependent stimulation of human alveolar macrophages: significance in type 1 hypersensitivity. *Clin. Exp. Immunol.* **65** (2), 416–426.

Howell, C.J., Pujol, J.L., Crea, A.E., Davidson, R., Gearing, A.J., Godard, P. and Lee, T.H. (1989). Identification of an alveolar macrophage-derived activity in bronchial asthma which enhances LTD_4 generation by human eosinophils stimulated by ionophore (A23187) as granulocyte macrophage colony stimulating factor (GM–CSF). *Am. Rev. Respir. Dis.* **140** (5), 1340–1347.

Joseph, M., Tonnel, A.B., Torpier, G., Capron, A., Arnoux, B. and Benveniste, J. (1983). Involvement of immunoglobulin E in the secretory processes of alveolar macrophages from asthmatic patients. *J. Clin. Invest.* **71** (2), 221–230.

Kay, A.B., Diaz, P., Carmichaël, J. and Grant, I.W. (1981). Corticosteroid-resistant chronic asthma and monocyte complement receptors. *Clin. Exp. Immunol.* **44** (3), 576–580.

Melewicz, F.M., Zeiger, R.S., Mellon, M.H., O'Connor, R.D. and Spiegelberg, H.L. (1981). Increased peripheral blood monocytes with Fc receptors for IgE in patients with severe allergic disorders. *J. Immunol.* **126**, 1592–1595.

Melewicz, F.M., Kline, L.E., Cohen, A.B. and Spiegelberg, H.L. (1982). Characterization of Fc receptors for IgE on human alveolar macrophages. *Clin. Exp. Immunol.* **49A**(2), 364–370.

Metzger, W.J., Zavala, D., Richerson, H.B., Moseley, P., Iwamota, P., Monick, M., Sjoerdsma, K. and Hunninghake, G.W. (1987). Local allergen challenge and bronchoalveolar lavage of allergic asthmatic lungs. *Am. Rev. Respir. Dis.* **135**, 433–440.

Poston, R.N., Litchfield, T., Chanez, P., Lacoste, J.Y., Lee, T.H. and Bousquet, J. (1992). Immunohistochemical characterization of the cellular infiltration in asthmatic bronchi. *Am. Rev. Respir. Dis.* **145**, 918–921.

Poznansky, M.C., Gordon, A.C., Douglas, J.G., Krajewski, A.S., Wyllie, A.H. and Grant, I.W. (1984). Resistance to methylprednisolone in cultures of blood mononuclear cells from glucocorticoid-resistant asthmatic patients. *Clin. Sci.* **67** (6), 639–645.

Rankin, J.A., Hitchcock, M., Merrill, W., Bach, M.K., Brashler, J.R. and Askenase, P.W. (1982). IgE-dependent release of leukotriene C_4 from alveolar macrophages. *Nature* **297** (5864), 329–331.

Rankin, J.A. (1986). IgE immune complexes induce LTB release from rat alveolar macrophages. *Ann. Inst. Pasteur Immunol.* **137**, 364–367.

Spiegelberg, H.L. (1984). Structure and function of Fc receptors for IgE on lymphocytes, monocytes and macrophages. *Adv. Immunol.* **35**, 61–88.

Tonnel, A.B., Joseph, M., Gosset, P., Fournier, E. and Capron, A. (1983) Stimulation of alveolar macrophages in asthmatic patients after local provocation test. *Lancet* **1** (8339), 1406–1408.

Wilkinson, J.R., Crea, A.E., Clark, T.J. and Lee, T.H. (1989). Identification and characterization of a monocyte-derived neutrophil activating factor in corticosteroïd-resistant bronchial asthma. *J. Clin. Invest.* **84** (6), 1930–1941.

Discussion

C. Haslett

I think that some of the effects on modulating survival in eosinophils may be mediated by effects on programmed cell death or apoptosis. In our studies of macrophage influences on neutrophil-programmed cell death, we found a factor released by monocytes that inhibits programmed cell death, slows it down, and increases the survival of the neutrophil. There are very early suggestions that it is not a cytokine; we are not sure whether it is similar to Dr Lee's factor. When we look at monocytes maturing into macrophages, we find that it is produced at a very early stage, not really, surprisingly, as it matures into a full-blown macrophage, so it is a monocyte function. Have you any information on maturation?

T.H. Lee
This is a very interesting point. Survival has many factors. The secretion of molecules, like granulocyte–macrophage colony-stimulating factor (GM–CSF), from the monocyte macrophage which enhance survival occurs but inhibition of programmed death is also an important factor, as shown in your very elegant studies. In our studies, we are using supernatants, not macrophages in the cultures, so our system looks at only one end of it, but clearly the death end is also extremely important.

C. Haslett
Do mature macrophages produce your factor and also the lipid-soluble factor or is it very much a property of the immature monocyte?

T.H. Lee
The mature macrophages also make GM–CSF, but not the lipid-soluble factor.

B.B. Vargaftig
It is clear from your results and others that macrophages are upregulated in activation when they come from patients. In other conditions, we have results similar to those in animals. Can you give a general idea of what you think may be the cause: do you think it likely that, as we found, the "excitability" of the cyclic-AMP system in alveolar macrophages provided by patients is lowered with respect to stimulation by prostaglandin E_2 or salbutamol? The defect in this case would be in the ability of the cells to build up a sort of conservative mediator, which is cyclic-AMP. When they lack this, they are more excited in general and more able to produce the different substances which we have discussed.

T.H. Lee
There are a number of mechanisms whereby the cells may be primed, and it is a very important area of study. I do not have any data of our own to discuss, but the mechanism you describe is possible. The issue really is that in asthma there are many cell types, all of which appear to

have a greater releasability, ranging from the mast cell to the macrophage. Whatever mechanism is responsible probably is a general mechanism for cells in the asthmatic airway. I do not have any definitive answers at the moment, but it is clearly an important question to ask.

R. Dahl

You showed very elegantly that with corticosteroids one of the mechanisms of actions in asthma might be the inhibition of cytokine-mediated eosinophil survival. Have you studied other anti-asthma drugs on this effect?

T.H. Lee

The only other drug we have studied is nedocromil, which does not have any effect on survival induced by recombinant GM–CSF.

M.K. Church

I support you 100% in your statement that we ought to call this cell the lung macrophage as opposed to the alveolar macrophage.

15

Role of Monocytes–Macrophages in Bronchial Asthma

P. GODARD,* M. DAMON,‡ P. CHANEZ,* P. DEMOLY,* J. BOUSQUET* and F.B. MICHEL*

** Clinique des maladies respiratoires, Hôpital Arnaud de Villeneuve, 555 Route de Ganges, 34059 Montpellier, France*

‡ INSERM U 58 Avenue de Navacelle, 34100 Montpellier, France

Numerous cells have been implicated in the pathophysiology of bronchial asthma (Djukanovic *et al.*, 1990). Mast cells seem to be the most important ones because they bear high-affinity immunoglobulin E (IgE) receptors and they are able to release many inflammatory mediators; they are present in the airways, where they appear to be activated (Peters, 1990). Eosinophils also play a central role and asthma has been defined as an eosinophilic chronic bronchitis. Eosinophils are recruited in great numbers during asthma and have two effects. On one hand they are able to counteract the deleterious actions of numerous mediators, but on the other hand, they release great quantities of inflammatory mediators which are responsible for many deleterious effects on the bronchi (Bousquet *et al.*, 1990). Other cells have also been implicated: lymphocytes (Corrigan and Kay, 1991), bronchial epithelial cells (Vachier *et al.*, 1990) and neutrophils.

Macrophages are resident cells, mainly located in the alveoli, but also in the airways (Rankin, 1989), where they are involved in the defence against aerocontaminants. Increasing evidence suggests that they could

T-Lymphocyte and Inflammatory Cell Research in Asthma
ISBN 0-12-388170-6

play an important role in the pathophysiology of bronchial asthma (Rankin, 1989).

In this chapter we overview some of the abnormalities of monocytes and macrophages which have been described in bronchial asthma: monocytes are primed in blood; they are recruited into the alveoli and the airways; airway macrophages are activated and release great quantities of various mediators; they act in cooperation with other cells; cell death can be observed via necrosis and apoptosis.

Blood Monocytes

Blood monocytes display many abnormalities in experimental asthma as well as in acute or chronic asthma (Burke *et al.*, 1991a,b; Lane and Lee, 1991). It is clear now that they bear FcεRII receptors and their number is increased in allergic patients; that they appear to be activated as assessed by their capacity to form rosettes; and that they show increased complement receptor expression. Blood monocytes are able to release granulocyte–macrophage colony-stimulating factor (GM–CSF) (Burke *et al.*, 1991a) after stimulation and this capacity is enhanced in asthmatics (Fig. 15.1).

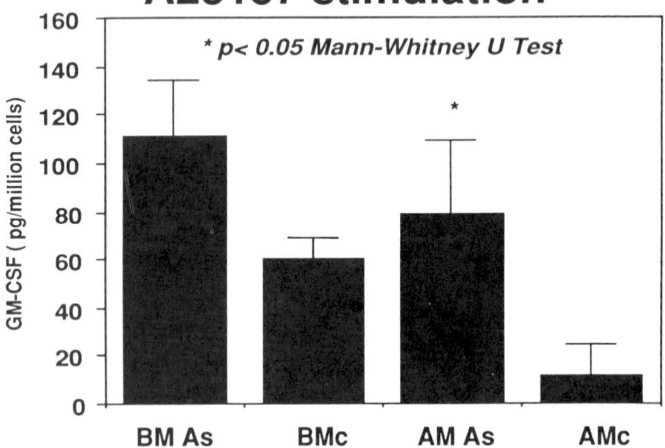

Fig. 15.1 Liberation of granulocyte–macrophage colony-stimulating factor (GM–CSF) by airway macrophages (AM) and blood monocytes (BM) from eight asthmatic patients (As) and six normal subjects (c). The cells were incubated for 3 days on adherence at 37°C in an incubator gassed with air and 5% CO_2 and stimulated by 1 ng/ml of phorbol myristate acetate (PMA) and 0.5 μM of A23186.

The releasability of blood monocytes can also be evaluated by studying the respiratory burst (Damon *et al.*, 1990). Superoxide anion accumulation was found to be higher in asthmatics as compared with non-asthmatics; the adherence by itself was able to activate the respiratory burst. Using lumino-enhanced chemiluminescence, which takes into account the whole set of oxygen species, blood monocytes from asthmatics display an increased capacity to generate oxygen radicals. In contrast to healthy subjects where a slow decrease of chemiluminescence was observed over time after the phorbol myristate acetate (PMA)-induced peak, a plateau was observed in asthmatics.

Blood monocytes appear to be primed in asthmatics. The exact mechanism is not known, although it is possible that immunoglobulin E (IgE) is involved in the process. Indeed, adding IgE to blood monocytes obtained from allergic rhinitis or asthmatics activated the cells to release O_2^-, as shown in Fig. 15.2.

Recruitment of Monocytes

There is no doubt that blood monocytes are recruited into the alveoli and into the airways in bronchial asthma. The number of peroxidase-

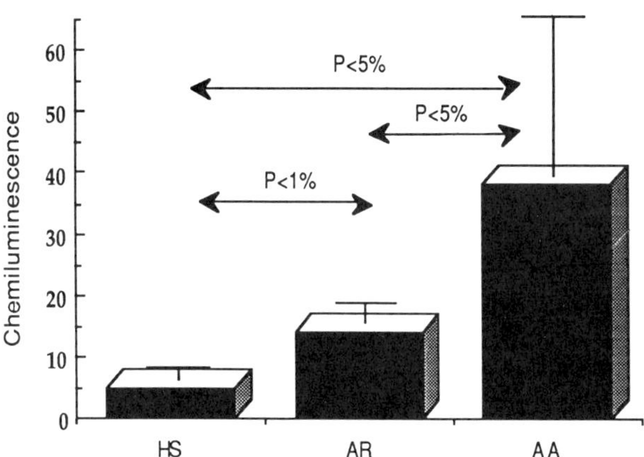

Fig. 15.2 Serum IgE induction of superoxide anion ($O_2{\cdot}^-$) release by peripheral blood monocytes of non-allergic healthy subjects (HS), allergic rhinitis (AR) and asthmatics (AA). Blood monocytes were recovered on Percoll gradients and purified by adherence. $O_2{\cdot}^-$ was measured before (background values) and after IgE (240 UI/ml) stimulation (peak), by lucigenin (10^{-5} M)-enhanced chemiluminescence in a photon-counting camera (Hamamatsu, Photonics). Results were expressed related to background values (CL peak/background values).

positive cells in bronchoalveolar lavage (BAL) fluid increases 48 h after antigen challenge in allergic asthmatics. In bronchial biopsies, using various monoclonal antibodies, Poston *et al.* (unpublished) observed the presence of a large number of monocytes in asthmatic patients.

Macrophages derive from blood monocytes; they are named lung or interstitial macrophages in the parenchyma, alveolar macrophages in the alveoli and airway macrophages in the bronchi. One of the best (and safest) ways to sample macrophages is to use the bronchoalveolar lavage technique. This has been widely used in asthmatics and guidelines have been proposed by NIH for research purposes (Hurd, 1991). BAL can be used to sample airway macrophages from the bronchoalveolar lumen and from the alveoli.

However the movements of blood monocytes and macrophages and the mechanisms which control them are not known.

Airway Macrophages

Increasing evidence is now available suggesting that airway macrophages are involved in the pathogenesis of asthma. In an elegant and important piece of work, R. Patterson demonstrated that bronchoalveolar cells obtained by BAL in sensitized monkeys and injected into the trachea of unsensitized syngenic monkeys were able to promote bronchial asthma after specific inhalation challenge (Patterson *et al.*, 1978). Since airway macrophages accounted for about 90–95% of the cells recovered by BAL, a potential role for the airway macrophages in asthma was suggested.

We would like to overview this involvement from three points of view: (1) the release of inflammatory mediators and cytokines from airway macrophages; (2) the interaction between airway macrophages and other cells which are involved in the asthmatic inflammatory process, namely lymphocytes, eosinophils and epithelial cells; (3) the heterogeneity of airway macrophages which could be related to the production of airway macrophages, ageing, necrosis or programmed cell death.

Mediator Release from Airway Macrophages

To prove that enhanced mediator release from airway macrophages is a hallmark of bronchial asthma, a two-step argument can be made:

Airway macrophages from asthmatics are different to those from healthy subjects and they release higher quantities of mediators.

Eicosanoids

Balter *et al.* (1988) did not find any intrinsic differences in basal or ionophore A23187-stimulated arachidonic acid release and eicosanoid synthesis by adherent airway macrophages obtained from normal and asthmatic subjects. On the other hand, Damon *et al.* (1990) demonstrated that airway macrophages from asthmatics generate large quantities of leukotrienes when compared with normal healthy volunteers (Damon *et al.*, 1987, 1989). These different results could be explained mainly by the differences in the severity of asthma in the patients studied.

Oxygen species

Airway macrophages are phagocytosing cells and a respiratory burst is observed in stimulated airway macrophages in the presence of phagocytosed particles (zymosan, opsonized zymosan). The release of oxygen species can be studied by luminol- or lucigenin-enhanced chemiluminescence (CL). Using these methods, it has been demonstrated that airway macrophages are more activated in asthmatic patients (Cluzel *et al.*, 1987; Kelly *et al.*, 1988) and that they can be stimulated via an IgE-dependent mechanism (Joseph *et al.*, 1980). Conflicting results have been obtained by others (McDermott and Fuller, 1988). Luminol-enhanced CL seems to be the consequence of phagocytosed eosinophil peroxidase, and a direct correlation between the total number of eosinophils in BAL fluid and luminol-enhanced CL has been described in asthmatics (Cluzel *et al.*, 1987).

Cytokines

Airway macrophages release various cytokines: interleukin-1 (IL-1) (Pujol *et al.*, 1990), GM–CSF (Howell *et al.*, 1989), IL-6 and tumour necrosis factor (TNF). Resting cells release equivalent quantities of IL-6 in healthy subjects and in asthmatics, but significantly higher quantities of IL-1, GM–CSF and TNF in asthmatics. After non-specific activation with lipopolysaccharide (LPS) during various periods of time (from 24 to 48 h), airway macrophages release higher quantities of IL-1, TNF, GM–CSF and IL-6 compared to resting cells; but in that situation the release of IL-1 was identical in asthmatics and in healthy subjects, whereas IL-6 was significantly higher in asthmatics. The significance of these different responses is not known.

Airway macrophage releasability corresponds to symptoms

Bronchial asthma is best defined by clinical symptoms and severity can be correctly assessed by clinical scores. Another main characteristic of asthma is bronchial hyperreactivity (BHR) as assessed by histamine or methacholine inhalation challenge test.

Kelly *et al.* (1988) observed an increased metabolic activity of airway macrophages and their results indicate that airway macrophage activity (lucigenin-enhanced CL) was directly related to the degree of airway responsiveness (Kelly *et al.*, 1988). In children it was shown that BHR was closely correlated to increased counts of eosinophils and macrophages in BAL fluid and to the ratio of eosinophils to macrophages (Ferguson and Wang, 1989; Kirby *et al.*, 1987); this however, has not been reported in adults.

In more severe asthmatics whose disease activity was assessed by the Aas' clinical score, the peak of opsonized zymosan-induced luminol-enhanced CL was directly correlated with the severity of asthma (Cluzel *et al.*, 1987).

Using a specific assay for γ-glutamyl transpeptidase (GT), it was shown that airway macrophage γ-GT activity was increased according to the local endobronchial inflammation as assessed by endoscopic score; this increased activity was correlated with the ability of airway macrophages to transform leukotriene (LT) C_4 into LTD_4 and LTE_4 (Damon *et al.*, 1988a).

The study of phosphatidylinositol turnover in airway macrophages from allergic asthmatics showed a continuous Li^+-sensitive production of IP_1, indicating that the cells were continuously activated (Damon *et al.*, 1988b).

The synthesis and release of TNF was observed only in asthmatics who developed a late asthmatic response after a specific allergen inhalation challenge, and not in asthmatics who developed only an early response (Tonnel *et al.*, 1990).

Cellular Inter-actions

Airway macrophages act in cooperation with other cells present in bronchoalveolar wall and lumen; in asthma, other cells such as lymphocytes and eosinophils can be recruited and the cellular interactions could amplify the inflammatory processes.

Airway macrophages and lymphocytes

During a bronchial asthma attack, there is an influx of lymphocytes into the bronchial wall as assessed by biopsy (Azzawi *et al.*, 1990) and in the deep lung as assessed by BAL (Godard *et al.*, 1987).

In healthy subjects the airway macrophages/lymphocytes ratio in BAL fluid is about 10/1 and it has been proved repeatedly that airway macrophages suppress the concanavalin A and phytohaemagglutinin (PHA) lymphoproliferative responses. In allergic asthma, this suppressive activity was significantly decreased (Aubas *et al.*, 1984).

Airway macrophages may interact with lymphocytes through the release of cytokines. Some conflicting results have been reported. Gosset and co-workers did not find any increased generation of IL-1 in allergic asthmatics as compared to healthy volunteers; moreover, they found that anti-IgE-stimulated airway macrophages released higher quantities of an IL-1 inhibitory factor (Gosset *et al.*, 1988). In contrast, it has been shown that in asthmatics, airway macrophages released higher quantities of IL-1 as assessed by a biologic assay (Pujol *et al.*, 1990).

Airway macrophages and eosinophils

Eosinophils play an important role in the pathophysiology of bronchial asthma. They are recruited by activated cells and mediators into the bronchoalveolar lumen and release their own mediators (LTC_4, possibly 15-HETE, cationic proteins, oxygen species and peroxidase), thereby amplifying inflammatory processes.

Airway macrophages recruit and activate eosinophils mainly via platelet activating factor, but also by LTB_4 and TNF. Incubation of eosinophils with airway macrophage supernatants isolated from asthmatic subjects followed by stimulation with calcium ionophore A23187 resulted in an enhancement of the capacity of the eosinophil to release LTC_4. The enhancing activity was heat- and trypsin-sensitive and was neutralized by a specific antibody. GM–CSF may play a role in the amplification of the eosinophilic inflammation in asthmatic airways (Howell *et al.*, 1989). Tonnel *et al.* showed that supernatants of cultured airway macrophages activated normodense eosinophils to release oxygen species as assessed by chemiluminescence (Tonnel *et al.*, 1985).

In the same way, airway macrophages were able to transform LTC_4 released by activated eosinophils and mast cells into LTD_4 and LTE_4. This transformation depended on the activation state of the airway macrophages and its intensity correlated with the local inflammatory process. Moreover, airway macrophages may also be able to transform

15-HPETE and 15-HETE released by eosinophils and epithelial cells into lipoxins and related compounds (Lee *et al.*, 1990; Kim, 1990). In several *in vitro* experiments, we observed that airway macrophages were able to release higher quantities of lipoxin A_4 and B_4 in stable asymptomatic asthmatics than in healthy subjects. On the other hand, activated eosinophils appear to be hypodense and release major basic protein (MBP) and eosinophil cationic protein (ECP) into the bronchoalveolar lumen and in the bronchial wall. In the BAL fluid, quantities of ECP were assessed by specific radioimmunoassay and correlated with clinical severity of asthma according to the Aas' score (Bousquet *et al.*, 1990). In bronchial biopsies, ECP was evidenced by specific monoclonal antibodies (EG1 and EG2); it was present in the areas of the bronchial tree where desquamation of epithelial cells was the most prominent (Bousquet *et al.*, 1990). MBP can be released in the BAL fluid and airway macrophages could phagocytose MBP granules. These observations could explain the decreased viability of airway macrophages in a 24 h culture according to the number of eosinophils (Godard *et al.*, 1982).

Airway macrophages and bronchial epithelial cells

The interactions between airway macrophages and bronchial epithelial cells can be considered from several points of view:

1) Airway macrophages release oxygen species which may be involved in the decreased viability of epithelial cells observed in asthmatics; this could contribute to the shedding of epithelium.
2) In contrast, bronchial epithelial cells release large quantities of 15-HETE in asthmatics; this compound could be metabolized into lipoxins by airway macrophages.
3) Airway macrophages may contribute to bronchial repair after an asthma attack. It is known that airway macrophages from healthy subjects release growth factors, but this has to be evaluated in asthmatics. However, on the other hand, airway macrophages may enhance bronchial fibrosis.

Airway Macrophage Heterogeneity

By comparison with eosinophils, it could be hypothesized that airway macrophage activation corresponds to heterogeneity. Using Percoll density fractionation airway macrophages from asthmatics were mainly recovered in the lower density fractions (1.03 and 1.04 g/ml) whereas airway macrophages from normal subjects were in the higher density fractions (1.07 g/ml). Electron microscopy studies have shown that low-density airway macrophages have the morphological characteristics of activated cells (Chanez *et al.*, 1991). However, no definitive observations have been made as regards the releasability of airway macrophages. Necrotic and apoptotic airway macrophages (as assessed by electron microscopy) have been observed in asthmatics but further studies are required.

Conclusion

The ability of airway macrophages to release pro-inflammatory mediators could be used to study the effect of various drugs in the treatment of asthma. However, only a few studies have been performed in asthmatics. Most of them were done *in vitro*. Damon and co-workers found that nedocromil decreased the generation of LTB_4 and 5-HETE from airway macrophages in asthmatic patients (Damon *et al.*, 1989), and Kakuta and colleagues found that ketotifen inhibited in a dose-dependent manner the PMA-induced chemiluminescence of airway macrophages in non-asthmatic patients (Kakuta *et al.*, 1988). *In vitro* it is well known that dexamethasone inhibits the release of arachidonic acid metabolites; however treatment of healthy subjects with dexamethasone resulted in a non-significant inhibition of the release of these metabolites from macrophages triggered *ex vivo* (Yoss *et al.*, 1990). This could be explained by a low diffusion of the drug in the deep lung. In healthy smokers, inhaled glucocorticoids decreased the synthesis and release of angiotensin-converting enzyme (ACE) and fibronectin, but modified neither the generation of oxygen species nor the LTB_4 production (Bergstrand *et al.*, 1990).

Between the various stimuli inducing an asthma attack and the target organ, i.e. the bronchi, exist resident cells such as mast cells and alveolar macrophages, but also epithelial cells, which are stimulated to release mediators and induce the inflammatory cascade which leads to the airway obstruction. Increased mediator release could be one mechanism in the pathophysiology of bronchial asthma and justifies much attention and therapeutic consideration. Mediators released from airway macrophages may be involved in asthma and by use of their phagocytic capacity drugs can be specifically targeted to these cells in order to assess their relative importance.

References

Aubas, P., Cosso, B., Godard, Ph., Michel, F.B. and Clot, J. (1984). Decreased suppressor cell activity of alveolar macrophages in bronchial asthma. *Am. Rev. Respir. Dis.* **130**, 875–878.

Azzawi, M., Bradley, B., Jeffrey, P.K., Frew, A.J., Wardlaw, A.J., Knowles, G., Assoufi, B., Collins, J.V., Durham, S.R. and Kay, A.B. (1990). Identification of activated T lymphocytes and eosinophils in bronchial biopsies in stable atopic asthma. *Am. Rev. Respir. Dis.* **142**, 1407–1413.

Balter, M.S., Eschenbacher, W.L. and Peters-Golden, M. (1988). Arachidonic acid metabolism in cultured alveolar macrophages from normal, atopic and asthmatic subjects. *Am. Rev. Respir. Dis.* **138**, 1134–1142.

Bergstrand, H., Bjornson, A., Blaschke, E., Brattsand, R., Eklund, A., Larsson, K. and Linden, M. (1990). Effects of an inhaled corticosteroid budesonide, on alveolar macrophage function in smokers. *Thorax* **45**, 362–368.

Bousquet, J., Chanez, P., Lacoste, J.Y., Barnéon, G., Ghavanian, N., Enander, I., Venge, P., Ahlstedt, S., Simonylafontaine, J., Godard, Ph. and Michel, F.B. (1990). Eosinophilic inflammation in asthma. *New Engl. J. Med.* **323**, 1033–1039.

Burke, L.A., Hallsworth, M.P., Litchfield, T.M., Davidson, R. and Lee, T.H. (1991a). Identification of the major activity derived from cultured human peripheral blood mononuclear cells, which enhances eosinophil viability, as granulocyte macrophage colony-stimulating factor (GM–CSF). *J. Allergy Clin. Immunol.* **88**, 226–235.

Burke, L.A., Wilkinson, J.R.W., Howell, C.J. and Lee, T.H. (1991b). Interactions of macrophages and monocytes with granulocytes in asthma. *Eur. Respir. J.* **4**, S85–S90.

Chanez, P., Bousquet, J., Couret, I., Cornillac, L., Barnéon, G., Vic, P., Michel, F.B. and Godard, Ph. (1991). Increased number of hypodense alveolar macrophages in patients with bronchial asthma. *Am. Rev. Respir. Dis.* **144**, 923–930.

Chavis, C., Godard, Ph., Michel, F.B., Crastes de Paulet, A. and Damon, M. (1991). Sulfidopeptide leukotrienes contribute to human alveolar macrophage activation in asthma. *Prost. Leuk. Fatty Acid* **42**, 95–100.

Cluzel, M., Damon, M., Chanez, P., Crastes de Paulet, A., Michel, F.B. and Godard, Ph. (1987). Enhanced alveolar cell luminol-dependent chemiluminescence in asthma. *J. Allergy Clin. Immunol.* **80**, 195–201.

Corrigan, C.J. and Kay, A.B. (1991). The roles of inflammatory cells in the pathogenesis of asthma and of chronic obstructive pulmonary disease. *Am. Rev. Respir. Dis.* **143**, 1165–1168.

Damon, M., Chavis, C., Crastes de Paulet, A., Michel, F.B. and Godard, Ph. (1987). Arachidonic acid metabolism in alveolar macrophages. A comparison of cells from healthy subjects, allergic asthmatics and chronic bronchitis patients. *Prostaglandins* **34**, 291–309.

Damon, M., Chavis, C., Le Doucen, Ch., Crastes de Paulet, A., Michel, F.B. and Godard, Ph. (1988a). Gamma glutamyl transpeptidase activity of alveolar macrophages. *Proc. XIII ICACI Montreux* **9**, A98.

Damon, M., Vial, H., Crastes de Paulet, A. and Godard, Ph. (1988b). Phosphoinositide breakdown and superoxide anion release in formyl-peptide-stimulated human alveolar macrophages. Comparison between quiescent and activated cells. *FEBS Letts.* **239**, 169–173.

Damon, M., Chavis, C., Daurès, J.P., Crastes de Paulet, A., Michel, F.B. and Godard, Ph. (1989). Increased generation of the arachidonic metabolites LTB4 and 5HETE by human alveolar macrophages in patients with asthma; effect *in vitro* of nedocromil sodium. *Eur. Respir. J.* **2**, 202–209.

Damon, M., Vachier, I., Le Doucen, CH., Godard, Ph. and Nicolas, J.C. (1990). Video imaging of blood monocyte chemiluminescence: application to asthma. *In* "Biolum. Chemilum. Current Status" (P.E. Stanley and L.J. Kricka, eds) pp. 345–349. John Wiley, New York.

Djukanovic, R., Roche, W.R., Wilson, J.W., Beasley, C.R.W., Twentyman, O.P., Howarth, P.H. and Holgate, S.T. (1990). Mucosal inflammation in asthma. *Am. Rev. Respir. Dis.* **142**, 434–457.

Ferguson, A.C. and Wong, F.W.M. (1989). Bronchial hyperresponsiveness in asthmatic children. Correlation with macrophages and eosinophils in broncholavage fluid. *Chest* **96**, 988–991.

Godard, Ph., Chaintreuil, J., Damon, M., Coupe, M., Flandre, O., Crastes de Paulet, A. and Michel, F.B. (1982). Functional assessment of alveolar macrophages: comparison of cells from asthmatic and normal subjects. *J. Allergy Clin. Immunol.* **70**, 88–93.

Godard, Ph., Bousquet, J., Lebel, B. and Michel, F.B. (1987). Lavage bronchoalvéolaire de l'asthmatique. *Bull. Europ. Physiopath. Resp.* **23**, 73–83.

Gosset, Ph., Lassalle, Ph., Tonnel, A.B., Dessaint, J.P., Wallaert, B., Prin, L., Pestel, J. and Capron, A. (1988). A production of an interleukine-1 inhibitory factor by human alveolar macrophages in normal and allergic asthmatic patients. *Am. Rev. Respir. Dis.* **138**, 40–46.

Howell, C.J., Pujol, J.L., Crea, A.E.G., Davidson, R., Gearing, A.J.H., Godard, Ph. and Lee, T.H. (1989). Identification of an alveolar macrophage derived activity in bronchial asthma that enhances LTC4 generation by human eosinophils stimulated by A23187 as a granulocyte macrophage colony stimulating factor. *Am. Rev. Respir. Dis.* **140**, 1340–1347.

Hurd, S.S. (1991). Special Article. Workshop summary and guidelines. Investigative use of bronchoscopy, lavage and bronchial biopsies in asthma and other airways diseases. *Clin. Exp. Allergy* **21**, 533–539.

Joseph, M., Tonnel, A.B., Capron, A. and Voisin, C. (1980). Enzyme release and superoxyde anion production by human alveolar macrophages stimulated with IgE. *Clin. Exp. Immunol.* **40**, 416–422.

Kakuta, Y., Kato, T., Sasaki, H. and Takishima, T. (1988). Effect of ketotifen on human alveolar macrophages. *J. Allergy Clin. Immunol.* **81**, 469–474.

Kelly, C.A., Ward, C., Stenton, C.S., Bird, G., Hendrick, D.J. and Walters, E.H. (1988). Number and activity of inflammatory cells in bronchoalveolar lavage fluid in asthma and their relation to airway responsiveness. *Thorax* **43**, 684–692.

Kim, S.J. (1990). Elevated formation of lipoxins in viral antibody-positive rat alveolar macrophages. *Am. J. Respir. Cell Molec. Biol.* **3**, 113–118.

Kirby, J.G., Hargreave, F.E., Gleich, G.J. and O'Byrne, P.M. (1987). Bronchoalveolar cell profiles of asthmatic and non-asthmatic subject. *Am. Rev. Respir. Dis.* **136**, 379–383.

Lane, S.J. and Lee, T.H. (1991). Glucocorticoid receptor characteristics in monocytes of patients with corticosteroid resistant bronchial asthma. *Am. Rev. Respir. Dis.* **143**, 1020–1024.

Lee, T.H., Crea, A.E.G., Gant, V., Spur, B.W., Marron, B.E., Nicolaou, K.C., Reardon, E., Brezinski, M. and Serhan, C.N. (1990). Identification of lipoxin A4 and its relationship to the sulfidopeptide leukotrienes C4, D4 and E4 in the bronchoalveolar lavage fluids obtained from patients with selected pulmonary diseases. *Am. Rev. Respir. Dis.* **141**, 1453–1458.

McDermott, J. and Fuller, R.W. (1988). *In* "Macrophages in Asthma: Basic Mechanism and Clinical Management" (P.J. Barnes, I.W. Rodger and N.C. Thomson, eds), pp. 97–114. Academic Press, London.

Patterson, R., Susko, I.M. and Harris, K.E. (1978). The *in vivo* transfer of antigen induced airway reactions by bronchial lumen cells. *J. Clin. Invest.* **61**, 519–524.

Peters, S.P. (1990). Mast cells and histamine in asthma. *J. Allergy Clin. Immunol.* **86**, 642–646.

Pujol, J.L., Cosso, B., Daurès, J.P., Clot, J., Michel, F.B. and Godard, Ph. (1990). Interleukin-1 release by alveolar macrophages in asthmatic patients and healthy subjects. *Int. Arch. Allergy Appl. Immunol.* **91**, 207–210.

Rankin, J.A. (1989). The contribution of alveolar macrophages to hyperreactive airway disease. *J. Allergy Clin. Immunol.* **83**, 722–729.

Tonnel, A.B., Prin, L., Capron, M., Wallaert, B. and Capron, A. (1985). Infiltrats pulmonaires à éosinophiles. Etude comparée des éosinophiles sanguins et alvéolaires. *In* "Traitement de l'Asthme" (P. Godard, ed.), pp. 21–30. Masson, Paris.

Tonnel, A.B., Gosset, P. and Lasalle, P. (1990). Involvement of alveolar macrophages in the pathophysiology of allergic asthma. *Eur. Respir. J.* 272S (abst.).

Vachier, I., Godard, Ph., Michel, F.B., Descomps, B. and Damon, M. (1990). Aberrant expression of antigen HLA-DR of Class-II MHC in bronchial epithelial cells from asthmatic patients. *Comptes rendus de l'Académie des Sciences série III. Sciences* **311**, 341–346.

Yoss, E.B., Spannhake, E.W., Flynn, J.T., Fish, J.E. and Peters, S.P. (1990). Arachidonic acid metabolism in normal human alveolar macrophages: stimulus specificity for mediator release and phospholipid metabolism, and pharmacologic modulation *in vitro* and *in vivo*. *Am. J. Respir. Cell. Molec. Biol.* **2**, 69–80.

Discussion

B.B. Vargaftig

You mentioned the interesting observation that arachidonic acid is incorporated more effectively in asthmatic macrophages and mainly in phosphatidylinositol. This may only be a detail, but how long were the macrophages exposed to arachidonic acid before the experiment? If this is done very quickly, the incorporation is mainly in phosphatidylcholine; if it is done for 18–24 h, it is more in phosphatidylethanolamine.

P. Godard

The alveolar macrophages were incubated for 24 h, and cultured without any stimulus.

B.B. Vargaftig

By doing that, I think the arachidonic acid escapes from the main source of lipid mediators and goes to phosphatidylethanolamine. If there is still an increasing incorporation in phosphatidylinositol, this is an interesting observation because it would point to phosphatidylinositol phospholipase C rather than to phospholipase A_2.

P. Godard

The culture was stopped at 6, 12, 18 and 24 h, and no difference was observed in the incorporation on phosphatidylinositol between 6 and 24 h. Incorporation on phosphatidylinositol was higher all the time.

T.H. Lee

I do not fully understand the density of the macrophages. The data appear to show some difference. How do we interpret this, and does it correlate with anything?

P. Godard

It appears that macrophages with low density were mainly aged macrophages because they were not able to suppress lymphocyte stimulation, which is why I asked about apoptosis. We checked the functional activity of these different macrophages, but they were identical.

M.K. Church

From the pharmaceutical point of view, it is obviously necessary to know the effect of drugs upon macrophages. You described many experiments which, added together, suggest that the macrophage can support other cells in their life and in programmed death afterwards. Is it known what is the drug modulation, say by β-stimulants, nedocromil or any other type of drugs (you mentioned steroids briefly), upon this?

P. Godard

Some work has been done on the modulation of macrophage activation by drugs. With a high dose of nedocromil, if all the subjects were pooled there was, as a general rule, a slight inhibition of LTB_4 and 5-hydroxyeicosatetraenoic acid (HETE) synthesis by alveolar macrophages, mainly in asthmatic patients and not in healthy subjects. But some patients appear to be responders, and others non-responders to nedocromil, in exactly the same way as is observed with steroid-resistant asthmatic patients. We cannot predict whether or not an individual patient will respond to the treatment. A correlation between the *in vitro* and *in vivo* observations has not yet been made. [*M.K. Church*: And β-stimulants?] β-stimulants have not been checked.

T.H. Lee

I was interested in the lipoxin results because there are not many of us working in this area. Were sulphidopeptide leukotrienes measured in the same supernatants as lipoxins? [*P. Godard*: No.]

If I understood correctly, the asymptomatic asthmatics had the most lipoxin? [*P. Godard*: Yes – it is surprising.] It is not really surprising. I do not know how much people are aware of these molecules, which were described by Serhan and Samuelson 6 or 7 years ago. They are products of arachidonic acid produced through a double lipoxygenation by the 5- and the 15-lipoxygenases acting on arachidonic acid. They can be formed through a 5-lipoxygenase, but the 15-lipoxygenase, which is present in eosinophils and also other granulocytes, can also be produced by platelets because the platelet has a 12-lipoxygenase which can have a C-15 specificity and work on the carbon at position 15. Thus, lipoxins are made through a double lipoxygenation. There are two isomers, lipoxin A_1 and lipoxin B_4.

Most of the work done previously was *in vitro*, in test-tubes, in which arachidonic acid was added to mixed granulocyte suspensions. Activation with calcium ionophore then produced these molecules, but their function was not really established. About 2 years ago we felt it was important to try to find out whether lipoxins are in fact present *in vivo*. The lung makes a lot of 15-lipoxygenase products, so if lipoxins are going to be made it will be in the lung. In a study with Serhan, we were able to identify lipoxins in bronchoalveolar lavage fluid using gas chromatography, and mass spectrometry with selective ion monitoring.

Some recent, and intriguing, data suggest that lipoxin A_4 at least may work through a sulphidopeptide leukotriene receptor. Sven-Erik Dahlen, at the Karolinska Institute, is able to inhibit LTC_4-induced bronchial contractions of human airways *in vitro* using lipoxin A_4, which suggests that lipoxin A_4 may be an endogenous sulphidopeptide leukotriene antagonist.

Very recently, using synthetic material we have made, this has been studied *in vivo*. There is little doubt that if lipoxin A_4 is inhaled, LTC_4 dose–response curves can be displaced to the right. This suggests that it does indeed displace LTC_4 from the receptor or inhibit LTC_4-induced contraction.

I was therefore very interested in Dr Godard's data showing that lipoxin A_4 was made in greater quantities in the asymptomatic asthmatic patients, because this is what might have been anticipated based on the data on LTC_4.

P. Godard

But the results concerning the patients with steroids are not encouraging because we stop this . . .

T.H. Lee (*interrupting*)
The steroids do so many different things. I did not mean to give a lecture on lipoxins, but they are very intriguing and an area which has not really been discussed yet.

Could you summarize Tonnel's interesting work with the late phase response and tumour necrosis factor (TNF) production by the macrophages?

P. Godard
If I remember rightly, he studied TNF release by alveolar macrophages in asthmatic patients after challenge. In asthmatics who develop a late phase reaction, there is an increased release of TNF, but not in patients who develop only an early asthmatic response.

T.H. Lee
He suggested that the TNF release is increasing adhesion molecule expression on the endothelial cells? This may in part be responsible for the cellular recruitment in a late phase response.

P. Godard
It is only speculation, and it has to be demonstrated.

16

Mast Cells and their Role in Inflammation

E. BRZEZIŃSKA-BŁASZCZYK and M.K. CHURCH

Clinical Pharmacology, Centre Block, Southampton General Hospital, Southampton SO9 4XY, UK

Introduction

In 1878 Paul Ehrlich identified mast cells in human tissues by observing the metachromatic staining properties of their prominent cytoplasmic granules. The fascinating feature of mast cells is that some aspects of their behaviour as a component of the immune system are very well understood, whilst others still remain a mystery. The essential role of mast cells acting as critical effector cells in immediate hypersensitivity reactions has been established beyond reasonable doubt. The receptor for immunoglobulin E (IgE) ($Fc_{\epsilon}RI$) present on the mast cell membrane which binds IgE with high affinity is one of the key molecules involved in triggering these reactions (Metzger, 1991). In sensitized individuals $Fc_{\epsilon}RI$ cross-linkage by multivalent antigens, or allergens as they are termed when initiating an allergic response, induces the redistribution of IgE-receptor complex in the cell membrane, which in turn triggers the release of preformed and newly generated mediators which are responsible for allergic symptoms (Ishizaka and Ishizaka, 1984).

There is growing evidence that mast cells participate not only in immediate hypersensitivity reactions but also in many other physiological and pathological processes. The range of functions in which mast cells may participate is the subject of intense speculation and controversy. It is widely accepted that IgE-dependent mast cell activation represents a central pathogenic event in certain host responses to parasites (Miller

T-Lymphocyte and Inflammatory Cell Research in Asthma
ISBN 0-12-388170-6

and Jarrett, 1971; Gustowska *et al.*, 1983; Reed, 1989). Morphological studies suggest that mast cells may also participate in a broad spectrum of biological processes which do not necessarily involve IgE-dependent initiation of their secretory mechanisms. These include many protective or pathological immune responses (Askenase *et al.*, 1980; Farram and Nelson, 1980), a variety of disorders associated with persistent chronic inflammation (Lloyd *et al.*, 1975; Strobel *et al.*, 1983), tissue remodelling (Lindholm and Lindholm, 1970), development of pathological fibrosis (Kischer *et al.*, 1978; Goto *et al.*, 1984; Hawkins *et al.*, 1985), and host reactions to certain neoplasms (Goto *et al.*, 1984). It has also been suggested that the mast cell is involved in angiogenesis (Kessler *et al.*, 1976; Azizkhan *et al.*, 1980; Crowle and Starkey, 1989) and nerve regeneration (Bienenstock *et al.*, 1989). Furthermore, studies indicate that mast cells play an important role in the control of blood flow, vascular permeability and leukocyte infiltration. It should be pointed out, however, that the specific role and significance of mast cells in most of the above reactions have been assigned on purely circumstantial evidence.

We may consider the mast cell, therefore, to be a pro-inflammatory cell with widespread functions in inflammatory situations of either an allergic or non-allergic basis. In this review we consider the basic structure and function of the mast cell and explore how its two-way communications with inflammatory cells and sensory nerves may influence the development of inflammation.

The Origin of Mast Cells

It has been suggested that mast cells are derived from T-lymphocytes, fibroblasts or macrophages (Zucker-Franklin *et al.*, 1981; Czarnetzki *et al.*, 1982). It is now accepted, however, that mast cells are most likely to be derived from pluripotential haematopoietic cells in the bone marrow. This was demonstrated by Kitamura and colleagues with *in vivo* experiments using genetically mast cell-deficient (W/W^v) mutant mice and their congeneic normal littermates (Kitamura *et al.*, 1978, 1989; Kitamura and Go, 1979). It was also shown that mast cells originate from cells less differentiated than those precursors committed either to the neutrophil–macrophage or erythropoid cell lineages (Sonoda *et al.*, 1983). Mast cell precursors comprise only a small fraction of the total precursor cell pool, the number in the bone marrow being estimated to be between 10 and 68 cells per 10^5 bone marrow cells (Sonoda *et al.*, 1982; Thompson *et al.*, 1990) while splenic cells contain only around 2 mast cell progenitors per 10^5 cells (Sonoda *et al.*, 1983). On leaving the bone marrow, mast cell precursors migrate, using the blood as a carrier, to the site of their final deposition where they mature into tissue mast cells. Circulating mouse mast cell precursors, which cannot be identified as mast cells by morphology and are only described as non-granulated cells with a density of 1.060–1.070 g/ml (Jarboe *et al.*, 1989), are present in normal blood in small numbers, 1–2 cells per 10^5 nucleated cells (Nakano *et al.*, 1987).

In vitro studies with murine mast cells have been instrumental in the identification of growth factors involved in the proliferation and maturation of mast cells. Studies with the cytokine interleukin, IL-3, which stimulates the formation of colonies of nearly all haematopoietic lineages (Ihle *et al.*, 1983), showed that it stimulated the proliferation of mast cells, some 30% of colonies containing demonstrable mast cells (Lanotte *et al.*, 1986). A further interleukin, IL-4, which has little or no ability to sustain the proliferation of mouse mast cells in isolation (Lee *et al.*, 1986), acts cooperatively with IL-3 to promote murine mast cell maturation *in vitro* (Hamaguchi *et al.*, 1987). On the other hand, granulocyte–macrophage colony-stimulating factor (GM–CSF) inhibits the growth of IL-3-dependent mast cells (Bressler *et al.*, 1989). Recently, a new mast cell growth factor has been identified (Zsebo *et al.*, 1990). This factor, stem cell factor (SCF), is a pluripotential colony-stimulating factor on normal mouse bone marrow, giving rise to colonies of granulocytes, macrophages, megakaryocytes and eosinophils, and in combination with erythropoietin, erythroid bursts. The gene encoding this factor has been cloned and its product found to be identical to the ligand for c-kit tyrosine kinase receptor (Zsebo *et al.*, 1990).

Acquisition of IgE receptors appears to occur early in the development of mast cells, before many exhibit the morphological characteristics of the mature cell; after 1 week of culture in the presence of IL-3 one-third of mouse bone marrow cells have been reported to have this receptor, and by 3 weeks all cells were positive (Prystowsky *et al.*, 1984; Razin *et al.*, 1984). Thus, early bone marrow-derived mast cells can be identified by their IgE receptors. The early appearance of IgE receptors during mast cell differentiation may be important for proliferation and for maturation.

In contrast to the murine mast cell system, growth factors and microenvironment required for the differentiation and proliferation of human mast cells are less well understood; the development of culture techniques so far producing disappointing results. While it was shown that recombinant human IL-3 promoted a transient, selective differentiation of human basophils in suspension cultures of bone marrow and cord blood cells (Saito *et al.*, 1988; Dvorak *et al.*, 1989), prolongation of the culture to 4 weeks resulted in the majority of non-adherent cells becoming eosinophils. No mast cells were detected. Furthermore, recombinant human IL-4 failed to promote the differentiation of basophils or mast cells in the suspension culture of cord blood cells (Saito *et al.*, 1988; Dvorak *et al.*, 1989). Taken together, these results suggest that differentiation of human mast cells may require a feeder layer or cytokine(s) from non-T cells. It has been shown recently that a long-term co-culture of mononuclear cells of human umbilical cord blood with mouse embryo-derived 3T3 fibroblasts resulted in the development of mast cells (Levi-Schaffer *et al.*, 1985, 1987; Furitsu *et al.*, 1989), but the majority of the cells developed in an 11-week co-culture of cord blood cells with human fibroblasts were basophils and eosinophils (Furitsu *et al.*, 1989).

The mast cells obtained by co-culture of cord blood cells with mouse 3T3 fibroblasts contained metachromatic granules and have been termed M cells (Furitsu *et al.*, 1989). These cells contain a large oval or round nucleus with partially condensed chromatin, narrow surface folds characteristic of mast cells, a limited number of lipid bodies, numerous membrane-bound granules and granules of various substructural patterns which had been described in human mast cells (Craig *et al.*, 1988). M cells contain 1.4–2.8 μg histamine per 10^6 cells (Furitsu *et al.*, 1989). Examination of these cells by sequential double staining procedures and by immunofluorescence revealed that granules of almost all cells contain tryptase, and that granules in over 84% cells contain both tryptase and chymase (Schwartz, 1985; Castells *et al.*, 1987). In immunofluorescence, the majority of mature M cells were clearly stained with the YB5 B8 monoclonal antibody, specific for surface markers on human mast cells (Mayrhofer *et al.*, 1987). Finally, the presence of FcεRI on M cells was demonstrated by immunofluorescence and by the binding of ^{125}I-labelled human E myeloma protein (Kirshenbaum *et al.*, 1989). All these studies indicate that M cells are indeed human mature mast cells.

Recent studies have clearly shown that differentiation of human mast cell progenitors did not require direct contact with 3T3 fibroblasts, and that soluble factor(s) released from these fibroblasts are sufficient for the development of mast cells (Ishizaka *et al.*, 1991). The nature of this growth factor(s) is still unknown.

Mast Cells: Distribution and Functional Properties

Mast cells are distributed throughout normal human tissues, where they are often associated with mucosal surfaces, situated adjacent to blood and lymphatic vessels or near or within nerves (Galli *et al.*, 1984). In the lung, mast cells are situated at the luminal mucosal surface of the bronchi, where they may interact with the external environment and in the parenchyma (Metcalfe *et al.*, 1981). In the urinary tract, mast cells are predominantly situated between the epithelial cells. Skin mast cells are found in the dermis rather than in the epidermis (Eady *et al.*, 1979) with large variations being observed between their numbers in various anatomical sites (Binazzi and Rampichini, 1959), with an average number around 7×10^3 mast cells/mm^3 (Hellstrom and Holmgreen, 1950; Mikhail and Miller-Milinska, 1964). In the lung they occur in concentrations of 1–7×10^6 cells/g lung tissue (Wasserman, 1980) and constitutes as much as 2% of alveolar tissue (Fox *et al.*, 1981).

Regardless of their source, mast cells share many common characteristics. Mast cells dispersed from human tissues have a similar spectrum of size, being 5–18 μm in diameter, show metachromatic staining with basic dyes, and have a capacity to release many biologically active substances, so-called mediators, after immunological IgE-dependent activation (Ishizaka and Ishizaka, 1984).

A characteristic feature of mast cells is the presence of modified lysosomal granules in which the preformed mediators are packed and from where they are released into the external microenvironment following cell activation. Of these mediators histamine and tryptase are ubiquitous occurring in all human mast cells regardless of the anatomical localization. The mast cells dispersed from lung, skin, colonic mucosa, and colonic submucosa have a similar histamine content, the mean values ranging from 1 to 2 pg/cell (Schwartz *et al.*, 1987). A second neutral protease, chymase, is found only in a population of mast cells which is normally associated with connective or fibrous tissues (Irani *et al.*, 1986). The recent availability of specific antibodies against the mast cell neutral proteases, tryptase and chymase, has allowed a division of human mast cells into two different subpopulations according to their immunocytochemical characteristics (Irani and Schwartz, 1990). One population, containing only tryptase, is designated MC_T and the second, containing both tryptase and chymase, is designated MC_{TC} (Irani *et al.*, 1986). At the present time it seems that cytoplasmic granule protease content is the most attractive, currently available potential marker for the discrimination of human mast cell subpopulations.

In the lung and small intestinal mucosa the majority of the mast cells contain only tryptase (MC_T) (Irani *et al.*, 1986) and, like mucosal mast cells of the rat, appear to be dependent on T-lymphocyte products for their development and maturation (Aldenborg and Enerback, 1985). The majority of mast cells in the skin and small intestinal submucosa contain both tryptase and chymase (MC_{TC}) (Craig *et al.*, 1986) and appear, like rodent connective tissue mast cells, to be independent of T-lymphocyte-derived factors for their proliferation (Mayrhofer and Fisher, 1979). It should be emphasized, however, that most anatomical sites contain a mixture of the two subpopulations (Schwartz, 1989) and that respective numbers of each may change with disease indicating that microenvironmental factors also influence the migration and maturation of mast cells. Thus human mast cells cannot be classified as MC_T or MC_{TC} based on tissue localization alone.

Transmission electron microscopic studies of human mast cells have established that their cytoplasmic granules can exhibit a variety of substructural patterns (Craig *et al.*, 1988). The MC_T population contains characteristic crystalline scrolls, lattices and gratings formed by the interaction of tryptase with the proteoglycan backbone. The MC_{TC} are more electron dense because of their extra protease content (Irani and Schwartz, 1990). Also, the clear crystalline structures within the granule are less obvious because chymase, carboxypeptidase and cathepsin G associated with the proteoglycan in a non-crystalline amorphous complex (Schwartz *et al.*, 1981b). Furthermore, the granules of MC_{TC} are larger than those of MC_T (Craig *et al.*, 1988).

Activation of mast cells results in the release of a variety of mediators, all of which have the capability to influence the function of adjacent cells or to alter the constitution of the extracellular matrix of connective tissue. Mast cell mediators can be categorized into three groups: the preformed intragranular mediators, the newly generated, primarily lipid membrane-derived mediators, and cytokines (Robinson, 1988; Schwartz, 1988).

To the first group belong the biogenic amines, histamine and serotonin (the latter only in rodent mast cells) (Riley and West, 1953; Benditt *et al.*, 1955), heparin and/or chondroitin sulphate proteoglycans (Schiller and Dorfman, 1959; Razin *et al.*, 1982), neutral proteases (Schwartz *et al.*, 1981a; Schechter *et al.*, 1983; Meier *et al.*, 1985; Goldstein *et al.*, 1989), chemotactic factors (eosinophil chemotactic factor of anaphylaxis, ECF-A (Goetzl and Austen, 1975; Boswell *et al.*, 1978) and high molecular weight neutrophil chemotactic factor of anaphylaxis, NCF-A (Atkins *et al.*, 1977; O'Driscoll *et al.*, 1983)), arylsulphatase A (Lynch *et al.*, 1978), peroxidase (Henderson and Kaliner, 1979), superoxide dismutase (Henderson and Kaliner, 1978), and several exoglycosidases (Schwartz and Austen, 1984). These preformed mediators are held together by close ionic attraction of the basic elements, namely histamine and proteases, with the highly acidic heparin or chondroitin sulphate. The dominant acidity of the proteoglycan ensures that the enzymes are stored in a form in which they are inactive. Also, the ionic attraction between the more highly charged neutral proteases, chymase and carboxypeptidase, prevents their diffusion and slows the rate of inactivation of these enzymes once they are released from granules (Yurt and Austen, 1977; Schwartz *et al.*, 1981b).

To the second, or newly generated, group of mediators belong prostaglandin $(PG)D_2$, leukotrienes (LT) C_4 and D_4, and platelet-activating factor (PAF) (Holgate *et al.*, 1984; Robinson, 1988). These products of arachidonate metabolism are synthesized *de novo* by appropriate stimulation of the cell. Arachidonic acid, generated from membrane lipids by the actions of phospholipase A_2 or diacylglycerol (DAG) lipase (Kennerly *et al.*, 1979), may be metabolized via one of two major enzymatic pathways, the cyclooxygenase pathway to generate the PGD_2 or the lipoxygenase pathway to generate the leukotrienes (Dahlen *et al.*, 1980; Lewis and Austen, 1984; Robinson *et al.*, 1989).

Mast Cell Mediators and Immediate Hypersensitivity

Mast cell-derived mediators are able to exert many different actions, and thereby participate in many physiological and pathological reactions. Consideration of every biological effect of all mast cell-associated substances would require a separate review and is beyond the scope of the present paper. However, the major effects of mast cell mediators in immediate hypersensitivity reactions and the development of allergic inflammation are summarized below.

The effects of histamine are mediated primarily through H_1 and H_2 receptors (Ash and Schild, 1966; White and Eiser, 1983). Histamine H_1 receptor-mediated effects include contraction of airways and gastro-intestinal tract smooth muscle, increased vasopermeability, nasal mucus production, pruritus and cutaneous vasodilation. In allergic responses, the results of H_2 receptor stimulation include increased vasopermeability and vasodilation and modulation of leukocyte function. Prostaglandin D_2 injected intradermally causes vasodilation, increased vasopermeability and a prolonged non-pruritic wheal-and-flare reaction accompanied by an inflammatory cell infiltrate (Beasley *et al.*, 1987a). When inhaled, PGD_2 produces bronchoconstriction (Beasley *et al.*, 1987b). Platelet-activating factor is a potent inducer of platelet aggregation (O'Donnell *et al.*, 1979) and when injected intradermally, is 1000 times more potent than histamine at eliciting a wheal-and-flare response. It is also a potent bronchoconstrictor, and a potent chemotactic agent for eosinophils and, to a lesser extent, neutrophils (Wardlaw *et al.*, 1986).

Inhalation of LTs results in a slowly evolving, sustained constriction of both central and peripheral airways, LTC_4 and LTD_4 being up to 1000 times more potent bronchoconstrictor agents than histamine. The sulphidopeptide LTs are also potent stimulants of mucus secretion (Parker, 1989).

Despite the recognition of four mast cell neutral proteases, difficulty in obtaining them in sufficient quantities for large-scale studies of their biological properties has meant that we still know little of their biological role. Experiments using dog enzymes have shown that tryptase is capable of degrading the bronchoconstrictor neuropeptide, vasoactive intestinal peptide (VIP) but not its bronchodilator counterpart substance P (Tam and Caughey, 1990). Furthermore, canine tryptase has also been shown to have direct effects on dog bronchial muscle by directly increasing its sensitivity to contractile agonists such as histamine and serotonin (Sekizawa *et al.*, 1989). The actions of tryptase on neuropeptide metabolism and on myocyte function would both indicate a pro-asthmatic role for the neutral protease in the lung. It has also been shown that chymase can degrade substance P (Caughey *et al.*, 1988) and this may have an important regulatory effect in mast cell–nerve interactions, for example during neurogenic inflammation in the skin.

It is now accepted that the early phase of immediate hypersensitivity reactions is largely the result of the release and actions of the mast cell mediators histamine, PGD_2, LTC_4/D_4, and PAF. The action of these mediators may be supplemented by the generation of kinins by the actions of tryptase and TAME-esterases released by mast cells and by neuropeptide release following nerve stimulation. In the lungs these mediators induce bronchoconstriction, oedema of the airway walls and secretion of mucus. In the nose mast cell mediators induce rhinorrhoea, nasal blockage and sneezing by a combination of actions on the vasculature and sensory nerve endings, and in the skin local vasodilation and oedema.

Allergic late phase responses (LPR) are delayed-in-time responses and are recognized in the lung as airway obstruction, in the skin as erythema and oedema, in the nose as blockage and itching, and in the conjunctiva as oedema and itching. LPRs occur some 3–12 h after exposure to the relevant allergen and persist for several hours. The pathogenesis of the LPR remains unresolved although a number of mechanisms have been proposed to explain it. The role of mast cells and mast cell-derived products in late phase reaction is controversial, and, in general, it is thought that this cell does not play a primary mediator-secreting role. Moreover, it appears that the late phase reaction cannot be attributed to the action of a single mediator or a single type of cell, but it is rather thought to be a consequence of infiltration and activation of various cells, including eosinophils, basophils, neutrophils and macrophages. Also T-lymphocyte infiltration is a feature of the late phase response to allergen in atopic individuals in both the skin and lung (Frew and Kay, 1988; Metzger *et al.*, 1987). This may have particular relevance as the TH_2-lymphocyte has been suggested to coordinate the function of other cells at this stage (Mosmann and Coffman, 1989). Because of the participation of so many pro-inflammatory cells, our current understanding of the late phase reaction is that its chronic aspects are best considered as representing an inflammatory process, particularly chronic allergic inflammation.

Although mast cells are thought not to contribute directly to the LPR, they are involved in the recruitment of inflammatory cells, especially eosinophils, to the reaction site during allergic inflammation. While histamine and a number of peptides, varying from tetramers to oligomers, may attract eosinophils, the most potent stimulus would appear to be PAF (Wardlaw *et al.*, 1986). It should be pointed out that none of these substances is specific for eosinophils but will attract neutrophils as well. Simultaneously, mast cell-derived histamine and PGD_2 cause increased vasopermeability, leukotrienes increase the adherence of leukocytes to the vascular endothelium, and neutral proteases degrade blood vessel basement membrane, all events which are facilitatory to the influx of inflammatory cells. The recognition that IgE-dependent stimulation of human mast cells results in the generation of cytokine interleukins is of essential importance and provides a new mechanism whereby mast cells could contribute to the selective recruitment of eosinophils and mononuclear cells.

Mast Cell–Leukocyte Interactions

If mast cells and leukocytes both contribute to the development of allergic inflammation then it would seem logical for there to be a two-way dialogue between them, each contributing to the development and maturation of the other.

The primary stimulus for the induction of cellular influx and maturation is the generation, and subsequent effects, of cytokine interleukins. While T-lymphocytes are currently thought to be the main source of cytokines, the observations that mast cells can also generate these substances would suggest that they may also influence the development of allergic inflammation. Experiments with rodent mast cells and mast cell lines have shown that mast cells have the capacity to generate various cytokines including IL-3, IL-4, IL-5, IL-6 and granulocyte–macrophage colony-stimulating factor (GM–CSF) (Plaut *et al.*, 1989; Gordon *et al.*, 1990). It has also been shown that activated cultured mast cells express and release mRNA for multiple cytokines, including interferon-γ (IFN-γ) (Brown *et al.*, 1987). Human skin mast cells have recently been reported to contain and release tumour necrosis factor-α/cachectin (TNF-α) (Walsh *et al.*, 1991). It has been also shown not only that preformed immunoreactive IL-4 in nasal and bronchial biopsies is contained within mast cells but also that up to 80% of mast cells contain this interleukin (Bradding *et al.*, 1992). In addition to examining biopsies, the presence of this cytokine was also demonstrated in dispersed mast cells. These observations that mast cells are a source of cytokine interleukins are of crucial importance to understanding mast cell participation in many reactions, including inflammatory processes. Cytokines are pleotropic, exhibiting multiple biological activities, and interact with one another in a regulatory "network". In this network, a single cytokine can simultaneously induce itself or other cytokines, modulate cell-surface cytokine receptors, and act in a synergistic, additive or antagonistic manner, all of which result in modulation/regulation of cellular function. IL-3 is a haematopoietic growth factor affecting the earliest stages of maturation of a variety of cell lineages, including granulocytes, eosinophils, megakaryocytes, erythrocytes, macrophages and mast cells (Ihle and Weinstein, 1986). IL-4 appears to have a major role in the regulation of B cell immunoglobulin isotype switching to the heavy chain constant region ϵ and γ genes, thereby inducing the preferential production of IgE and IgG subclasses (Coffman *et al.*, 1986; Snapper *et al.*, 1988) and has recently been reported to induce expression of the adhesion proteins endothelial leukocyte adhesion molecule-1 (ELAM-1) and vascular cell adhesion molecule-1 (VCAM-1) (Schleimer *et al.* 1992). IL-5 is essential for terminal differentiation of the eosinophils from their committed precursors (Clutterbuck *et al.*, 1989) and also primes mature eosinophils for more efficient effector cell functions (Lopez *et al.*, 1988; Sher *et al.*, 1990). Thus, IL-5 could lead to the specific recruitment of eosinophils, enhanced eosinophil cytotoxicity and prolonged eosinophil survival. IL-6 displays growth factor activity, playing an important role in the regulation of normal haematopoiesis by acting synergistically with IL-3 to sustain proliferation of progenitor stem cells (Ikebuchi *et al.*, 1987).

The concept that mast cells may store preformed cytokines, particularly IL-4, which they release on immunological activation, is particularly attractive as an initiating factor in allergic inflammation. It is now established that TH_2 cells need a pulse of IL-4 to proliferate and generate their spectrum of cytokines (Le Gros *et al.*, 1990; Teper *et al.*, 1990). The explosive release of IL-4 from activated mast cells would provide this pulse and thus act as the initiating signal to TH_2 cell involvement in the response. Also, the rapid accumulation of inflammatory leukocytes in the airways which occurs within minutes of allergen challenge is not readily explicable by the *de novo* synthesis of cytokines by lymphocytes but would be explained by such a release of cytokines by mast cells.

The accumulation and activation of eosinophils at the site of provocation is characteristic of the allergic response. This cell has an armoury of preformed and newly generated mediators which are implicated in causing the chronic tissue damage in asthma. Of particular note are the basic granule-associated proteins which interact with eosin to give the cell its typical staining properties (Gleich and Adolphson, 1986). These proteins include major basic protein (MBP), eosinophil cationic protein (ECP), eosinophil peroxidase (EPO) and eosinophil-derived neurotoxin (EDN) (Peters *et al.*, 1986). In addition to causing secretion of these preformed proteins, eosinophil activation initiates the *de novo* production of LTC_4, PAF, 15-hydroxyeicosatetraenoic acid (15-HETE) and active species of oxygen (Lee *et al.*, 1984; Foegh *et al.*, 1986; Kanofsky *et al.*, 1988; Sigal *et al.*, 1988). Eosinophils have also been suggested to be a source of enzymes such as histaminase, arylsulphatase and phospholipase D (Archer and Hirsch, 1963; Zeiger *et al.*, 1976a,b) and neuropeptides, particularly substance P and a truncated form of VIP (Aliakbari *et al.*, 1987; Weinstock *et al.*, 1988). These products act in concert to produce many of the cytotoxic effects associated with the eosinophil.

The interrelationships between the mast cell and the eosinophil are particularly pertinent to this review. As stated above, mast cell-derived chemoattractants PAF, ECF-A and histamine all promote eosinophil accumulation (Clark *et al.*, 1975; Wardlaw *et al.*, 1986) while IL-3, IL-5 and GM–CSF will assist in the maturation and priming of eosinophils (Sanderson *et al.*, 1985; Lopez *et al.*, 1988). PAF will also serve to activate eosinophils for the generation of both preformed and newly generated mediators (Kroegel *et al.*, 1988). In reverse, MBP has been reported to release histamine from rodent mast cells by a temperature-dependent, energy-requiring, non-cytotoxic process (O'Donnell *et al.*, 1983; Zheutlin *et al.*, 1984). It does not, however, have a similar effect on human mast cells but preliminary results suggest that it may have a small priming effect on human skin mast cells for IgE-dependent histamine release while inhibiting release induced by substance P (Okayama and Church, unpublished observations). The EPO-hydrogen peroxidase-halide system and ECP have also been reported to induce histamine release from rodent mast cells (Henderson *et al.*, 1980). In contrast, eosinophil enzymes, particularly histaminase, will aid in the inactivation of mast cell products (Zeiger *et al.*, 1976b). It was reported that eosinophil-derived arylsulphatase was capable of degrading LTC_4 (Wasserman *et al.*, 1975) but discriminating experiments *in vitro* suggest that this is unlikely.

A field of study which has attracted much recent interest is the ability of mononuclear cells and neutrophils to interact with histamine-releasing cells by production of specific histamine-releasing factors (HRFs) and histamine release inhibitory factors (HRIFs). However, almost all these studies have been performed on basophils rather than mast cells.

Histamine-releasing factor was first described by Thueson and colleagues (1979a,b) as a factor synthesized by human mononuclear cells which induced histamine release from human basophils. Since that time, many HRFs have been reported to be generated from a variety of cell sources including alveolar macrophages (Schulman *et al.*, 1985), platelets (Orchard *et al.*, 1986), B- and T-lymphocytes (Sedgwick *et al.*, 1981; Haak-Frendscho *et al.*, 1988b), neutrophils (White and Kaliner, 1987; White *et al.*, 1989) and eosinophils (O'Donnell *et al.*, 1983). Furthermore, HRFs have been found in fluids obtained from nasal lavages (Sim *et al.*, 1990), late phase blister fluids (Warner *et al.*, 1986) and bronchoalveolar lavage fluids (Gittlen *et al.*, 1988; Alam *et al.*, 1990). All these HRFs induce non-cytotoxic, calcium-dependent histamine release from human basophils (Thueson *et al.*, 1979b; Dvorak *et al.*, 1984) and those which have been examined also induce the release of LTD_4 (Ezeamuzie and Assem, 1985). Relatively few studies have been reported on the effect of HRFs on mast cell mediator release. Human lung mast cells degranulate when exposed to HRF produced by macrophages (Ezeamuzie and Assem, 1983; Schulman *et al.*, 1985). HRF from mononuclear cells isolated from asthmatic patients causes histamine release from human lung mast cells obtained by bronchoalveolar lavage (Kuna *et al.*, 1992). The synovial mast cells are also activated to release histamine by mononuclear cell-derived HRF (Gruber *et al.*, 1986). The secretion of histamine from murine, rat and guinea-pig mast cells induced by HRF from human lymphocytes has also been observed (Brzezinska-Blaszczyk *et al.*, 1988).

The synthesis of a histamine release inhibitory factor (HRIF) by human mononuclear cells has also been observed (Alam *et al.*, 1988). The generation of human HRIF is increased by physiological concentrations of histamine, suggesting a mechanism for feedback inhibition of histamine secretion (Alam *et al.*, 1988). HRIF is synthesized in greater quantities by B cells, followed by T cells and monocytes (Alam *et al.*, 1989).

The exact mechanisms by which HRFs induce histamine release is still unknown but they are likely to be diverse. It has been suggested recently that HRFs derived from alveolar macrophages, platelets and nasal washings stimulate basophil mediator release by interacting with surface-bound IgE (Liu *et al.*, 1986; Orchard *et al.*, 1986; MacDonald *et al.*,

1987). Furthermore, it has been postulated that this HRF binds only a more highly glycosylated species of IgE which has been designated as IgE+ (MacDonald *et al.*, 1987; Lichtenstein, 1988). Lichtenstein (1988) has proposed that IgE+ molecules occur only in atopic individuals, that the presence of IgE+ is related to the late phase reaction and that HRFs are responsible for the mediator release from human basophils that occurs at this time. More recently it has been shown that the interleukin, IL-3, may also act as a histamine-releasing factor from human basophils (Haak-Frendscho *et al.*, 1988a), and that the mechanism of action of this cytokine is interaction with membrane-bound IgE+ (Okayama and Church, 1992). IL-3 does not, however, release histamine from human mast cells (Valent *et al.*, 1990).

Histamine-releasing factors are a heterogeneous family of molecules varying in molecular size, stability when heated, in their capability to bind to IgE and, probably, in their requirement for interactions with surface-bound IgE. Some HRFs do not appear to release histamine in an IgE-dependent manner (Baeza *et al.*, 1988; Broide *et al.*, 1990). At least part of this heterogeneity may be accounted for by variability in the cellular source of HRFs. Whatever the mechanism is, it should be pointed out that there are indeed many processes in which activation of basophil/mast cell by HRFs may have an essential role. The production of HRFs by cells known to be involved in inflammatory responses strongly suggests a fundamental role of this factor in inflammation. Thus, the relationship between mast cells and leukocytes is complex and bidirectional, the subtleties of such interactions are as yet poorly understood, however.

Mast Cell–Nerve Interactions

There is increasing evidence that neural mechanisms may also participate in the inflammatory response in several tissues and that there is a close interaction between inflammatory cells and nerves (Barnes, 1986; Bienenstock *et al.*, 1989). The neurotransmitters released from the nerves may influence the inflammatory response, either enhancing or suppressing the degree of inflammation. This sequence of events, known as neurogenic inflammation, mimics various manifestations of diseases. Neuropeptides, small amino acid components that are localized particularly to sensory neurones, are capable of affecting inflammatory cell function. For example, substance P causes T-lymphocytes to proliferate (Payan *et al.*, 1983), macrophages to release pro-inflammatory and immunomodulatory substances (Hartung *et al.*, 1986), enhanced phagocytosis by macrophages and by neutrophils (Bar-Shavit *et al.*, 1980) and enhanced production of immunoglobulins by B-lymphocytes (Stanisz *et al.*, 1986). Both substance P and neurokinin A (NKA) stimulate the release of IL-4, TNF-α, and IL-6 from human blood monocytes (Lotz *et al.*, 1988). In contrast, vasoactive intestinal peptide (VIP) has been demonstrated to have various anti-inflammatory actions. VIP inhibits human natural killer cell activity, lymphocyte traffic and lymphocyte proliferation (Drew and Shearman, 1985; Stanisz *et al.*, 1986, 1988). In the airways, substance P is bronchoconstrictor and VIP is bronchodilator.

It is now clear that communication between nerves and mast cells exists (Skofitsch *et al.*, 1985; Bienenstock *et al.*, 1987, 1989), and is bidirectional, neuropeptides being capable of stimulating mast cell mediator secretion, while mast cell mediators have the capability of initiating neuronal reflexes and of metabolizing neuropeptides.

It has been established that several basic neuropeptides including substance P, VIP and somatostatin induce histamine release from rat and murine mast cells (Johnson and Erdos, 1973; Pearce and Thompson, 1986). It has also been shown that these neuropeptides induce histamine release from human mast cells dispersed from the skin (Lowman *et al.*, 1988a) but not those dispersed from lung, intestinal mucosa, intestinal submucosa, adenoids and tonsils which appear to be unresponsive to neuropeptide stimulation (Lowman *et al.*, 1988b; Rees *et al.*, 1988). It is now well documented with dispersed human skin mast cells that substance P, VIP and somatostatin all induce a similar, concentration-dependent release of histamine (Benyon *et al.*, 1987; Lowman *et al.*, 1988a; Church *et al.*, 1991). Release of histamine is rapid and a transient elevation of intracellular calcium is observed, but the calcium is mobilized from intracellular stores, probably the endoplasmic reticulum or the inner leaflet of the cell membrane (Benyon *et al.*, 1987). Stimulation with neuropeptides causes only minimal eicosanoid generation in skin mast cells (Benyon *et al.*, 1989). The activation of mast cells by substance P is not mediated via a classical tachykinin receptor, but rather by interaction with a site of a low affinity and low specificity for neuropeptides which is distinct from those involved in IgE-dependent mast cell activation (Lowman *et al.*, 1988a). The nature of the activation site on skin mast cells has not been elucidated although it has been suggested that neuropeptides may interact directly with membrane-associated G proteins (Penner, 1988; Mousli *et al.*, 1990).

The ability of mast cell mediators to induce sensory stimulation can be demonstrated by examination of the wheal-and-flare response. Injection of histamine intradermally induces a local oedematous wheal surrounded by a large erythema, the flare, which may be prevented by the administration of histamine H_1 antagonists or by the injection of local anaesthetic into the skin. The proposed mechanism of this response is the stimulation of H_1 receptors on the sensory nerve endings of non-myelinated nerve fibres to initiate a local antidromic generation of neuropeptides from another branch of the same nerve. The secondary release of neuropeptides at a site distinct from the wheal results in vasodilation, either by a direct effect on the blood vessels or secondary to neuropeptide-induced mast cell degranulation.

A major factor in the modulation of neurogenic inflammation is the metabolism of neuropeptides. Numerous peptidases have been described as being capable of fulfilling this function, including neural endopeptidase (NEP), angiotensin-converting enzyme (ACE) (Erdos and Skidgel, 1989) and mast cell proteases (Caughey *et al.*, 1988; Franconi *et al.*, 1989). Of these, NEP in particular has been suggested to be axial in the modulation of neurogenic inflammation (Nadel, 1991). This enzyme is localised to epithelial cells, fibroblasts and neutrophils, with little activity found in endothelial cells (Painter *et al.*, 1988; Erdos and Skidgel, 1989). When epithelium is intact and healthy, production of NEP limits the amplitude of neurogenic inflammation by its proteolytic actions. However, when airway epithelium is shed or damaged, as is often the case in severe asthma, there is a relative reduction of NEP and thus the effects of tachykinins are markedly potentiated. The recognition that mast cell-derived neural proteases chymase and tryptase can degrade neuropeptides (Caughey *et al.*, 1988; Franconi *et al.*, 1989) suggests a role for mast cells also in modulation of neurogenic inflammation. Comparison of substrate specificities suggests that mast cell tryptase and NEP may cooperate in degrading neuropeptides, substance P and NKA being the preferential substrates for NEP (Hooper *et al.*, 1985; Katayama *et al.*, 1990), with VIP and calcitonin gene-related peptide (CGRP) being degraded avidly by mast cell tryptase. However, an imbalance of these enzymes, as has been purported to occur in asthma, would result in the selective survival of specific tachykinins. For example, deficiency of NEP together with the activation of MC_T would result in the preferential degradation of the bronchodilator neuropeptide VIP while the broncho-constrictor peptides substance P and NKA would exert their effects unopposed. This would result in increased airway smooth muscle tone and hyperreactivity, oedema, plasma extravasation and mucus hypersecretion, all features of asthma. In addition, substance P-immuno-reactive nerves have been reported to proliferate in asthmatic airways particularly in the submucosa (Ollerenshaw *et al.*, 1989). Neurogenic inflammation is readily demonstrated to contribute to airway inflammatory responses in animal airways where capsaicin pretreatment reduces the vasodilator response to allergen in pig airways (Alving *et al.*, 1988) and the microvascular leakage which follows exposure of rats to toluene diisocyanate (Thompson *et al.*, 1987). The mechanism of neurogenic inflammation in human airways, however, remains to be elucidated.

Evidence that neurogenic inflammation may be involved in inflammatory reactions in the skin derives from studies of the effects of neuropeptides injected intradermally and from the use of capsaicin to deplete the neuropeptides from primary sensory afferents. Substance P, somatostatin, and VIP all induce a wheal-and-flare reaction when injected into human skin (Anand *et al.*, 1983; Foreman *et al.*, 1983), and this correlates with their ability to release histamine from isolated skin mast cells. On the other hand, CGRP and NKA which do not induce histamine release from human skin mast cells, cause a local persistent erythema (CGRP) or local vasodilation (NKA), neither of which are accompanied by flare reactions (Brain *et al.*, 1986). The flare or vasodilatory component of the triple response is blocked by nerve section, local anaesthesia or depletion of neuropeptides by pretreatment of the skin with capsaicin (Anand *et al.*, 1983; Foreman *et al.*, 1983). Histamine H_1 antagonists also markedly reduce the flare (Foreman *et al.*, 1983; Saria and Lundberg, 1983), suggesting that histamine is involved in its development. Furthermore, evidence for a direct link between neuropeptides, mast cells and some forms of urticaria has also been presented (Kaplan *et al.*, 1975; Toth-Kasa *et al.*, 1983; Heavey *et al.*, 1986).

Conclusion

It is well established that mast cells are ordinarily distributed throughout normal human tissues and that they are the source of a variety of mediators which are able to exert many different actions. The mast cell-derived mediators are released after activation and can all influence adjacent cells, surrounding matrix tissues and neuropeptides. Moreover, there are many factors, both IgE-dependent and IgE-independent, which may cause activation of mast cells leading to the release of their mediators.

The mast cell is now considered to play a pivotal role not only in allergic responses but also in a number of inflammatory disorders. Inflammation is defined as a localized or systemic protective response elicited by injury to cells or tissues, and serves to destroy, dilute or wall off both injurious agents and the injured tissues. Acute allergic inflammation which is evoked during immediate hypersensitivity reactions totally or in part by IgE-dependent mast cell activation, is of short duration. Chronic allergic inflammation is of longer duration, is characterized by infiltration with many various cells, and is thought to be a consequence of cooperation between these cells. Moreover, it seems that neuropeptides are also involved in evoking chronic inflammation, because of the multiple cell systems stimulated by neuropeptides and the wide array of stimuli that could activate the sensory nerves to release their mediators. However, the exact role of neurogenic inflammation remains to be elucidated. Having taken account of all the above information, it would appear that chronic allergic inflammation is evoked by a combination of actions of a variety of cells and nerve and that the mast cell has an important part to play in the process.

References

Alam, R., Grant, J.A. and Lett-Brown, M.A. (1988). Identification of a histamine release inhibitory factor produced by human mononuclear cells in vitro. *J. Clin. Invest.* **82**, 2056–2062.

Alam, R., Forsythe, P.A., Lett-Brown, M.A. and Grant, J.A. (1989). Study of the cellular origin of histamine release inhibitory factor using highly purified subsets of mononuclear cells. *J. Immunol.* **143**, 2280–2284.

Alam, R., Welter, J., Forsythe, P.A., Lett-Brown, M.A., Rankin, J.A., Boyars, M. and Grant, J.A. (1990). Detection of histamine release inhibitory factor- and histamine releasing factor-like activities in bronchoalveolar lavage fluids. *Am. Rev. Respir. Dis.* **141**, 666–671.

Aldenborg, F. and Enerback, L. (1985). Thymus dependence of connective tissue mast cells: a quantitative cytofluorometric study of the growth of peritoneal mast cells in normal and athymic rats. *Int. Arch. Allergy Appl. Immunol.* **78**, 277–282.

Aliakbari, J., Sreedharan, S.P., Turck, C.W. and Goetzl, E.J. (1987). Selective localization of vasoactive intestinal peptide and substance P in human eosinophils. *Biochem. Biophys. Res. Commun.* **148**, 1440–1445.

Alving, K., Matran, R., Lacroix, J.S. and Lundberg, J.M. (1988). Allergen challenge induces vasodilation in pig bronchial circulation via a capsaicin-sensitive mechanism. *Acta Physiol. Scand.* **134**, 571–572.

Anand, P., Bloom, S.R. and McGregor, G.P. (1983). Topical capsaicin pretreatment inhibits axon reflex vasodilation caused by somatostatin and vasoactive intestinal polypeptide in human skin. *Brit. J. Pharmacol.* **78**, 665–669.

Archer, G.T. and Hirsch, J.G. (1963). Isolation of granules from eosinophil leucocytes and study of their enzyme content. *J. Exp. Med.* **118**, 277–286.

Ash, A.S. and Schild, H.O. (1966). Receptors mediating some actions of histamine. *Brit. J. Pharmac. Chemother.* **27**, 427–437.

Askenase, P.W., Bursztajn, S., Gershon, M.D. and Gershon, R.K. (1980). T cell-dependent mast cell degranulation and release of serotonin in murine delayed-type hypersensitivity. *J. Exp. Med.* **152**, 1358–1374.

Atkins, P.C., Norman, M., Weiner, H. and Zweiman, B. (1977). Release of neutrophil chemotactic activity during immediate hypersensitivity reactions in humans. *Ann. Intern. Med.* **86**, 415–418.

Azizkhan, R.G., Azizkhan, J.C., Zetter, B.R. and Folkman, J. (1980). Mast cell heparin stimulates migration of capillary endothelial cells *in vitro*. *J. Exp. Med.* **152**, 931–944.

Baeza, M.L., Haak-Frendscho, M., Satnick, S. and Kaplan, A.P. (1988) Responsiveness to human mononuclear cell-derived histamine-releasing factor. Studies of allergic status and the role of IgE. *J. Immunol.* **141**, 2688–2692.

Barnes, P.J. (1986). Asthma as an axon reflex. *Lancet* **1**, 242–245.

Bar-Shavit, Z., Goldman, R., Stabinsky, Y., Gottlieb, P., Fridkin, M., Teichberg, V.I. and Blumberg, S. (1980). Enhancement of phagocytosis – a newly found activity of substance P residing in its N-terminal tetrapeptide sequence. *Biochem. Biophys. Res. Commun.* **99**, 1445–1451.

Beasley, C.R.W., Hovell, C.J., Mani, R., Robinson, C. and Holgate, S.T. (1987a). The comparative vascular effects of histamine, prostaglandin (PG) D2 and its metabolite 9α11b-PGF_2 in human skin. *Brit. J. Clin. Pharmacol.* **23**, 605P–606P.

Beasley, C.R.W., Varley, J., Robinson, C. and Holgate, S.T. (1987b). Direct and reflex bronchoconstrictor actions of prostaglandin (PG) D_2 and its initial metabolite 9α11b-PGF_2 in asthma. *Brit. J. Clin. Pharmacol.* **23**, 606P–607P.

Benditt, E.P., Wong, R.L., Arase, M. and Roeper, E. (1955). 5-hydroxytryptamine in mast cells. *Proc. Soc. Exp. Biol. Med.* **90**, 303–304.

Benyon, R.C., Lowman, M.A. and Church, M.K. (1987). Human skin mast cells: their dispersion, purification, and secretory characterization. *J. Immunol.* **138**, 861–867.

Benyon, R.C., Robinson, C. and Church, M.K. (1989). Differential release of histamine and eicosanoids from human skin mast cells activated by IgE-dependent and non-immunological stimuli. *Brit. J. Pharmacol.* **97**, 898–904.

Bienenstock, J., Blennerhassett, M., Kakuta, Y., MacQueen, G., Marshall, J., Perdue, M., Castells, M.C., Irani, A.-M. and Schwartz, L.B. (1987). Evaluation of human peripheral blood leukocytes for mast cell tryptase. *J. Immunol.* **138**, 2184–2189.

Bienenstock, J., Blennerhassett, M., Kakuta, Y., MacQueen, G., Marshall, J., Perdue, M., Siegel, S., Tsuda, T., Denburg, J. and Stead, R. (1989). Evidence for central and peripheral nervous system interaction with mast cells. *In* "Mast Cell and Basophil Differentiation in Health and Disease" (S.J. Galli and K.F. Austen, eds), pp. 275–284. Raven Press, New York.

Binazzi, M. and Rampichini, L. (1959). Investigations on the regional distribution of mast cells in human skin. *Ital. Gen. Rev. Dermatol.* **1**, 17–21.

Boswell, R.N., Austen, K.F. and Goetzl, E.J. (1978). Intermediate molecular weight eosinophil chemotactic factors in rat peritoneal mast cells. Immunologic release, granule association, and demonstration of structural heterogeneity. *J. Immunol.* **120**, 15–20.

Bradding, P., Feather, I.H., Howarth, P.H., Mueller, R., Roberts, J.A., Britten, K., Bews, J.P.A., Hunt, T.C., Okayama, Y., Heusser, C.H., Bullock, G.R., Church, M.K. and Holgate, S.T. (1992). Interleukin-4 is localised to and released by human mast cells. *J. Exp. Med.* **176**, 1381–1386.

Brain, S.D., Tippins, J.R., Morris, H.R., MacIntyre, I. and Williams, T.J. (1986). Potent vasodilator activity of calcitonin gene-related peptide in human skin. *J. Invest. Dermatol.* **87**, 533–536.

Bressler, R.B., Thompson, H.L., Keffer, J.M. and Metcalfe, D.D. (1989). Inhibition of the growth of IL-3-dependent mast cells from murine bone marrow by recombinant granulocyte macrophage-colony-stimulating factor. *J. Immunol.* **143**, 135–139.

Broide, D.H., Smith, C.M. and Wasserman, S.I. (1990). Mast cells and pulmonary fibrosis. Identification of a histamine releasing factor in bronchoalveolar lavage. *J. Immunol.* **145**, 1838–1844.

Brown, M.A., Pierce, J.H., Watson, C.J., Falco, J., Ihle, J.N. and Paul, W.E. (1987). B cell stimulatory factor-1/interleukin-4 mRNA is expressed by normal and transformed mast cells. *Cell* **50**, 809–818.

Brzezinska-Blaszczyk, E., Czuwaj, M. and Kuna, P. (1988). Histamine release from mast cells of various species induced by histamine releasing factor from human lymphocytes. *Agents Actions* **21**, 26–31.

Castells, M.C., Irani, A.M. and Schwartz, L.B. (1987). Evaluation of human peripheral blood leucocytes for mast cell tryptase. *J. Immunol.* **138**, 2184–2189.

Caughey, G.H., Leidig, F., Viro, N.F. and Nadel, J.A. (1988). Substance P and vasoactive intestinal peptide degradation by mast cell tryptase and chymase. *J. Pharmacol. Exp. Ther.* **244**, 133–137.

Church, M.K., El Lati, S. and Okayama, Y. (1991). Biological properties of human skin mast cells. *Clin. Exp. Allergy* **21** (suppl. 3), 1–9.

Clark, R.A.F., Gallin, J.I. and Kaplan, A.P. (1975). The selective eosinophil chemotactic activity of histamine. *J. Exp. Med.* **142**, 1462–1476.

Clutterbuck, E.J., Hirst, E.M.A. and Sanderson, C.J. (1989). Human interleukin-5 (IL-5) regulates the production of eosinophils in human bone marrow cultures: Comparison and interaction with IL-1, IL-3, IL-6, and GMCSF. *Blood* **73**, 1504–1512.

Coffman, R.L., Ohara, J., Bond, M.W., Carty, J., Zlotnik, A. and Paul, W.E. (1986). B cell stimulatory factor-1 enhances the IgE response of lipopolysaccharide-activated B cells. *J. Immunol.* **136**, 4538–4541.

Craig, S.S., DeBlois, G. and Schwartz, L.B. (1986). Mast cells in human keloid, small intestine, and lung by an immunoperoxidase technique using a murine monoclonal antibody against tryptase. *Am. J. Pathol.* **124**, 427–435.

Craig, S.S., Schechter, N.M. and Schwartz, L.B. (1988). Ultrastructural analysis of human T and TC mast cells identified by immunoelectron microscopy. *Lab. Invest.* **58**, 682–691.

Crowle, P.K. and Starkey, J.R. (1989). Mast cells and tumor-associated angiogenesis. *In* "Mast Cell and Basophil Differentiation and Function in Health and Disease" (S.J. Galli and K.F. Austen, eds), pp. 307–315. Raven Press, New York.

Czarnetzki, B.M., Sterry, W., Bazin, H. and Kalveram, K.J. (1982). Evidence that tissue mast cells derive from mononuclear phagocytes. *Int. Arch. Allergy Appl. Immunol.* **67**, 44–48.

Dahlen, S.E., Hedqvist, P., Hammarstrom, S. and Samuelsson, B. (1980). Leukotrienes are potent constrictors of human bronchi. *Nature* **288**, 484–486.

Drew, P.A. and Shearman, D.J. (1985). Vaso-active intestinal peptide: a neurotransmitter which reduces human NK cell activity and increases Ig synthesis. *Aust. J. Exp. Biol. Med. Sci.* **63**, 313–318.

Dvorak, A.M., Lett-Brown, M.A., Thueson, D.O., Pyne, K., Raghuprased, P.K., Galli, S.J. and Grant, J.A. (1984). Histamine-releasing activity (HRA). III. HRA induces human basophil histamine release by provoking noncytotoxic granule exocytosis. *Clin. Immunol. Immunopathol.* **32**, 142–150.

Dvorak, A.M., Saito, H., Estrella, P., Kissell, S., Arai, N. and Ishizaka, T.

(1989). Ultrastructure of eosinophils and basophils stimulated to develop in human cord blood mononuclear cell cultures containing recombinant human interleukin-5 or interleukin-3. *Lab. Invest.* **61**, 116–132.

Eady, R.A.J., Cowen, T., Marshall, T.F., Plummer, V. and Greaves, M.W. (1979). Mast cell population density, blood vessel density and histamine content of normal human skin. *Brit. J. Dermatol.* **100**, 623–633.

Ehrlich, P. (1878). Beiträge zur Theorie und Praxis der histologischen Färbung. Leipzig Thesis.

Erdos, E.G. and Skidgel, R.A. (1989). Neutral endopeptidase 24.11 (enkephalinase) and related regulators of peptide hormones. *FASEB J.* **3**, 145–151.

Ezeamuzie, I.C. and Assem, E.S. (1983). A study of histamine release from human basophils and lung mast cells by products of lymphocyte stimulation. *Agents Actions* **13**, 222–230.

Ezeamuzie, I.C. and Assem, E.S. (1985). Release of slow reacting substance (SRS) from human leucocytes by lymphokine. *Int. J. Immunopharmacol.* **7**, 533–542.

Farram, E. and Nelson, D.S. (1980). Mouse mast cells as anti-tumor effector cells. *Cell Immunol.* **55**, 294–301.

Foegh, M.L., Maddox, Y.T. and Ramwell, P.W. (1986). Human peritoneal eosinophils and formation of arachidonate cyclooxygenase products. *Scand. J. Immunol.* **23**, 599–603.

Foreman, J.C., Jordan, C.C., Oehme, P. and Renner, H. (1983). Structure-activity relationships for some substance P-related peptides that cause wheal and flare reactions in human skin. *J. Physiol. (Lond.)* **335**, 449–465.

Fox, B., Bull, T.B. and Guz, A. (1981). Mast cells in the human alveolar wall: an electromicroscopic study. *J. Clin. Pathol.* **34**, 1333–1342.

Franconi, G.M., Graf, P.D., Lazarus, S.C., Nadel, J.A. and Caughey, G.H. (1989). Mast cell tryptase and chymase reverse airway smooth muscle relaxation induced by vasoactive intestinal peptide in the ferret. *J. Pharmacol. Exp. Ther.* **248**, 947–951.

Frew, A.J. and Kay, A.B. (1988). The relationship between infiltrating CD4+ lymphocytes, activated eosinophils, and the magnitude of the allergen-induced late phase cutaneous reaction in man. *J. Immunol.* **141**, 4158–4164.

Furitsu, T., Saito, H., Dvorak, A.M., Schwartz, L.B., Irani, A.-M.A., Burdick, J.F., Ishizaka, K. and Ishizaka, T. (1989). Development of human mast cells *in vitro*. *Proc. Natl. Acad. Sci. U.S.A.* **86**, 10039–10043.

Galli, S.J., Dvorak, A.M. and Dvorak, H.F. (1984). Basophils and mast cells: morphologic insights into their biology, secretory patterns, and function. *Progr. Allergy* **34**, 1–141.

Gittlen, S.D., MacDonald, S.M., Bleecker, E.R., Liu, M.C., Kagey-Sobotka, A. and Lichtenstein, L.M. (1988). An IgE-dependent histamine releasing factor (HRF) in human bronchoalveolar lavage (BAL) fluid. *FASEB J.* **2**, A1232.

Gleich, G.J. and Adolphson, C.R. (1986). The eosinophilic leukocyte: Structure and function. *Adv. Immunol.* **39**, 177–253.

Goetzl, E.J. and Austen, K.F. (1975). Purification and synthesis of eosinophilotactic tetrapeptides of human lung tissue: Identification as eosinophil chemotactic factor of anaphylaxis. *Proc. Natl. Acad. Sci. U.S.A.* **72**, 4123–4127.

Goldstein, S.M., Kaempfer, C.E., Kealey, J.T. and Wintroub, B.U. (1989).

Human mast cell carboxypeptidase. Purification and characterization. *J. Clin. Invest.* **83**, 1630–1636.

Gordon, J.R., Burd, P.R. and Galli, S.J. (1990). Mast cells as a source of multifunctional cytokines. *Immunol. Today* **11**, 458–464.

Goto, T., Befus, D., Low, R. and Bienenstock, J. (1984). Mast cell heterogeneity and hyperplasia in bleomycin-induced pulmonary fibrosis of rats. *Am. Rev. Respir. Dis.* **130**, 797–802.

Gruber, B., Poznansky, M., Boss, E., Partin, J., Gorevic, P. and Kaplan, A.P. (1986). Characterization and functional studies of rheumatoid synovial mast cells. Activation by secretagogues, anti-IgE, and a histamine-releasing lymphokine. *Arthr. Rheum.* **29**, 944–955.

Gustowska, L., Ruitenberg, E.J., Elgersma, A. and Kociecka, W. (1983). Increase of mucosal mast cells in the jejunum of patients infected with Trichinella spiralis. *Int. Arch. Allergy Appl. Immunol.* **71**, 304–308.

Haak-Frendscho, M., Arai, N., Arai, K., Baeza, M.L., Finn, A. and Kaplan, A.P. (1988a). Human recombinant granulocyte-macrophage colony-stimulating factor and interleukin-3 cause basophil histamine release. *J. Clin. Invest.* **82**, 17–20.

Haak-Frendscho, M., Sarfati, M., Delespesse, G. and Kaplan, A.P. (1988b). Comparison of mononuclear cell and B-lymphoblastoid histamine-releasing factor and their distinction from an IgE-binding factor. *Clin. Immunol. Immunopathol.* **49**, 72–82.

Hamaguchi, Y., Kanakura, Y., Fujita, J., Takeda, S.-I., Nakano, T., Tarui, S., Honjo, T. and Kitamura, Y. (1987). Interleukin-4 as an essential factor for in vitro clonal growth of murine connective tissue-type mast cells. *J. Exp. Med.* **165**, 268–273.

Hartung, H.-P., Wolters, K. and Toyka, K.V. (1986). Substance P: binding properties and studies on cellular responses in guinea pig macrophages. *J. Immunol.* **136**, 3856–3863.

Hawkins, R.A., Claman, H.N., Clark, R.A.F. and Steigerwald, J.C. (1985). Increased dermal mast cell populations in progressive systemic sclerosis: a link in chronic fibrosis? *Ann. Intern. Med.* **102**, 182–186.

Heavey, D.J., Kobza-Black, A., Barrow, S.E., Chappell, C.G., Greaves, M.W. and Dollery, C.T. (1986). Prostaglandin D_2 and histamine release in cold urticaria. *J. Allergy Clin. Immunol.* **78**, 458–461.

Hellstrom, B. and Holmgreen, H. (1950). Numerical distribution of mast cells in the human skin and heart. *Acta Anat. (Basel)* **10**, 81–107.

Henderson, W.R. and Kaliner, M. (1978). Immunologic and nonimmunologic generation of superoxide from mast cells and basophils. *J. Clin. Invest.* **61**, 187–196.

Henderson, W.R. and Kaliner, M. (1979). Mast cell granule peroxidase: location, secretion, and SRS-A inactivation. *J. Immunol.* **122**, 1322–1328.

Henderson, W.R., Chi, E.Y. and Klebanoff, S.J. (1980). Eosinophil peroxidase-induced mast cell secretion. *J. Exp. Med.* **152**, 265–279.

Holgate, S.T., Burns, G.B., Robinson, C. and Church, M.K. (1984). Anaphylactic- and calcium-dependent generation of prostaglandin D_2 (PGD_2), thromboxane B_2, and other cyclooxygenase products of arachidonic acid by dispersed human lung cells and relationship to histamine release. *J. Immunol.* **133**, 2138–2144.

Hooper, N.M., Kenny, A.J. and Turner, A.J. (1985). The metabolism of neuropeptides. Neurokinin A (substance K) is a substrate for endopeptidase-

24.11 but not for peptidyl dipeptidae A (angiotensin-converting enzyme). *Biochem. J.* **231**, 357–361.

Ihle, J.N. and Weinstein, Y. (1986). Immunological regulation of hematopoietic/lymphoid stem cell differentiation by interleukin β. *Adv. Immunol.* **39**, 1–50.

Ihle, J.N., Keller, J., Oroszlan, S., Henderson, L.E., Copeland, T.D., Fitch, F., Prystowsky, M.B., Goldwasser, E., Schrader, J.W., Palaszynski, E., Dy, M. and Lebel, B. (1983). Biologic properties of homogeneous interleukin 3. I. Demonstration of WEHI-3 growth factor activity, mast cell growth factor activity, P cell stimulating factor activity, colony-stimulating factor activity, and histamine-producing cell-stimulating factor activity. *J. Immunol.* **131**, 282–287.

Ikebuchi, K., Wong, G.G., Clark, S.C., Ihle, J.N., Hirai, Y. and Ogawa, M. (1987). Interleukin-6 enhancement of interleukin-3-dependent proliferation of multipotential hematopoietic progenitors. *Proc. Natl. Acad. Sci. U.S.A.* **84**, 9035–9039.

Irani, A.-A. and Schwartz, L.B. (1990). Neutral proteases as indicators of human mast cell heterogeneity. *In* "Neutral Proteases of Mast Cells" (L.B. Schwartz, ed.), pp. 146–162. *Monogr. Allergy* 27, Karger, Basel.

Irani, A.A., Schechter, N.M., Craig, S.S., DeBlois, G. and Schwartz, L.B. (1986). Two types of human mast cells that have distinct neutral protease compositions. *Proc. Natl. Acad. Sci. U.S.A.* **83**, 4464–4468.

Ishizaka, T. and Ishizaka, K. (1984). Activation of mast cells for mediator release through IgE receptors. *Progr. Allergy* **34**, 188–235.

Ishizaka, T., Furitsu, T. and Inagaki, N. (1991). *In vitro* development and functions of human mast cells. *Int. Arch. Allergy Appl. Immunol.* **94**, 116–121.

Jarboe, D.L., Marshall, J.S., Randolph, T.R., Kukolja, A. and Huff, T.F. (1989). The mast cell-committed progenitor. I. Description of a cell capable of IL-3-independent proliferation and differentiation without contact with fibroblasts. *J. Immunol.* **142**, 2405–2417.

Johnson, A.R. and Erdos, E.G. (1973). Release of histamine from mast cells by vasoactive peptides. *Proc. Soc. Exp. Biol. Med.* **142**, 1252–1256.

Kanofsky, J.R., Hoogland, H., Wever, R. and Weiss, S.J. (1988). Singlet oxygen production by human eosinophils. *J. Biol. Chem.* **263**, 9692–9696.

Kaplan, A.P., Gray, L., Shaff, R.E., Horakova, Z. and Beaven, M.A. (1975). In vivo studies of mediator release in cold urticaria and cholinergic urticaria. *J. Allergy Clin. Immunol.* **55**, 394–402.

Katayama, M., Bunnett, N.W., Keki, I.F., Nadel, J.A. and Borsen, D.B. (1990). Recombinant human neutral endopeptidase (NEP) cleaves calcitonin gene-related peptide (CGRP). *FASEB J.* **4**, A999.

Kennerly, D.A., Sullivan, T.J., Sylwester, P. and Parker, C.W. (1979). Diacylglycerol metabolism in mast cells: A potential role in membrane fusion and arachidonic acid release. *J. Exp. Med.* **150**, 1039–1044.

Kessler, D.A., Langer, R.S., Pless, N.A. and Folkman, J. (1976) Mast cells and tumor angiogenesis. *Int. J. Cancer* **18**, 703–709.

Kirshenbaum, A.S., Dreskin, S.C. and Metcalfe, D.D. (1989). A staphylococcal protein A rosetting assay for the demonstration of high affinity IgE receptors on rIL-3 dependent human basophil-like cells grown in mixed cell cultures. *J. Immunol. Meth.* **123**, 55–62.

Kischer, C.W., Bunce, H. and Shetlar, M.R. (1978). Mast cell analyses in hypertrophic scars, hypertrophic scars treated with pressure and mature scars. *J. Invest. Dermatol.* **70**, 355–357.

Kitamura, Y. and Go, S. (1979). Decreased production of mast cells in Sl/Sl^d anemic mice. *Blood* **53**, 492–497.

Kitamura, Y., Go, S. and Hatanaka, K. (1978). Decrease of mast cells in W/W^v mice and their increase by bone marrow transplantation. *Blood* **52**, 447–452.

Kitamura, Y., Nakayama, H. and Fujita, J. (1989). Mechanism of mast cell deficiency in mutant mice of W/W^v and Sl/Sl^d genotype. *In* "Mast Cell and Basophil Differentiation and Function in Health and Disease" (S.J. Galli and K.F. Austen, eds), pp. 15–25. Raven Press, New York.

Kroegel, C., Yukawa, T., Dent, G., Chanez, P., Chung, K.F. and Barnes, P.J. (1988). Platelet-activating factor induces eosinophil peroxidase release from purified human eosinophils. *Immunology* **64**, 559–562.

Kuna, P., Brzezinska-Blaszczyk, E., Gaik, A. and Rozniecki, J. (1992). Histamine release from basophils and mast cells from bronchoalveolar lavage (BAL-MC): effect of histamine releasing factors (HRF), anti-IgE and allergen. *Ann. Allergy* **68**, 75.

Lanotte, M., Arock, M., Lacaze, N. and Guy-Grand, D. (1986). Murine basophil-mast differentiation: toward optimal conditions for selective growth and maturation of basophil-mast or allied cells. *J. Cell. Physiol.* **129**, 199–226.

Lee, F., Yokota, T., Otsuka, T., Meyerson, P., Villaret, D., Coffman, R., Mosmann, T., Renninck, D., Roehm, N., Smith, C., Zlotnik, A. and Arai, K.-I. (1986). Isolation and characterization of a mouse interleukin cDNA clone that expresses B-cell stimulatory factor 1 activities and T-cell- and mast-cell-stimulating activities. *Proc. Natl. Acad. Sci. U.S.A.* **83**, 2061–2065.

Lee, T., Lenihan, D.J., Malone, B., Roddy, L.L. and Wasserman, S.I. (1984). Increased biosynthesis of platelet-activating factor in activated human eosinophils. *J. Biol. Chem.* **259**, 5526–5530.

Le Gros, G., Ben-Sasson, S.Z., Seder, R., Finkelman, F.D. and Paul, W.E. (1990). Generation of interleukin-4 (IL-4)-producing cells *in vivo* and *in vitro*: IL-2 and IL-4 are required for in vitro generation of IL-4-producing cells. *J. Exp. Med.* **172**, 921–929.

Levi-Schaffer, F., Austen, K.F., Caulfield, J.P., Hein, A., Bloes, W.F. and Stevens, R.L. (1985). Fibroblasts maintain the phenotype and viability of the rat heparin-containing mast cell in vitro. *J. Immunol.* **135**, 3454–3462.

Levi-Schaffer, F., Austen, K.F., Caulfield, J.P., Hein, A., Gravallese, P.M. and Stevens, R.L. (1987). Co-culture of human lung-derived mast cells with mouse 3T3 fibroblasts: Morphology and IgE-mediated release of histamine, prostaglandin D2, and leukotrienes. *J. Immunol.* **139**, 494–500.

Lewis, R.A. and Austen, K.F. (1984). The biologically active leukotrienes. Biosynthesis, metabolism, receptors, functions, and pharmacology. *J. Clin. Invest.* **73**, 889–897.

Lichtenstein, L.M. (1988). Histamine-releasing factors and IgE heterogeneity. *J. Allergy Clin. Immunol.* **81**, 814–820.

Lindholm, R.V. and Lindholm, T.S. (1970). Mast cells in endosteal and periosteal bone repair. A quantitative study on callus tissue of healing fractures in rabbits. *Acta Orthop. Scand.* **41**, 129–133.

Liu, M.C., Proud, D., Lichtenstein, L.M., MacGlashan, D.W. Jr., Schleimer, R.P., Adkinson, N.F. Jr., Kagey-Sobotka, A., Schulman, E.S. and Plaut, M.

(1986). Human lung macrophage-derived histamine-releasing activity is due to IgE-dependent factors. *J. Immunol.* **136**, 2588–2595.

Lloyd, G., Green, F.H.Y., Fox, H., Mani, V. and Turnberg, L.A. (1975). Mast cells and immunoglobulin E in inflammatory bowel disease. *Gut* **16**, 861–866.

Lopez, A.F., Sanderson, C.J., Gamble, J.R., Campbell, H.D., Young, I.G. and Vadas, M.A. (1988). Recombinant human interleukin-5 is a selective activator of human eosinophil function. *J. Exp. Med.* **167**, 219–224.

Lotz, M., Vaughan, J.H. and Carson, D.A. (1988). Effect of neuropeptides on production of inflammatory cytokines by human monocytes. *Science* **241**, 1218–1221.

Lowman, M.A., Benyon, R.C. and Church, M.K. (1988a). Characterization of neuropeptide-induced histamine release from human dispersed skin mast cells. *Brit. J. Pharmacol.* **95**, 121–130.

Lowman, M.A., Rees, P.H., Benyon, R.C. and Church, M.K. (1988b). Human mast cell heterogeneity: Histamine release from mast cells dispersed from skin, lung, adenoids, tonsils, and colon in response to IgE-dependent and nonimmunological stimuli. *J. Allergy Clin. Immunol.* **81**, 590–597.

Lynch, S.M., Austen, K.F. and Wasserman, S.I. (1978). Release of arylsulfatase A but not B from rat mast cells by noncytotoxic secretory stimuli. *J. Immunol.* **121**, 1394–1399.

MacDonald, S.M., Lichtenstein, L.M., Proud, D., Plaut, M., Naclerio, R.M., MacGlashan, D.W. and Kagey-Sobotka, A. (1987). Studies of IgE-dependent histamine releasing factors: heterogeneity of IgE. *J. Immunol.* **139**, 506–512.

Mayrhofer, G. and Fisher, R. (1979). Mast cells in severely T-cell depleted rats and the response to infestation with *Nippostrongylus brasiliensis*. *Immunology* **37**, 145–155.

Mayrhofer, G., Gadd, S.J., Spargo, L.D. and Ashman, L.K. (1987). Specificity of a mouse monoclonal antibody raised against acute myeloid leukemia cells for mast cells in human mucosal and connective tissues. *Immunol. Cell Biol.* **65**, 241–250.

Meier, H.L., Heck, L.W., Schulman, E.S. and MacGlashan, D.W. Jr. (1985). Purified human mast cells and basophils release human elastase and cathepsin G by an IgE-mediated mechanism. *Int. Arch. Allergy Appl. Immunol.* **77**, 179–183.

Metcalfe, D.D., Kaliner, M. and Donlon, M.A. (1981). The mast cell. *CRC Crit. Rev. Immunol.* **1**, 23–74.

Metzger, M. (1991). The high affinity receptor for IgE on mast cells. *Clin. Exp. Allergy* **21**, 269–279.

Metzger, W.J., Zavala, D., Richerson, H.B., Moseley, P., Iwamota, P., Monick, M., Sjoerdsma, K. and Hunninghake, G.W. (1987). Local allergen challenge and bronchoalveolar lavage of allergic asthmatic lungs. Description of the model and local airway inflammation. *Am. Rev. Respir. Dis.* **135**, 433–440.

Mikhail, G.R. and Miller-Milinska, A. (1964). Mast cell population in human skin. *J. Invest. Dermatol.* **43**, 249–254.

Miller, H.R.P. and Jarrett, W.F.H. (1971). Immune reactions in mucous membranes. I. Intestinal mast cell response during helminth expulsion in the rat. *Immunology* **20**, 277–288.

Mosmann, T.R. and Coffman, R.L. (1989). Heterogeneity of cytokine secretion patterns and functions of helper T cells. *Adv. Immunol.* **46**, 111–147.

Mousli, M., Bronner, C., Bockaert, J., Roust, B. and Landry, Y. (1990).

Interaction of substance P, compound 48/80, and mastopyran with the α-subunit C-terminus of G protein. *Immunol. Lett.* **25**, 355–358.

Nadel, J.A. (1991). Neutral endopeptidase modulates neurogenic inflammation. *Eur. Respir. J.* **4**, 745–754.

Nakano, T., Kanakura, Y., Nakahata, T., Matsuda, H. and Kitamura, Y. (1987). Genetically mast cell-deficient W/W^v mice as a tool for studies of differentiation and function of mast cells. *Fed. Proc.* **46**, 1920–1923.

O'Donnell, M.C., Henson, P.M. and Fiedel, B.A. (1979). Activation of human platelets by platelet activating factor (PAF) derived from sensitized rabbit basophils. *Immunology* **35**, 953–958.

O'Donnell, M.C., Ackerman, S.J., Gleich, G.J. and Thomas, L.L. (1983). Activation of basophil and mast cell histamine release by eosinophil granule major basic protein. *J. Exp. Med.* **157**, 1981–1991.

O'Driscoll, R.B.C., Lee, T.H., Cromwell, O. and Kay, A.B. (1983). Immunologic release of neutrophil chemotactic activity from human lung tissue. *J. Allergy Clin. Immunol.* **72**, 695–701.

Okayama, Y. and Church, M.K. (1992). IL-3 primes and evokes histamine release from human basophils. *Int. Arch. Allergy Appl. Immunol.* **99**, 343–345.

Ollerenshaw, S.L., Jarvis, D.L., Woolcock, A.J., Scheibner, T. and Sullivan, C.E. (1989). Substance P immunoreactive nerve fibres in airways from patients with and without asthma. *Am. Rev. Respir. Dis.* **139**, A237.

Orchard, M.A., Kagey-Sobotka, A., Proud, D. and Lichtenstein, L.M. (1986). Basophil histamine release induced by a substance from stimulated human platelets. *J. Immunol.* **136**, 2240–2244.

Painter, R.G., Dukes, R., Sullivan, J., Carter, R., Erdos, E.G. and Johnson, A.R. (1988). Function of neutral endopeptidase on the cell membrane of human neutrophils. *J. Biol. Chem.* **263**, 9456–9461.

Parker, C.W. (1989). Leukotrienes and other arachidonic acid metabolites. *In* "Progress in Allergy and Clinical Immunology" (W.J. Pichler, B.M. Stadler, C.A. Dahinden, A.R. Pecoud, P. Frei, C.H. Schneider and A.L. de Weck, eds), pp. 28–32. Hogrefe & Huber, Toronto, Lewiston, New York, Bern, Göttingen, Stuttgart.

Payan, D.G., Brewster, D.R. and Goetzl, E.J. (1983). Specific stimulation of human T lymphocytes by substance P. *J. Immunol.* **131**, 1613–1615.

Pearce, F.L. and Thompson, H.L. (1986). Some characteristics of histamine secretion from rat peritoneal mast cells stimulated with nerve growth factor. *J. Physiol. (Lond.)* **372**, 379–393.

Penner, R. (1988). Multiple signaling pathways control stimulus-secretion coupling in rat peritoneal mast cells. *Proc. Natl. Acad. Sci. U.S.A.* **85**, 9856–9860.

Peters, M.S., Rodriguez, M. and Gleich, G.J. (1986). Localization of human eosinophil granule major basic protein, eosinophil cationic protein, and eosinophil-derived neurotoxin by immunoelectron microscopy. *Lab. Invest.* **54**, 656–662.

Plaut, M., Pierce, J.H., Watson, C.J., Hanley-Hyde, J., Nordan, R.P. and Paul, W.E. (1989). Mast cell lines produce lymphokines in response to cross-linkage of Fc$_\epsilon$RI or to calcium ionophores. *Nature* **339**, 64–67.

Prystowsky, M.B., Otten, G., Naujokas, M.F., Vardiman, J., Ihle, J.N., Goldwasser, E. and Fitch, F.W. (1984). Multiple hematopoietic lineages are found after stimulation of mouse bone marrow precursor cells with interleukin 3. *Am. J. Pathol.* **117**, 171–179.

Razin, E., Stevens, R.L., Akiyama, F., Schmid, K. and Austen, K.F. (1982). Culture from mouse bone marrow of a subclass of mast cells possessing a distinct chondroitin sulfate proteoglycan with glycosaminoglycans rich in N-acetylgalactosamine-4,6-disulfate. *J. Biol. Chem.* **257**, 7229–7236.

Razin, E., Ihle, J.N., Seldin, D., Mencia-Huerta, J.-M., Katz, H.R., Leblanc, P.A., Hein, A., Caulfield, J.P., Austen, K.F. and Stevens, R.L. (1984). Interleukin 3: a differentiation and growth factor for the mouse mast cell that contains chondroitin sulfate E proteoglycan. *J. Immunol.* **132**, 1479–1486.

Reed, N.D. (1989). Function and regulation of mast cells in parasite infections. *In* "Mast Cell and Basophil Differentiation and Function in Health and Disease" (S.J. Galli and K.F. Austen, eds), pp. 205–215. Raven Press, New York.

Rees, P.H., Hillier, K. and Church, M.K. (1988). The secretory characteristics of mast cells isolated from the human large intestinal mucosa and muscle. *Immunology* **65**, 437–442.

Riley, J.F. and West, G.B. (1953). The presence of histamine in tissue mast cells. *J. Physiol. (Lond.)* **120**, 528–537.

Robinson, C. (1988). Mast cells and newly-generated lipid mediators. *In* "Mast Cells, Mediators and Disease" (S.T. Holgate, ed.), pp. 149–174. Kluwer Academic, Dordrecht, Boston, London.

Robinson, C., Benyon, R.C., Holgate, S.T. and Church, M.K. (1989). The IgE- and calcium-dependent release of eicosanoids and histamine from human purified cutaneous mast cells. *J. Invest. Dermatol.* **93**, 397–404.

Saito, H., Hatake, K., Dvorak, A.M., Leiferman, K.M., Donnenberg, A.D., Arai, N., Ishizaka, K. and Ishizaka, T. (1988). Selective differentiation and proliferation of hematopoietic cells induced by recombinant human interleukins. *Proc. Natl. Acad. Sci. U.S.A.* **85**, 2288–2292.

Sanderson, C.J., Warren, D.J. and Strath, M. (1985). Identification of a lymphokine that stimulates eosinophil differentiation *in vitro*. Its relationship to interleukin-3, and functional properties of eosinophils produced in cultures. *J. Exp. Med.* **162**, 60–74.

Saria, A. and Lundberg, J.M. (1983). Capsaicin pretreatment inhibits heat-induced oedema in the rat skin. *Naunyn Schmiedeberg's Arch. Pharmacol.* **323**, 341–342.

Schechter, N.M., Fraki, J.E., Geesin, J.C. and Lazarus, G.S. (1983). Human skin chymotryptic proteinase. Isolation and relation to cathepsin G and rat mast cell proteinase I. *J. Biol. Chem.* **258**, 2973–2978.

Schiller, S. and Dorfman, A. (1959). The isolation of heparin from mast cells of the normal rat. *Biochim. Biophys. Acta* **31**, 278–280.

Schleimer, R.P., Sterbinsky, S.A., Kaiser, J., Bickel, C.A., Klunk, D.A., Tomioka, K., Newman, W., Luscinskas, F.W., Gimbrone, M.A. Jr., McIntyre, B.W. and Bochner, B.S. (1992). IL-4 induces adherence of human eosinophils and basophils but not neutrophils to endothelium. Association with expression of VCAM-1. *J. Immunol.* **148**, 1086–1092.

Schulman, E.S., Liu, M.C., Proud, D., MacGlashan, D.W. Jr., Lichtenstein, L.M. and Plaut, M. (1985). Human lung macrophages induce histamine release from basophils and mast cells. *Am. Rev. Respir. Dis.* **131**, 230–235.

Schwartz L.B. (1985). Monoclonal antibodies against human mast cell tryptase demonstrate shared antigenic sites on subunits of tryptase and selective localization of the enzyme to mast cells. *J. Immunol.* **134**, 526–531.

Schwartz, L.B. (1988). Preformed mediators of human mast cells and basophils. *In* "Mast Cells, Mediators and Disease" (S.T. Holgate, ed.), pp. 129–147. Kluwer Academic, Dordrecht, Boston, London.

Schwartz, L.B. (1989). Heterogeneity of mast cells in humans. *In* "Mast Cell and Basophil Differentiation and Function in Health and Disease" (S.J. Galli and K.F. Austen, eds), pp. 93–105. Raven Press, New York.

Schwartz, L.B. and Austen, K.F. (1984). Structure and function of the chemical mediators of mast cells. *Progr. Allergy* **34**, 271–321.

Schwartz, L.B., Lewis, R.A. and Austen, K.F. (1981a). Tryptase from human pulmonary mast cells. Purification and characterization. *J. Biol. Chem.* **256**, 11939–11943.

Schwartz, L.B., Riedel, C., Caulfield, J.P., Wasserman, S.I. and Austen, K.F. (1981b). Cell association of complexes of chymase, heparin proteoglycan, and protein after degranulation of rat mast cells. *J. Immunol.* **126**, 2071–2078.

Schwartz, L.B., Irani, A.A., Roller, K., Castells, M.C. and Schechter, N.M. (1987). Quantification of histamine, tryptase, and chymase in dispersed human T and TC mast cells. *J. Immunol.* **138**, 2611–2615.

Sedgwick, B.D., Holt, P.G. and Turner, B. (1981). Production of a histamine-releasing lymphokine by antigen- or mitogen-stimulated human peripheral T cells. *Clin. Exp. Immunol.* **45**, 409–412.

Sekizawa, K., Caughey, G.H., Lazarus, S.C., Gold, W.M. and Nadel, J.A. (1989). Mast cell tryptase causes airway smooth muscle hyperresponsiveness in dogs. *J. Clin. Invest.* **83**, 175–179.

Sher, A., Coffman, R.L., Hieny, S., Scott, P. and Cheever, A.W. (1990). Interleukin 5 is required for the blood and tissue eosinophilia but not granuloma formation induced by infection with Schistosoma mansoni. *Proc. Natl. Acad. Sci. U.S.A.* **87**, 61–65.

Sigal, E., Grunberger, D., Cashman, J.R., Craig, C.S., Caughey, G.H. and Nadel, J.A. (1988). Arachidonate 15-lipoxygenase from human eosinophil-enriched leukocytes: partial purification and properties. *Biochem. Biophys. Res. Commun.* **150**, 376–383.

Sim, T.C., Forsythe, P.A., Alam, R., Welter, J.B., Lett-Brown, M.A. and Grant, J.A. (1990). Evaluation of histamine releasing factor (HRF) in nasal washings from individual subjects. *J. Allergy Clin. Immunol.* **85**, 156.

Skofitsch, G., Savitt, J.M. and Jacobowitz, D.M. (1985). Suggestive evidence for a functional unit between mast cells and substance P fibers in the rat diaphragm and mesentery. *Histochemistry* **82**, 5–8.

Snapper, C.M., Finkelman, F.D. and Paul, W.E. (1988). Differential regulation of IgG1 and IgE synthesis by interleukin-4. *J. Exp. Med.* **167**, 183–196.

Sonoda, T., Ohno, T. and Kitamura, Y. (1982). Concentration of mast-cell progenitors in bone marrow, spleen and blood of mice determined by limiting dilution analysis. *J. Cell. Physiol.* **112**, 136–140.

Sonoda, T., Kitamura, Y., Haku, Y., Hara, H. and Mori, K.J. (1983). Mast-cell precursors in various hematopoietic colonies of mice produced *in vivo* and in vitro. *Brit. J. Hematol.* **53**, 611–620.

Stanisz, A.M., Befus, D. and Bienenstock, J. (1986). Differential effects of vasoactive intestinal peptide, substance P, and somatostatin on immunoglobulin synthesis and proliferation by lymphocytes from Peyer's patches, mesenteric lymph nodes, and spleen. *J. Immunol.* **136**, 152–156.

Stanisz, A.M., Scicchitano, R. and Bienenstock, J. (1988). The role of vasoactive intestinal peptide and other neuropeptides in the regulation of the immune response *in vitro* and *in vivo*. *Ann. N.Y. Acad. Sci.* **527**, 478–485.

Strobel, S., Busuttil, A. and Ferguson, A. (1983). Human intestinal mucosal mast cells: expanded population in untreated coeliac disease. *Gut* **24**, 222–227.

Tam, E.K. and Caughey, G.H. (1990). Degradation of airway neuropeptides by human lung tryptase. *Am. J. Respir. Cell Molec. Biol.* **3**, 27–32.

Teper, R.I., Levinson, D.A., Stanger, B.Z., Campos-Torres, J., Abbas, A.K. and Leder, P. (1990). IL-4 induces allergic-like inflammatory disease and alters T-cell development in transgenic mice. *Cell* **62**, 457–467.

Thompson, H.L., Metcalfe, D.D. and Kinet, J.-P. (1990). Early expression of high affinity receptor for immunoglobulin E ($Fc_{\epsilon}RI$) during differentiation of mouse mast cells and human basophils. *J. Clin. Invest.* **85**, 1227–1233.

Thompson, J.E., Scypinski, L.A., Gordon, T. and Sheppard, D. (1987). Tachykinins mediate the acute increase in airway responsiveness caused by toluene diisocyanate in guinea pigs. *Am. Rev. Respir. Dis.* **136**, 43–49.

Thueson, D.O., Speck, L.S., Lett-Brown, M.A. and Grant, J.A. (1979a). Histamine-releasing activity (HRA). I. Production by mitogen- or antigen-stimulated human mononuclear cells. *J. Immunol.* **123**, 626–632.

Thueson, D.O., Speck, L.S., Lett-Brown, M.A. and Grant, J.A. (1979b). Histamine-releasing activity (HRA). II. Interaction with basophils and physicochemical characterization. *J. Immunol.* **123**, 633–639.

Toth-Kasa, I., Jancso, G., Obal, F., Husz, S. and Simon, N. (1983). Involvement of sensory nerve endings in cold and heat urticaria. *J. Invest. Dermatol.* **80**, 34–36.

Valent, P., Besemer, J., Sillaber, C., Butterfield, J.H., Eher, R., Majdic, O., Kishi, K., Klepetko, W., Eckersberger, F., Lechner, K. and Bettelheim, P. (1990). Failure to detect IL-3 binding sites on human mast cells. *J. Immunol.* **145**, 3432–3437.

Walsh, L.J., Trinchieri, G., Waldorf, H.A., Whitaker, D. and Murphy, G.F. (1991). Human dermal mast cells contain and release tumor necrosis factor α, which induces endothelial leukocyte adhesion molecule 1. *Proc. Natl. Acad. Sci. U.S.A.* **88**, 4220–4224.

Wardlaw, A.J., Moqbel, R., Cromwell, O. and Kay, A.B. (1986). Platelet-activating factor. A potent chemotactic and chemokinetic factor for human eosinophils. *J. Clin. Invest.* **78**, 1701–1706.

Warner, J.A., Pienkowski, M.M., Plaut, M., Norman, P.S. and Lichtenstein, L.M. (1986). Identification of histamine releasing factor(s) in the late phase of cutaneous IgE-mediated reactions. *J. Immunol.* **136**, 2583–2587.

Wasserman, S.I. (1980). The lung mast cell: its physiology and potential relevance to defence of the lung. *Environ. Health Perspect.* **35**, 153–164.

Wasserman, S.I., Goetzl, E.J. and Austen, K.F. (1975). Inactivation of slow reacting substance of anaphylaxis by human eosinophil arylsulphatase. *J. Immunol.* **114**, 645–649.

Weinstock, J.V., Blum, A., Walder, J. and Walder, R. (1988). Eosinophils from granulomas in murine *Schistosomiasis mansoni* produce substance P. *J. Immunol.* **141**, 961–966.

White, J. and Eiser, N.M. (1983). The role of histamine and its receptors in the pathogenesis of asthma. *Brit. J. Dis. Chest* **77**, 215–226.

White, M.V. and Kaliner, M.A. (1987). Neutrophils and mast cells. I. Human neutrophil-derived histamine-releasing activity. *J. Immunol.* **139**, 1624–1630.

White, M.V., Baer, H., Kubota, Y. and Kaliner, M. (1989). Neutrophils and mast cells: Characterization of cells responsive to neutrophil-derived histamine-releasing activity (HRA-N). *J. Allergy Clin. Immunol.* **84**, 773–780.

Yurt, R. and Austen, K.F. (1977). Preparative purification of the rat mast cell chymase. Characterization and interaction with granule components. *J. Exp. Med.* **146**, 1405–1419.

Zeiger, R.S., Twarog, F.J. and Colten, H.R. (1976a). Histaminase release from human granulocytes. *J. Exp. Med.* **144**, 1049–1061.

Zeiger, R.S., Yurdin, D.L. and Colten, H.R. (1976b). Histamine metabolism. II. Cellular and subcellular localization of the catabolic enzymes, histaminase and histamine methyl transferase, in human leukocytes. *J. Allergy Clin. Immunol.* **58**, 172–179.

Zheutlin, L.M., Ackerman, S.J., Gleich, G.J. and Thomas, L.L. (1984). Stimulation of basophil and rat mast cell histamine release by eosinophil granule-derived cationic proteins. *J. Immunol.* **133**, 2180–2185.

Zsebo, K.M., Martin, F.H., Suggs, S.V., Wypych, J., Lu, H.S., McNiece, I., Medlock, E., Morris, F., Sachollev, R., Tung, W., Birkett, N., Smith, K., Yuschenkoff, V., Mendiaz, E.M., Jacobsen, F.W. and Langley, K.E. (1990). Biological characterization of a unique early acting hematopoietic growth factor. *Exp. Hematol.* **18**, 703 (A583).

Zucker-Franklin, D., Grusky, G., Hirayama, N. and Schnipper, E. (1981). The presence of mast cell precursors in rat peripheral blood. *Blood* **58**, 544–551.

Part IV

New Perspectives in Asthma

17

Novel Therapeutic Approaches in Asthma

A.G. ALEXANDER* and N.C. BARNES‡

*Department of Allergy and Clinical Immunology, National Heart and Lung Institute, London SW3 6ZY, UK

‡ The London Chest Hospital, Bonner Road, London E2 9JX, UK

Introduction

There are five major classes of drugs currently used in the treatment of asthma (see Table 17.1). With the partial exception of β_2-agonists, these drugs have been developed from folk remedies, e.g. anticholinergics, or from testing newly available therapeutic agents in asthma without a clear idea of any underlying theoretical justification, e.g. the Medical Research Council trials of corticosteroids in chronic asthma (1956a) and acute severe asthma (1956b).

All of these classes of drugs were in use 15 years ago. The change in

Table 17.1
Major classes of drugs currently used in treatment of asthma

β_2-Agonists	Salbutamol, terbutaline
Anticholinergics	Ipratropium bromide
Corticosteroids	
Systemic	Hydrocortisone, prednisolone
Inhaled	Beclomethasone dipropionate, budesonide
Methylxanthines	Theophylline
Disodium cromoglycate/nedocromil sodium	

T-Lymphocyte and Inflammatory Cell Research in Asthma
ISBN 0-12-388170-6

treatment of asthma since then has been due to changes in the way these drugs are formulated and used. We now use inhaled steroids at an earlier stage, high-dose inhaled steroids have been introduced, better delivery systems have been developed, e.g. dry powder inhalers and spacer devices for metered dose inhalers and slow-release preparations of tablets. Improvement in existing classes of drugs have been made, i.e. longer duration of action (salmeterol and formoterol), or decreased side-effects (fluticasone).

Over this 15-year period, there has been an explosion of research into the basic pathophysiology and pharmacology of asthma. The unifying theme of much of this research effort has been that asthma should be considered as an inflammatory disease of the airways (Barnes and Costello, 1987). Consideration of asthma as an inflammatory disease has led to research into the chemical mediators, inflammatory cells, neurological pathways and, more recently, adhesion molecules which may play an important part in this process. The various theories as to the pathogenesis of asthma have identified new sites of therapeutic intervention so that pharmaceutical companies have been able to develop drugs which affect a particular mediator or cell. Because the pathophysiology of asthma still remains unclear, the investigation of these new drugs in animal models, human models of asthma and in clinical asthma becomes a vital part of the investigation of the pathophysiology of asthma. While none of these new approaches has yet achieved widespread clinical usage and some are still only being investigated in clinical models of asthma, they are already contributing a great deal to our understanding of asthma. Many of these drugs have been tested in animal models of asthma but not yet in man. This review will concentrate on those which have been investigated in man.

Animal and Human Models of Clinical Asthma

No animal suffers a disease resembling human asthma. Animal models have been developed which attempt to mimic certain features of asthma, e.g. the early and late response to allergen inhalation or exercise-induced bronchospasm, but no animal model has approached the full complexity of human asthma (Smith, 1989). Because of the variable nature of clinical asthma with sufferers ranging from toddlers to the elderly, and the severity ranging from infrequent attacks requiring occasional treatment to prolonged impaired lung function with wheeze and shortness of breath, despite maximum regular treatment, there has been a search for controlled human models of asthma. A variety of these models have been used to evaluate new therapeutic agents. They include the early response to antigen challenge, the late response to antigen challenge, the increase in bronchial hyperresponsiveness occurring after antigen challenge, cold air-induced bronchoconstriction, exercise-induced asthma, the investigation of non-specific bronchial hyperresponsiveness and a variety of indirect challenges, such as metabisulphite and hypertonic and hypotonic saline solutions. As the predictive value of these clinical human models to chronic asthma is far from clear, the investigation of new pharmacological agents also becomes a test of the models.

Antihistamines

Antihistamines are included in the drugs to be considered because histamine was the first asthmatic mediator to be recognized and the evaluation of antihistamines demonstrates some of the pitfalls which can occur when anti-asthmatic drugs are investigated. Histamine was first described as a mediator of anaphylaxis by Dale and Laidlaw (1910). It plays an important role in the acute response of the guinea-pig airways to allergen challenge. In man, histamine is a potent bronchoconstrictor, causes cough (Mills *et al.*, 1969), is thought to open up tight junctions in the airway epithelium (Majno, 1964), can be shown to be released during the early response to allergen challenge and may have some weak chemoattractant properties for eosinophils (Clark *et al.*, 1975).

From these considerations, it would seem that antihistamines would be useful in asthma. The early antihistamines were shown to be effective in allergic rhinitis, but when used in asthma had a number of disadvantages. Their potency was relatively poor, they also crossed the blood–brain barrier and had central nervous system (CNS) effects, principally sedation. This meant that high doses of the drug could not be given to determine whether histamine was playing a fundamental role in asthma. Furthermore, many of these drugs also had anticholinergic activity, and it was often argued that any therapeutic effects were due largely to their anticholinergic rather than to their antihistaminic properties.

The recent development of newer, more potent antihistamines, which do not have CNS or anticholinergic actions, has led to a re-investigation of the role of antihistamines in asthma (Holgate *et al.*, 1985). Terfenadine and astemizole are very potent oral antihistamines, which produce large shifts in histamine dose–response curves in man. Studies in clinical models of asthma have shown them to block approximately 50% of the early response to allergen challenge (Rafferty *et al.*, 1987), to produce partial protection against cold air- (Badier *et al.*, 1988) and exercise-induced bronchoconstriction. Acutely, the antihistamines cause a small degree of bronchodilatation but this effect wears off with chronic dosage (Gould *et al.*, 1988). They appear to have no effect on non-specific bronchial hyperresponsiveness (Gould *et al.*, 1988). Studies of these drugs in clinical asthma have produced disappointing results. They have either been shown to be completely ineffective or to have a marginal effect in very mild asthma (Taytard *et al.*, 1987; Gould *et al.*, 1988; Ulbrich and Nowak, 1990). Doubt has recently been cast on whether these effects are due to histamine H_1 receptor antagonism, as some of these drugs may have additional effects on calcium channels and possibly release of other inflammatory mediators from mast cells (Nabe *et al.*, 1989, Naclerio *et al.*, 1990). Thus, to illustrate the problem of drug development in this field, histamine would appear to be an important mediator in allergic responses in both animals and man, and yet the results of studies in challenge models in man do not translate into benefit in chronic asthma.

Drugs Affecting the Cyclooxygenase Pathway

Following the elucidation of the mode of action of aspirin as being due to interference with the cyclooxygenase enzyme, there was interest in the potential for drugs affecting prostanoid pathways as therapies in asthma. However, interest waned when it became apparent that cyclooxygenase inhibitors generally had no effect in asthma (Fish *et al.*, 1981), although a small percentage of asthmatics seem to be aspirin-sensitive, and bronchoconstrict after aspirin (Szczeklik *et al.*, 1975) and a tiny minority improve with cyclooxygenase inhibitors.

Further investigation of the effects of prostanoids in man showed that prostaglandin D_2 and $F_{2\alpha}$ were potent bronchoconstrictors to which asthmatics were hypersensitive (Smith *et al.*, 1975; Hardy *et al.*, 1984) and that inhaled prostanoids would increase airway hyperresponsiveness to histamine (Heaton *et al.*, 1984). In animal models, these prostanoids were also shown to have effects in promoting inflammation. Interest in the role of prostanoids in asthma increased when the hypothesis was put forward that in man all the bronchoconstrictor prostanoids had their effect by binding to a common thromboxane A_2 receptor (Coleman and Sheldrick, 1989). Thus, it would be possible to block the effect of all the bronchoconstrictor prostanoids with a single thromboxane antagonist and leave the potentially beneficial bronchodilator prostaglandins E_1, E_2 and prostacyclin unaffected. If prostanoids were involved in promoting bronchial hyperresponsiveness, this would be an attractive target for drug development. Studies of thromboxane receptor antagonists have shown that they block PGD_2-induced bronchoconstriction in normal and asthmatic subjects while having no effect on histamine- or methacholine-induced bronchoconstriction (Beasley *et al.*, 1989). Investigation of the thromboxane antagonist GR 32191 has shown a small protective effect on the early response to antigen challenge (Beasley *et al.*, 1989). Studies of cyclooxygenase inhibitors have produced differing results with some groups showing no effect on the early or late response to antigen challenge, but blockade of the increase in bronchial hyperresponsiveness occurring after antigen challenge, and others showing a small protective effect against the early response to antigen challenge, but no additive effect when these drugs are combined with antihistamines (Curzen *et al.*, 1987). There have been no reports of these drugs being investigated in chronic asthma but the small effects they have shown in challenge models do not make them look promising. Recent studies with more potent thromboxane antagonists, such as BAYμ3405, suggest greater effects in allergen and exercise challenges compared with earlier drugs (Gardiner, 1992).

Drugs Affecting the Lipoxygenase Pathway

Of all the chemical mediators which have been considered to have a role in asthma, most attention has focused on the 5-lipoxygenase pathway. Studies of drugs acting against this pathway are already at an advanced stage in man. The cysteinyl leukotrienes C_4, D_4 and E_4 are potent bronchoconstrictor agents in normal and asthmatic subjects (Barnes *et al.*, 1984a; Adelroth *et al.*, 1986), and some studies have suggested they may increase sensitivity to other inflammatory mediators (Barnes *et al.*, 1984b; Bel *et al.*, 1987; Arm *et al.*, 1988). Cysteinyl leukotrienes have been shown to be released during the early response to allergen challenge (Taylor *et al.*, 1989) and to be present during acute severe asthma attacks (Taylor *et al.*, 1989). The role, if any, of the dihydroxyacid leukotriene B_4 is less clear. It seems to be present in the sputum of patients suffering from a variety of diseases in which airflow obstruction is present (Zakrzewski *et al.*, 1987) and has been found in bronchoalveolar lavage fluid from asthmatics. However, LTB_4 showed no biological effect when inhaled by normal subjects (Black *et al.*, 1988).

A number of different cysteinyl leukotriene antagonists have now been investigated. These have been given by the oral, inhaled and intravenous routes, and have a variety of different molecular structures. When account is taken of their differing potencies and durations of action, it becomes apparent that the effects seen with leukotriene antagonists are consistent. Their different structures would suggest that the activity seen was due to leukotriene antagonism and not to some other unrecognized effect of the drugs. The first drug of this type to be investigated in man was the SRS-A antagonist, FPL55712. This was developed before the structure of leukotrienes had been elucidated. Bioavailability was poor and only a limited number of investigations were done, but these suggested some effect on antigen challenge (Ahmed *et al.*, 1981), and a possible effect in chronic asthma (Lee *et al.*, 1981).

The next generation of leukotriene antagonists studied were based on the structure of FPL55712 but with better bioavailability (Fleisch *et al.*, 1985; Young, 1988). They caused shifts of between four- and eightfold in the leukotriene D_4 dose–response curve (Barnes and Costello, 1987; Phillips *et al.*, 1987; Evans *et al.*, 1989), and so they were analogous to the early antihistamines in having only limited potency. They showed activity in partially protecting against the early response to antigen challenge (Britton *et al.*, 1987; Fuller *et al.*, 1988) and cold air-induced bronchoconstriction (Israel *et al.*, 1988). LY117883 also showed some activity in chronic asthma (Cloud *et al.*, 1989) with a small improvement in lung function, and in a subgroup analysis a decrease in β_2-agonist requirement in those taking more than 25 puffs of their bronchodilator per week. However, this class of drugs suffered from the problem of gastrointestinal side-effects and some liver toxicity. Interpretation of the study in chronic asthma was complicated because LY117883 is a phosphodiesterase inhibitor which may have accounted for some of its activity (Fleisch *et al.*, 1985).

The newer generation of leukotriene antagonists (Hay *et al.*, 1987; Jones *et al.*, 1989; Krell *et al.*, 1990) have been much more potent, producing around 50-fold shifts in leukotriene D_4 dose–response curves in man (Evans *et al.*, 1988; Smith *et al.*, 1990; Kips *et al.*, 1990). This has translated into improved effects in models of asthma. SK&F 104353, ICI 204,219 and MK 571 have all been shown to block about 80% of the early response to antigen challenge (Kips *et al.*, 1990; Taylor *et al.*, 1991), and when they have been combined with an antihistamine there has been almost total blockade of the early response to antigen challenge. ICI 204,219 and MK 571 have also been shown to block approximately 50% of the late response to antigen challenge (Kips *et al.*, 1990; Taylor *et al.*, 1991) and to attenuate the increase in bronchial hyperresponsiveness, which occurs after antigen challenge (Taylor *et al.*, 1991).

Effects on cold air- and exercise-induced bronchoconstriction (Manning *et al.*, 1990) have also been seen with these drugs. In clinical asthma, ICI 204,219 (Hui *et al.*, 1991a) and MK 571 (Gaddy *et al.*, 1990) have both been shown to bronchodilate wheezy asthmatics. This observation on its own might not be of great interest as similar results have been seen with antihistamines, but the intriguing observation, which was totally unexpected, was that this bronchodilatation was additive to that of salbutamol. Even with established bronchodilators, such as ipratropium bromide and theophyllines, it has proved difficult to get such clear-cut additive bronchodilatation when large doses of β_2-agonist are given.

The mechanism for this additive action is unclear; possibilities include that leukotriene-induced bronchodilatation is due to smooth muscle spasm which cannot be reversed by a β_2-agonist or that the bronchodilatation by leukotriene antagonist is due to mechanisms other than smooth muscle spasm, for instance oedema formation. This additive effect was not predicted from any animal studies. Preliminary results of the study of these drugs in chronic asthma has suggested that they may improve lung function (Margolskee *et al.*, 1991). Apart from some minor hepatic enzyme induction, this new class of drugs has been free of side-effects.

5-Lipoxygenase inhibitors have proved more difficult to develop than leukotriene receptor antagonists, but have the theoretical advantage that they will also block the production of leukotriene B_4. An oral 5-lipoxygenase inhibitor, Zileutin, has been shown to affect cold air-induced bronchoconstriction (Israel *et al.*, 1990), and to have a minor effect on the early response to antigen challenge (Hui *et al.*, 1991). However, its inability to block completely the production of cysteinyl leukotrienes after antigen challenge (Hui *et al.*, 1991b) would suggest that, unless with chronic dosage leukotriene production is more completely abolished, this drug will not be of clinical value.

An intriguing drug has been MK 886. This compound was shown to block the production of leukotrienes but investigations showed that it was not directly a 5-lipoxygenase inhibitor. In an elegant series of studies, (Ford-Hutchinson, 1992) it was shown that this drug binds to a previously undescribed protein 5-lipoxygenase-activation protein (FLAP). It is necessary for 5-lipoxygenase to bind to FLAP before it can be active. MK 886 probably binds to FLAP and prevents the enzyme binding. This has provided another target for drug development.

Drugs Acting Against Platelet-Activating Factor (PAF)

Platelet-activating factor (PAF) is an inflammatory mediator with a wide variety of actions. It recruits and activates inflammatory cells and can promote oedema formation (Barnes *et al.*, 1988). Interest in PAF as an asthmatic mediator was considerably heightened when Cuss *et al.* (1986) reported that not only was PAF a bronchoconstrictor in man but that it could increase bronchial hyperresponsiveness and this increased bronchial hyperresponsiveness could last up to 2 weeks. This increase in bronchial hyperresponsiveness has not been confirmed by other groups who studied PAF (Lai *et al.*, 1990) but the interest generated has persisted.

Three very potent PAF antagonists (WEB 2086, MK 287, UK 74,505) have now been studied in man. They are much more potent than the original leukotriene antagonists which were studied or the equivalent thromboxane antagonists. They have been shown to block completely exogenous PAF platelet aggregation (Adamus *et al.*, 1988) and to block the acute bronchoconstriction caused by inhaled PAF (O'Connor *et al.*, 1991). The effects of two of these drugs, WEB 2086 and MK 287, on antigen challenge has now been reported and no activity has been found (Wilkens *et al.*, 1991; Freitag *et al.*, 1991; Bel *et al.*, 1991).

Studies in chronic asthma are currently underway but the results of the antigen challenge studies do not look promising.

Immunosuppressants

There have been a number of studies going back to the 1970s of immunosuppressant agents in asthma. However, most of these studies were small scale, short term and produced negative or inconclusive results. Recently interest in this area has increased again. Mullarkey's work (Mullarkey *et al.*, 1988, 1990) on methotrexate showed that it was a steroid-sparing agent in asthma and controlled trials of gold have now been reported. From studies of basic mechanisms of asthma in man, Professor Kay and his group (Corrigan *et al.*, 1988; Corrigan and Kay, 1990) have implicated the activated T-lymphocyte in asthma and the subsequent demonstration that cyclosporin A (CsA), which is thought to have its principal mode of action on the T-cell, is effective in chronic severe steroid-dependent asthma has strengthened this hypothesis.

Methotrexate

Much is owed to the observation of Mullarkey that an asthmatic patient being treated with methotrexate for another condition improved and her oral steroid requirements fell. He subsequently performed a double-blind placebo-controlled, crossover study of methotrexate in a group of severe steroid-dependent asthmatics (Mullarkey *et al.*, 1988). This study demonstrated that patients' requirements for oral steroids fell while on methotrexate without any loss of control of asthma. A larger open series by Mullarkey *et al.* (1990) has added weight to this observation. The original study has been criticized because many of the patients were on unrepresentatively high doses of oral steroids and details of their other treatment, including high-dose inhaled steroids, were not given.

A further double-blind placebo-controlled parallel group design study has been performed by Shiner *et al.* (1990). In this study, a group of severe steroid-dependent asthmatics were treated for 28 weeks with either methotrexate 15 mg per week or matching placebo. There was a 14% fall in oral steroid requirement in the placebo-treated group with a highly significant 50% fall in prednisolone dosage in the methotrexate-treated group. Several other features of the study are of interest. First, the prednisolone requirements of the placebo and active treatment groups did not diverge until 12 weeks into the study; secondly, the methotrexate-treated group was still improving at the end of the study; and thirdly, on stopping methotrexate, the oral steroid requirement went back to baseline over the course of the next 10 weeks. This illustrates some of the problems of performing clinical studies with drugs of this type in asthma.

The place of methotrexate in the treatment of severe asthma is still unclear. Methotrexate has effects on all dividing cells, and therefore its mechanism of action in asthma is not clear. Increasing use of the drug has raised questions about both long-term efficacy and side-effects. It is recognized in rheumatoid arthritis, where there is greater experience with methotrexate as a steroid-sparing agent, that the effectiveness of methotrexate tends to wear off. Anecdotal reports of this occurring in asthma are now apparent. An increasing number of side-effects have been recognized with low-dose methotrexate, including methotrexate-induced asthma (Jones *et al.*, 1991), methotrexate-induced pneumonitis and *Pneumocystis carinii* pneumonia occurring both in patients with rheumatoid arthritis and, more recently, in patients with asthma (Kuitert and Harrison, 1991).

Gold

Gold has been used as a treatment for asthma in Japan for many years but properly controlled trials have been lacking. Open studies have suggested that it causes improved symptoms, a decrease in bronchial hyperresponsiveness (Bernstein *et al.*, 1988) and a decrease in steroid requirement (Klaustermeyer *et al.*, 1987). More recently, there have been preliminary reports of a trial of oral gold in a group of steroid-dependent asthmatics. This has shown a small decrease in oral prednisolone dosage without any loss of control of asthma (Nierop *et al.*, 1991). The mechanism of action of gold is not certain but it is of interest that in rheumatoid arthritis it is thought that, at least part of its action is by interference with T-lymphocyte function.

Azathioprine

Azathioprine has been the subject of short-term studies but the duration of treatment was probably insufficient in light of the evidence for the onset of action of methotrexate.

Hydroxychloroquine

Hydroxychloroquine has been shown to be a steroid-sparing agent in rheumatoid arthritis and a recent open study of hydroxychloroquine in steroid-dependent asthma has been reported (Charous, 1990). This has produced impressive results, but obviously double-blind placebo-controlled trials are now awaited.

Cyclosporin A

The rationale for investigating cyclosporin A in chronic asthma came partly from the work of Professor A.B. Kay and his group on the role of the T-lymphocyte in asthma. Studies of bronchial biopsies in asthmatics have shown that one of the prominent cells in the biopsy is the activated T-lymphocyte (Jeffrey *et al.*, 1989; Azzawi *et al.*, 1990). Corrigan and co-workers demonstrated that in patients with acute severe asthma there was an increase in activated $CD4^+$ T-lymphocytes in peripheral blood, which fell with effective treatment (Corrigan *et al.*, 1988; Corrigan and Kay, 1990). The phenomenon of corticosteroid-resistant asthma has also implicated the T-cell in the pathogenesis of asthma. It has been shown that in a group of asthmatic patients, who have been well documented as resistant to the effects of corticosteroids at normal therapeutic doses, the normal suppression of lymphocyte proliferation and IL-2 elaboration *in vitro* by exogenous corticosteroids does not occur. The clinical corticosteroid resistance is not due to any defect in prednisolone absorption or metabolism, and the cellular defect is not due to lack of ability of corticosteroids to bind to the T-lymphocyte (Corrigan *et al.*, 1991a,b).

Cyclosporin A (CsA) is a cyclo-undecapeptide whose use has revolutionized the effectiveness of organ transplantation. More recently, CsA has been shown to be effective in a variety of "autoimmune" disorders, including psoriasis, atopic dermatitis, Crohn's disease and rheumatoid arthritis. As the principal mode of action of CsA is thought to be to prevent the $CD4^+$ cell becoming activated, a trial of CsA in severe steroid-dependent asthma was performed to test further the hypothesis that the T-lymphocyte was important in asthma. A group of severe asthmatics dependent on maintenance oral corticosteroids in addition to high-dose inhaled steroids and bronchodilators were investigated. The subjects were all lifelong non-smokers with no evidence of other significant lung disease. They all showed conventional criteria of asthma with either spontaneous or pharmacologically induced improvements in airway function. Cyclosporin A given over a 12-week period improved lung function significantly, and also decreased the number of rescue courses of prednisolone required (Alexander *et al.*, 1992). This suggests that CsA may be able not only to improve lung function but also act as a steroid-sparing agent. Although it is now apparent that CsA does have actions on other inflammatory cells, apart from the T-lymphocyte, it is still thought that the major therapeutic action of cyclosporin A is due to its action on lymphocytes. The demonstration that a drug affecting T-lymphocyte function can have a therapeutic benefit in asthma points to a new and potentially exciting area for drug development, targeting either the T-lymphocyte or the cytokines which it produces. It is possible that much of the therapeutic action of steroids is based on their effects on lymphocyte function.

Conclusion

In the last 15 years, no fundamentally new drugs for the treatment of asthma have achieved widespread clinical use. However, research into the basic pathophysiology and pharmacology of asthma has identified many potential targets for drug development and some of these drugs are now being investigated in man. With any treatment, a balance must be struck between clinical effectiveness and side-effects. While some of these drugs may, therefore, not be as potent as inhaled or oral corticosteroids, if they are free of side-effects, or suitable for a particular group of asthmatics, e.g. children, they may find a use in clinical practice. Of the mediator antagonists so far studied, the leukotriene antagonists and, by implication, 5-lipoxygenase inhibitors look the most promising. Studies of steroid-sparing agents in asthma and the recent investigation of cyclosporin A have also indicated another potential target for drug development. While the toxicity of these immunosuppressant drugs means that, at present, they may only be suitable for a minority of severe and steroid-dependent asthmatics, reduction of side-effects by, for instance, inhalation or the specific design of safe and effective anti-lymphocyte drugs for the lung may mean that this approach can be extended to many more asthmatics. In investigating these new classes of drugs in asthma, important observations on the underlying pathophysiology of asthma will be made and the relevance of various animal and clinical models of asthma to chronic asthma will become clearer.

References

Adamus, W.S., Heuer, H., Meade, C.J. and Brecht, H.M. (1988). Effect of peroral WEB 2086 on ex-vivo platelet activating factor induced platelet aggregation in man. *Prostaglandins* **35**, 836.

Adelroth, E., Morris, M.M., Hargreave, P.E. and O'Byrne, P.M. (1986). Airway responsiveness to leukotrienes C4 and D4 and to methacholine in patients with asthma and normal controls. *New Engl. J. Med.* **314**, 480–484.

Ahmed, T., Greenblatt, D.W., Birch, S., Marchette, B. and Wanner, A. (1981). Abnormal mucociliary transport in allergic patients with antigen-induced bronchospasm; slow reacting substance of anaphylaxis. *Am. Rev. Respir. Dis.* **124**, 110–114.

Alexander, A.G., Barnes, N.C. and Kay, A.B. (1992). Trial of cyclosporin in corticosteroid-dependent chronic severe asthma. *Lancet* **339**, 324–328.

Arm, J.P., Spur, B.W. and Lee, T.W. (1988). The effects of inhaled leukotriene E4 on the airways responsiveness to histamine in subjects with asthma and normal subjects. *J. Allergy Clin. Immunol.* **82**, 654–660.

Azzawi, M., Bradley, B., Jeffrey, P.K. *et al.* (1990). Activated T-lymphocytes and eosinophils in bronchial biopsies in stable atopic asthma. *Am. Rev. Respir. Dis.* **142**, 1407–1413.

Badier, M., Beaumont, D. and Orehek, J. (1988). Attenuation of hyperventilation-induced bronchospasm by terfenadine; a new antihistamine. *J. Allergy Clin. Immunol.* **81**, 437–440.

Barnes, N.C. and Costello, J.F. (1987). Airway hyperresponsiveness and inflammation: mediators and mechanisms. *Brit. Med. Bull.* **43**, 445–459.

Barnes, N.C., Piper, P.J. and Costello, J.F. (1984). Comparative effects of inhaled leukotriene C4, leukotriene D4 and histamine in normal human subjects. *Thorax* **39**, 500–504.

Barnes, N.C., Watson, A., Koulouris, N., Piper, P.J. and Costello, J.F. (1984). The effect of pre-inhalation of leukotriene D4 on sensitivity to inhaled prostaglandin F2. *Thorax* **39**, 697.

Barnes, P.J., Chung, K.F. and Page, C.P. (1988). Platelet-activating factor as a mediator of allergic disease. *J. Allergy Clin. Immunol.* **81**, 919–934.

Beasley, R.G.W., Featherstone, R.L., Church, M.K. *et al.* (1989). Effect of a thromboxane antagonist on PGD2- and allergen-induced bronchoconstriction. *J. Appl. Physiol.* **66**, 1685–1693.

Bel, E.H., Van der Veen, H., Kramps, J.A., Dijkman, J.H. and Sterk, P.J. (1987). Maximal airway narrowing to inhaled leukotriene D4 in normal subjects. *Am. Rev. Respir. Dis.* **136**, 979–984.

Bel, E.H., De Smet, M., Rossing, T.H., Timmers, M.C., Dijkman, J.H. and Sterk, P.J. (1991). The effect of a specific oral PAF antagonist, on antigen induced early and late asthmatic reactions in man. *Am. Rev. Respir. Dis.* **143**, A811 (abst.).

Bernstein, D.I., Bernstein, I.L. Bodenheimer, S.J. and Pietrusko, R.G. (1988). An open study of auranofin in the treatment of steroid-dependent asthma. *J. Allergy Clin. Immunol.* **81**, 6–16.

Black, P.N., Fuller, R.W., Taylor, G.W., Barnes, P.J. and Dollery, C.T. (1988). Bronchial reactivity is not increased after inhalation of leukotriene B4 and prostaglandin D2. *Brit. J. Clin. Pharmacol.* **25**, 667P (abst.).

Britton, J.R., Hanley, S.P. and Tattersfield, A.E. (1987). The effect of an oral leukotriene D4 antagonist L649,923 on the response to inhaled antigen in asthma. *J. Allergy Clin. Immunol.* **79**, 811–816.

Charous, B.L. (1990). Open study of hydroxychloroquine in the treatment of severe symptomatic or corticosteroid-dependent asthma. *Ann. Allergy* **65**, 53–58.

Clark, R.A.F., Gallin, J.I. and Kaplan, A.P. (1975). The selective eosinophil chemotactic activity of histamine. *J. Exp. Med.* **142**, 1462–1476.

Cloud, M.L., Evans, G.C., Kemp, J., Platts-Mills, T., Altman, L.C., Townley, R.E. *et al.* (1989). A specific LTD4/LTE4 receptor antagonist improves pulmonary function in patients with mild chronic asthma. *Am. Rev. Respir. Dis.* **140**, 1336–1339.

Coleman, R.A. and Sheldrick, R.L.G. (1989). Prostanoid-induced contraction of human bronchial smooth muscle is mediated by TP-preceptors. *Brit. J. Pharmacol.* **90**, 688–692.

Corrigan, C.J. and Kay, A.B. (1990). CD4 T-lymphocyte activation in acute severe asthma: relationship to disease severity and atopic state. *Am. Rev. Respir. Dis.* **141**, 970–977.

Corrigan, C.J., Hartnell, A. and Kay, A.B. (1988). T-lymphocyte activation in acute severe asthma. *Lancet* **1**, 1129–1131.

Corrigan, C.J., Brown, P.H., Barnes, N.C. *et al.* (1991a). Glucocorticoid resistance in chronic asthma. Glucocorticoid pharmacokinetics, glucocorticoid receptor characteristics and inhibition of peripheral blood T-cell proliferation by glucocorticoids in vitro. *Am. Rev. Respir. Dis.* **144**, 1016–1025.

Corrigan, C.J., Brown, P.H., Barnes, N.C., Tsai, J.-J., Frew, A.J. and Kay, A.B. (1991b). Glucocorticoid resistance in chronic asthma. Peripheral blood T-lymphocyte activation and comparison of the T-lymphocyte inhibitory effects of glucocorticoids and cyclosporin A. *Am. Rev. Respir. Dis.* **144**, 1026–1032.

Curzen, N., Rafferty, P. and Holgate, S.T. (1987). Effects of a cyclooxygenase inhibitor, flurbiprofen, an H1 histamine receptor antagonist, terfenadine, alone and in combination on allergen-induced immediate bronchoconstriction in man. *Thorax* **42**, 946–952.

Cuss, F.M., Dixon, C.M.S. and Barnes, P.J. (1986). Effects of inhaled platelet-activating factor on pulmonary function and bronchial responsiveness in man. *Lancet* **2**, 189–192.

Dale, H.H. and Laidlaw, P.P. (1910). The physiological action of Biminazolylethamine. *J. Physiol.* **41**, 318–344.

Evans, J.M., Barnes, N.C., Zakrzewski, J.T., Glenny, H.P., Piper, P.J. and Costello, J.F. (1988). The activity of an inhaled leukotriene antagonist (SK&F 104,353–Z2) on bronchoconstriction induced by leukotriene D4 and histamine in man. *Brit. J. Clin. Pharmacol.* **26**, 677P–678P.

Evans, J.M., Barnes, N.C., Zakrzewski, J.T., Scibberas, D., Stahl, E., Piper,

P.J. and Costello, J.F. (1989). L648,051 a novel cysteinyl leukotriene antagonist is active by the inhaled route in man. *Brit. J. Clin. Pharmacol.* **28**, 125–135.

Fish, J.E., Ankin, M.G., Adkinson, N.F. and Peterman, V.I. (1981). Indomethacin modification of immediate-type immunologic airway responses in allergic asthmatic and non-asthmatic subjects. *Am. Rev. Respir. Dis.* **123**, 609–614.

Fleisch, J.H., Rinkema, L.E. and Haisch, K.D. (1985). [2-Hydroxy-3-propyl-4-(IH-tetrazol-5yl)butoxy]phenyl]ethanone an orally active leukotriene D4 antagonist. *J. Pharmacol. Exp. Ther.* **233**, 148–157.

Ford-Hutchinson, A.W. (1992). 5-Lipoxygenase inhibition. *In* "New Drugs for Asthma" (P.J. Barnes, ed.), vol. 2. IBC Technical Services Limited, Byfleet, United Kingdom.

Freitag, A., Watson, R.M., Matsar, G., Eastwood, C. and O'Byrne, P.M. (1991). The effect of treatment with an oral platelet activating factor antagonist (WEB 2086) on allergen induced asthmatic responses in human subjects. *Am. Rev. Respir. Dis.* **143**, A157.

Fuller, R.W., Black, P.N. and Dollery, C.T. (1988). Effect of oral LY171,883 on inhaled and intradermal antigen and LTD4 in atopic subjects. *Brit. J. Clin. Pharmacol.* **25**, 626P.

Gaddy, J., Bush, R.K., Margolskee, D., Williams, V.C. and Busse, W. (1990). The effects of a leukotriene D4 (LTD4) antagonist MK-571 in mild to moderate asthma. *Allergy Clin. Immunol.* **85**, A197.

Gardiner, P.J. (1992). Prostanoid agonists/inhibitors as new drugs for asthma. *In* "New Drugs for Asthma" (P.J. Barnes, ed.). IBC Technical Services Limited, Byfleet, United Kingdom.

Gould, C.A.L., Ollier, S., Aurich and Davies, J.R. (1988). A study of the clinical efficacy of azelastine in patients with extrinsic asthma and its effect on airway responsiveness. *Brit. J. Clin. Pharmacol.* **26**, 515–525.

Hardy, C.C., Robinson, C., Tattersfield, A.E. and Holgate, S.T. (1984). The bronchoconstrictor effect of inhaled prostaglandin D2 in normal and asthmatic men. *New Engl. J. Med.* **311**, 209–213.

Hay, W.P., Muccitelli, R.M. and Tucker, S.S. (1987). Pharmacologic profile of SK&F 104,353: a novel, potent and selective peptido-leukotriene receptor antagonist in guinea pig and human airways. *J. Pharmacol. Exp. Ther.* **243**, 474–487.

Heaton, R.W., Henderson, A.F., Dunlop, L.S. and Costello, J.F. (1984). The influence of pre-treatment with prostaglandin $F_{2\alpha}$ on bronchial sensitivity to inhaled histamine and methacholine in normal subjects. *Brit. J. Dis. Chest* **78**, 168–173.

Holgate, S.T., Emanuel, M.B. and Howarth, P. (1985). Astemizole and other H1-antihistamine drug treatment of asthma. *J. Allergy Clin. Immunol.* **76**, 375–380.

Hui, K.P. and Barnes, N.C. (1991a) Lung function improvement in asthma with a cysteinyl-leukotriene receptor antagonist. *Lancet,* **337**, 1062–1063.

Hui, K.P., Taylor, I.K., Taylor, G.W., (1991b). Effect of a 5-lipoxygenase inhibitor on leukotriene generation and airway responses after allergen challenge in asthmatic patients. *Thorax* **46**, 184–189.

Israel, E., Juniper, E.F., Morris, M.M., Dowell, A.R., Hargreave, F.E. and Drazen, J.M. (1988). A leukotriene D4 (LTD4) receptor antagonist, LY171, 883, reduces the bronchoconstriction induced by cold air challenge in asthmatics: a randomised double-blind, placebo-controlled trial. *Am. Rev. Respir. Dis.*, **137** (Suppl. 4), A27.

Israel, E., Dermarkarian, R., Rosenberg, M. *et al.* (1990). The effects of a 5-lipoxygenase inhibitor on asthma induced by cold, dry air. *New Engl. J. Med.* **323**, 1740–1744.

Jeffery, P.K., Wardlaw, A.J., Nelson, F.C., Collins, J.V. and Kay, A.B. (1989). Bronchial biopsies in asthma: an ultrastructural, quantitative study and correlation with hyperreactivity. *Am. Rev. Respir. Dis.* **140**, 1734–1753.

Jones, G., Mierins, E. and Karsh, J. (1991). Methotrexate-induced asthma. *Am. Rev. Respir. Dis.* **143**, 179–181.

Jones, T.R., Zamboni, R., Belley, M., Champion, E., Charette, L. and Ford-Hutchinson, A.W. (1989). Pharmacology of L660,711 (MK-571); a novel potent and selective leukotriene D4 receptor antagonist. *Can. J. Physiol. Pharmacol.* **67**, 17–28.

Kips, J., Joos, G., Pauwels, R., Van der Straeten, M. and De Lepeleire, I. (1990). MK-571 (L660,711): a potent LTD4 antagonist in asthmatic men. *Am. Rev. Respir. Dis.* **141** (Suppl. 4), A117.

Klaustermeyer, W.B., Noritake, D.T. and Kwong, F.K. (1987). Chrysotherapy in the treatment of corticosteroid-dependent asthma. *J. Allergy Clin. Immunol.* **79**, 720–725.

Krell, R.D., Aharony, D., Buckner, C.K., Keith, R.A., Kusner, E.J., Synder, D.W. *et al.* (1990). The preclinical pharmacology of ICI 204,219, a peptide leukotriene antagonist. *Am. Rev. Respir. Dis.* **141**, 978–987.

Kuitert, L. and Harrison, A.C. (1991) *Pneumocystis carinii* pneumonia as a complication of methotrexate treatment of asthma. *Thorax,* **461**, 936–937.

Lai, C.K.W., Jenkins, J.R., Polosa, R. and Holgate, S.T. (1990). Inhaled PAF fails to induce airway hyperresponsiveness to methacholine in normal human subjects. *J. Appl. Physiol.* **68**, 919–926.

Lee, T.H., Walport, M.J., Wilkinson, A.H., Turner-Warwick, M. and Kay, A.B. (1981). Slow-reacting substance of anaphylaxis antagonist FPL55712 in chronic asthma. *Lancet* **2**, 304–305.

Majno, G. (1964). Mechanisms of abnormal vascular permeability in acute inflammation. *In* "Injury, Inflammation and Immunity" (L. Thomas, H.W. Uh, and L. Grant, eds), pp. 58–93. Williams & Wilkins, Baltimore.

Manning, P.J., Watson, R.M., Margolskee, D.J., Williams, V.C., Schwartz, J.I. and O'Byrne, P.M. (1990). Inhibition of exercise-induced bronchoconstriction by MK-571 a potent leukotriene D4 receptor antagonist. *New Engl. J. Med.* **323**, 1736–1739.

Margolskee, D., Bodman, S., Dockhorn, R. and Israel, E. (1991). The therapeutic effects of MK-571, a potent and selective leukotriene (LT)D4 receptor antagonist in patients with chronic asthma. *J. Allergy Clin. Immunol.* **87**, 309(A677).

Medical Research Council (1956a). Controlled trial of effects of cortisone acetate in chronic asthma. *Lancet* **2**, 798–803.

Medical Research Council (1956b). Controlled trial of cortisone acetate in status asthmaticus. *Lancet* **2**, 803–806.

Mills, J.E., Sellick, H. and Widdicombe, J.C.T. (1969). Activity of lung irritant receptors in pulmonary microembolism, anaphylaxis and drug-induced bronchoconstriction. *J. Physiol.* **203**, 337–357.

Mullarkey, M.F., Blumenstein, B.A., Andrade, W.P., Bailey, G.A., Olason, I. and Wetzel, C.E. (1988). Methotrexate in the treatment of corticosteroid-dependent asthma. A double-blind crossover study. *New Engl. J. Med.* **318**, 603–607.

Mullarkey, M.F., Lammert, J.E. and Blumenstein, B.A. (1990). Long-term methotrexate treatment in corticosteroid-dependent asthma. *Ann. Intern. Med.* **112**, 5777–5781.

Nabe, M., Agrawal, D.K., Sarmiento, E.V. and Townley, R.G. (1989). Inhibitory effect of terfenadine on mediator release from human blood basophils and eosinophils. *Clin. Exp. Allergy* **19**, 515–520.

Naclerio, R.M., Kagey-Sobotka, A., Lichtenstein, L.M., Freidhoff, L. and Proud, D. (1990). Terfenadine, an H1 antihistamine inhibits histamine release in vivo in the human. *Am. Rev. Respir. Dis.* **142**, 167–171.

Nierop, G., Gijzel, W.P., Bel, E.H., Zwinderman, K. and Dijkman, J.H. (1991). Oral gold (Auranofin) in the treatment of steroid-dependent asthma; a long-term prospective study. *Eur. Resp. J.* **4** (Suppl. 14), 343.

O'Connor, B.J., Ridge, S.M., Chen-Worsdell, Y.M., Uden, S., Barnes, P.J. and Chung, K.F. (1991). Complete inhibition of airway and neutrophil responses to inhaled platelet activating factor (PAF) by an oral antagonist UK-74,505. *Am. Rev. Respir. Dis.* **143**, A156.

Phillips, G.D., Rafferty, P. and Holgate, S.T. (1987). LY-171 883 as an oral leukotriene D4 antagonist in non-asthmatic subjects. *Thorax* **42**, 723.

Rafferty, P., Beasley, R., Southagel, P. and Holgate, S.T. (1987). The role of histamine in allergen and adenosine-induced bronchoconstriction. *Int. Arch. Allergy Appl. Immunol.* **82**, 292–294.

Shiner, R.J., Nunn, A.J., Chung, K.F. and Geddes, D.M. (1990). A randomised, double-blind, placebo-controlled trial of methotrexate in steroid-dependent asthma. *Lancet* **336**, 137–140.

Smith, A.P., Cuthbert, M.F. and Dunlop, L.S. (1975). Effects of inhaled prostaglandins E1, E2 and F2α on the airways resistance of healthy and asthmatic man. *Clin. Sci.* **48**, 421–430.

Smith, L.J. (1989). Animal models of asthma. *Pulm. Pharmacol.* **2**, 59–74.

Smith, L.J., Geller, J., Elbright, L., Glass, M. and Thyrum, P.T. (1990). Inhibition of leukotriene D4-induced bronchoconstriction in normal subjects by the oral LTD4 receptor antagonist ICI 204,219. *Am. Rev. Respir. Dis.* **141**, 988–992.

Szczeklik, A., Gryglewski, R.J. and Czerniawska-Mysik, G. (1975). Relationship of inhibition of prostaglandin biosynthesis by analgesics to asthma attacks in aspirin sensitive patients. *Brit. Med. J.* **1**, 67–69.

Taylor, G.W., Taylor, I.K., Black, P., Maltby, N.H., Fuller, R.W. and Dollery, C.T. (1989). Urinary leukotriene E4 after antigen challenge and in acute asthma and allergic rhinitis. *Lancet* **1**, 584–588.

Taylor, I.K., O'Shaughnessy, K.M., Fuller, R.W. and Dollery, C.T. (1991). Effect of cysteinyl-leukotriene receptor antagonist ICI 204,219 on allergen-induced bronchoconstriction and airway hyperactivity in atopic subjects. *Lancet* **337**, 690–693.

Taytard, A. Beaumont, D., Pujet, J.C., Sapene, M. and Lewis, P.J. (1987). Treatment of bronchial asthma with terfenadine; a randomised controlled trial. *Brit. J. Clin. Pharmacol.* **24**, 743–746.

Ulbrich, E. and Nowak, M. (1990). Long term, multicentre study with azelastine in patients with intrinsic asthma. *Arzneimittelforschung* **40**, 1225–1230.

Wilkens, H., Wilkens, J.H., Bosse, S. *et al.* (1991). Effects of an inhaled PAF antagonist (WEB 2086BS) on allergen-induced early and late asthmatic responses and increased bronchial responsiveness to methacholine. *Am. Rev. Respir. Dis.* **143**, A812.

Young, R.N. (1988). The development of new anti-leukotriene drugs: L648,051 and L649,923, specific leukotriene D4 antagonists. *Drugs of the Future* **13**, 745–759.

Zakrzewski, J.T., Barnes, N.C., Costello, J.F. and Piper, P.J. (1987). Lipid mediators in cystic fibrosis and chronic obstructive pulmonary disease. *Am. Rev. Respir. Dis.* **136**, 779–782.

Discussion

C. Page

Do you think that because a drug does or does not work in early and late responses means that it will not work in asthma? Is it a good model to use?

N.C. Barnes

I do not think it is that good a model. We have such a limited number of drugs which are effective in asthma – essentially five, three of which are direct bronchodilators, with two of which direct bronchodilatation cannot be tested – so we might want to use some other model. These two happen to work in antigen challenge. This does not mean that other new classes of drugs will not be found which have no effect on antigen challenge but do affect asthma.

C. Page

It is clear from what we have heard today that one of the problems in asthma research generally is that everybody is looking at acute changes, whether it be in animals or in man. Whether PAF or antigen is taken as an example, there are very small changes that occur over 24 h to try to mimic a disease that may take years to come on or develop. We have to re-assess how we look at all these drugs generally.

N.C. Barnes

We cannot get somebody to take a drug for more than, say, 6 weeks unless it shows some effect. If a drug has to be taken for a year to get improvement, people will not take it. Some benefit has to be shown within a reasonable time frame.

C. Page
That is taking people with established disease, but surely the long-term aim of this area of research should be to identify people much earlier and try to stop them developing many of these changes.

N.C. Barnes
That assumes those changes are irreversible, but we do not know whether they are.

J.-A. Karlsson
I am interested in the role of the T cell. You said that cyclosporin may have many different actions, and you are treating with respectable doses of cyclosporin for quite a long time. Have you some other data to support a specific role for T cells?

N.C. Barnes
The data are inferential, in that they are another piece in the jigsaw – together with all the biopsy and acute severe asthma data – suggesting a role for T-lymphocytes. If a drug that appears in all diseases to have its major mode of action on the T-lymphocyte had failed this test, if it had not been effective in asthma, it would obviously have put a big question mark over the role of the T-lymphocytes in asthma. The fact that it has come through this test, must be of some support for the role of the lymphocyte.

J.-A. Karlsson
If there are the different subtypes of T cells that we have been discussing, cyclosporin would perhaps affect different subtypes, different types of T cells and also of other cells. How do your data fit with the idea that specifically the T helper 2 type lymphocyte would be incriminated in the disease?

N.C. Barnes
We have not investigated which particular subset it is. The only way in which it could be investigated would be to look at the changes in lymphocytes in bronchial biopsies. We discussed doing that at the beginning of this study, but decided that it was too much to put the patients through, but we are thinking of doing it in any subsequent trial.

I accept that there are other actions of cyclosporin, but even if it turns out that we are wrong and it is not the lymphocyte, its other actions are on cells expressing cytokines. Thus, even if it does not point to the lymphocyte, it points to cytokines as being very important.

J.-A. Karlsson

I certainly accept that. Another interesting point is that if it is accepted that the T cell is probably involved in early events, perhaps we should look at fairly recently established asthmatics to see if there is anything in the induction phase which would be affected even more.

N.C. Barnes

I think that is right. It would be fascinating to look at cyclosporin in much milder groups of asthmatics or in early stages of the disease. However, cyclosporin has a lot of side-effects, some of which are quite unpleasant, and it would not be ethically justified to use it in milder forms of disease. If a safer drug with a similar mode of action could be developed, or if the dose of cyclosporin could be decreased in some way, it would be fascinating to do that – and it obviously needs to be done.

A.R. Leff

Many of the criticisms (with which I agree) levelled against Mullarkey's work on methotrexate could be levelled against this work: relatively small changes not leading to a cure, an extremely expensive and toxic drug, certainly not for the everyday clinicians. As we look at drug strategies, the sort of anti-inflammatory agents we really want are drugs as safe as inhaled corticosteroids that anybody can take.

I am not sure, therefore, that this is the right direction to go – a toxic and extremely expensive anti-inflammatory drug – but perhaps it opens a book on the idea that drugs which may diminish the dose of prednisone *may* suggest pathways for intervention.

N.C. Barnes

I entirely accept that. There may be a very small number of patients with particularly bad side-effects on steroids or who have particularly bad asthma in whom the use of cyclosporin would be considered. Its importance is in opening a new therapeutic door, rather than in the drug itself. Its importance compared with methotrexate is, first, that methotrexate works on all dividing cells and, secondly, methotrexate does not improve lung function so patients are still left with their chronic disease – but with a lower dose of steroids. Cyclosporin, we think, improves lung function – it actually makes asthma better.

A.R. Leff

Is that based on the peak flow data that you showed? [*Dr Barnes*: Yes – and the FEV_1.] The changes in peak flow were something like 50 litres/min, which is negligible, even if significant.

N.C. Barnes

It cannot be said to be negligible. In the inhaled steroid studies that is the type of improvement in peak flow that was shown. With salmeterol, they are looking at smaller changes than that in morning peak flow. A lot of the studies on theophyllines in morning dipping show a 9% improvement in peak flow. The changes I presented are a bigger percentage than with those other drugs.

R. Dahl

In the leukotriene studies there was an additive effect to the β-agonist. Because you claim this effect is superimposed on the β_2-agonist response, the studies should probably be done the other way round to demonstrate the maximum β_2-agonist response, instead of giving the leukotriene antagonist first.

N.C. Barnes

I accept that – we did not expect the effect to be additive, so the study was not designed to look at it specifically. We are just about to start a study in which a β_2-agonist will be given first, then adding in the leukotriene antagonist.

An additive benefit of salbutamol and aminophylline can be shown if both are used at small doses but, with a big dose of salbutamol (which is what was used in the leukotriene study), aminophylline either has a small additive action or none.

S.T. Holgate

We have not talked much about the PAF antagonists. There has seldom been a research area promulgated throughout the world that was driven so much by animal pharmacology, with almost a negligible amount of human pharmacology to support why industry came so vehemently behind promoting this particular area in asthma. It has always been a mystery to me why industry responded in this way, particularly with the guinea-pig (which was the small model), with the view that hyperresponsiveness, as measured in an animal model acutely, has anything to do with the hyperresponsiveness measured in asthma. I find it extraordinary that a research project could have generated so many levels of enthusiasm on so few data based on the real disease.

My plea is that in future, learning possibly from mistakes in this field, the human model is used first – as Dr Barnes is doing – then developing the animal models to try to replicate as far as possible those aspects that we think we are trying to target, rather than the other way round.

N.C. Barnes
I completely agree – you are preaching to the converted.

J.M. Drazen
I would to some extent disagree. Of all the drugs which have been discovered in animal models, whether or not they work in human disease, as far as I know none has been found to work in human disease that does not work in animal models. We have to be willing to accept a level of false positives from the animal studies. It certainly makes sense: the leukotriene antagonists and the 5-lipoxygenase inhibitors, which look promising, were discovered in animal models. The bronchodilators, which are used commonly, were discovered and tested in animal models. The PAF antagonists were also discovered and tested in animal models, and it appears that they are not going to work – but there are no drugs that work in asthma that do not work in animal models.

It seems to me that the logical process to follow is basic discovery in animal models, then proceeding to clinical studies as soon as they are viable.

C. Page
I would also take issue with Professor Holgate, particularly about the PAF antagonists. We have seen single points of one dose of a PAF antagonist blocking exogenous PAF. People who have studied PAF for a long period of time know that one of the problems with many of the antagonists that have been discovered is that they do not penetrate membranes. We now know that the receptor for PAF inside the cell is completely different from the one on the surface, also that 90% of the PAF produced by cells after antigen provocation goes inside, as opposed to all the exogenous PAF.

Therefore, I think that in much of what has been done so far, a dose is chosen that blocks exogenous PAF – but if we look at the animal data carefully, much higher concentrations have to be used as is true in the lipoxygenase area. No one has actually shown in man shifts of the dose–response curve to know how potent these drugs are. Whether or not they work is irrelevant. At the moment, it is very misleading to say that one single dose that blocks PAF does not actually block antigen.

S.T. Holgate
I would disagree with Dr Drazen. In fact, many drugs that have gone into animal models are very effective against early and late phase reactions and hyperreactivity in animal models, but which have not stood the test of time in man. I can list a number of them, such as tranelast

and azelastine, which have trivial effects, if any, in humans, yet have powerful effects in the animal models.

J.M. Drazen
But we have to be willing to accept a level of false positives. Tell me of drugs that work in man that do *not* work in animals.

S.T. Holgate
I want to illustrate an iterative process here. The PAF story generated its own hypothesis that drove the programme far beyond the studies that were able to substantiate it in humans. If we are developing animal models, I think we need to keep an iterative process going whereby the human and the animals are feeding back on each other. I wanted to raise the point because it is controversial.

A.R. Leff
We are not taking a monolithic view here from the USA, but I would echo Dr Drazen's point. Many of the ideas for using the kind of immunosuppressive medication that Dr Barnes talked about came from studies in animals, in which compounds like hydroxyurea and cyclophosphamide were used in massive doses. Those were the first studies to suggest that suppressing granulocyte function (perhaps not lymphocyte function) might in some way possibly intervene in asthma. I am willing to accept the disappointments that Dr Drazen indicates we will have but, as an animal experimenter, I would like to see these studies, particularly with toxic drugs, begin in animals. What can be done in animals is to use very high doses, without getting into debates about how many units of peak flow changes are necessary to see something important. This becomes the screening process that Professor Holgate calls the iterative process that then can feed back and forth. I think we simply cannot start doing any study that comes to mind in humans.

N.C. Barnes
I accept that animal experimentation has to be done to look for mediators, to generate new hypotheses, but we have to have some evidence in man that something might be going on and might be working. PAF is an excellent example: it cannot be measured so we do not know it is there, its biological effects are purely bronchoconstriction because the bronchial hyperresponsiveness (the main point of interest) does not seem to exist as a real phenomenon, and drugs that work against it are developed – and they do not work. That is $2\frac{1}{2}$ of Koch's postulates for a mediator

which have disappeared, and yet people still say that PAF might be important.

We have to take a position on this. I would be extremely surprised – pleasantly surprised, because it would be nice to have a new drug in asthma – if PAF antagonists work. There is not a glimmer of any effect.

C. Page
Why was PAF studied in man? It was because it was studied in animals. We are not going suddenly to spray normal people with any mediator. We are hearing all the time at this meeting about cytokines – but there is less evidence that they do anything in man than there is with PAF.

N.C. Barnes
I accept that but, having done the studies in man, having done the PAF inhalation challenges and shown these very variable effects, there should have been a big question mark over the drug, especially when it was then shown to generate another mediator which could be blocked.

T.H. Lee
I think we all accept that leukotriene inhibitors and especially antagonists look interesting. We are, of course, interested in cyclosporin data and will be pleased to see the paper in the *Lancet* and look at the crossover analysis. We have inhaled steroids, β-agonists and all these other things. Where do you place leukotriene antagonists and cyclosporin? This is a difficult question, obviously, but can you put it into perspective?

N.C. Barnes
From the evidence so far, my feeling is that leukotriene antagonists will be active – I do not think there is any doubt about it – but less active than inhaled steroids. They may be additive in their actions with inhaled steroids and β_2-agonists. The evidence for the new ones is that they are very safe, so I have a feeling they may find a place, because they can be taken as a tablet, and can be added to other therapy. I cannot see them taking over from inhaled steroids, except perhaps in the very mildest asthmatics.

I think cyclosporin will have an extremely minor role. There will be a very small number of very bad asthmatics for whom it will be of importance. The approach of using drugs that work somewhere around the lymphocyte–cytokine axis is exciting. We have taken the toughest possible test for this drug: the worst asthmatics on high doses of known effective treatment, adding in this drug – and it works. This is a very tough test.

T.H. Lee
Were any of the asthmatics who were put on cyclosporin in your study steroid-resistant?

N.C. Barnes
We did not test whether they were steroid-resistant, but I suspect that a few of them may have been.

18

Anti-inflammatory Effects of Novel Selective Cyclic Nucleotide Phosphodiesterase Inhibitors

J.-A. KARLSSON, J. SOUNESS, D. RAEBURN,
M. PALFREYMAN and M. ASHTON

Rhône-Poulenc Rorer, Rainham Road South, Dagenham, Essex RM10 7XS, UK

Introduction

The asthmatic airway is characterized by a mucosal inflammation which seems to correlate with the severity of the disease and endows it with its peculiar characteristics such as variable airflow obstruction and hyperresponsiveness to bronchoconstrictor agents. One of the most prominent features of the bronchial inflammation is a pronounced eosinophilia, although the numbers of mast cells and sometimes lymphocytes and epithelial cells can also be increased in bronchoalveolar lavage (BAL) fluid and airway biopsies (Djukanovic *et al.*, 1990). A significant proportion of the inflammatory cells are degranulated in active disease and high levels of proteins such as eosinophil cationic protein (ECP), major basic protein (MBP) and mast cell tryptase can be detected together with albumin, other plasma proteins and a range of putative asthma mediators (Djukanovic *et al.*, 1990; Ädelroth *et al.*, 1990). The ongoing inflammatory process, which is also evident in patients between acute exacerbations and in subjects with only mild disease, is fuelled by such

T-Lymphocyte and Inflammatory Cell Research in Asthma
ISBN 0-12-388170-6

cytotoxic proteins and mediators and by extravasated pro-inflammatory proteins found in the inflamed mucosa.

Novel therapeutic agents with the potential of stabilizing inflammatory and immunocompetent cells, as for example through an interaction with intracellular signalling pathways, are actively being sought. Suppression of inflammatory and smooth muscle cell activity can be produced by raising intracellular levels of the cyclic nucleotide cyclic 3′,5′-adenosine monophosphate (cAMP). cAMP can be increased by stimulation of its synthesis by activation of adenylyl cyclase or by inhibition of its catabolism to 5′-AMP by cyclic AMP phosphodiesterase (PDE). Different PDE isozymes have been identified in various tissues and by use of selective inhibitors their relative importance in smooth muscle and inflammatory cells can now be assessed. Data obtained with the recently developed isozyme-selective PDE inhibitors suggest an important role for cyclic AMP-specific PDE (PDE IV) in these cells and agents which inhibit this activity may prove to be valuable drugs in the treatment of asthma.

Cyclic Nucleotide Phosphodiesterases

Cyclic nucleotide PDEs (EC 3.1.4.17) were discovered 30 years ago (Butcher and Sutherland, 1962). They hydrolyse the purine cyclic nucleotides (cAMP, cGMP) to the respective 5′-mononucleotides (5′-AMP, 5′-GMP) which do not activate cyclic nucleotide-dependent protein kinases. As a consequence of novel and improved biochemical separation techniques, multiple PDE isozymes with differing cell and tissue distributions have been identified. These have been categorized into five major families (Table 18.1). It is now clear from sequencing data that several subgroups exist within each family, giving the multiplicity of mammalian cyclic nucleotide PDEs a new dimension. The isolation of multiple PDE isoforms with differential tissue distribution has provided support for the view that they are involved in distinct tissue responses and a greater understanding of the roles of the individual PDE isozymes in different tissues and cells is emerging. A number of reviews which discuss the categorization of the PDE subtypes, based on biochemical, cloning and sequencing techniques, have recently appeared in the literature (Beavo and Reifsnyder, 1990; Thompson, 1991).

Pharmacological tools used in studies of PDE activity include the methylxanthines theophylline, caffeine and 3-isobutyl-1-methylxanthine (IBMX). These agents have been widely used but they are non-selective PDE inhibitors and, therefore, do not discriminate between isozymes. These xanthines are rather weak inhibitors, active only at

Table 18.1
Properties of phosphodiesterase families

PDE		Subfamilies reported	Effector	Preferred substrate(s)	Selective inhibitors
I	Ca^{2+} calmodulin-dependent	3–6	Ca^{2+}/calmodulin	cGMP	Vinpocetine
II	cGMP-stimulated	2–4	cGMP activate	cGMP = cAMP	None
III	cAMP-inhibited	2–4	cGMP inhibit	cAMP	Positive inotropes, e.g. SK&F 94836
IV	cAMP-specific	4	–	cAMP	Rolipram, Ro-20-1724
V	cGMP-specific	3–6	Light, cGMP	cGMP	Zaprinast, MY-5445

micromolar concentrations (Bergstrand, 1980), and much effort has been put into the search for more potent xanthine and non-xanthine PDE inhibitors.

Cyclic Nucleotide PDE Inhibitors Currently Used in Asthma Therapy

Theophylline has been long used in the treatment of asthma. In the last century, strong coffee (owing to its high content of caffeine) was suggested by Dr H.H. Salter as an effective remedy for acute shortness of breath (see Persson, 1985) but it was not until the middle of this century that xanthine pharmacology had been delineated and theophylline widely accepted in asthma therapy (see Persson, 1985). Theophylline effectively relaxes animal and human tracheobronchial smooth muscle *in vitro*, irrespective of which mediator has produced the contraction and is more effective than β_2-adrenoceptor agonists in highly contracted preparations (Finney *et al.*, 1985; Persson and Karlsson, 1987). A rapid improvement in airflow can be demonstrated in asthmatic patients which probably is due to relaxation of airway smooth muscle. Theophylline has a number of anti-inflammatory and immuno-modulatory effects (Persson *et al.*, 1988) and, indeed, it has been suggested that theophylline may act as a prophylactic agent. In clinical studies theophylline has been shown to inhibit acute and late phase bronchoconstrictor responses produced by antigen challenge (Pauwels *et al.*, 1985; Koëter *et al.*, 1989) and in severe asthma it may be a vital adjunct to glucocorticoid therapy (Brenner *et al.*, 1988). Theophylline seems, however, unable to reduce airway hyperresponsiveness in asthmatics (Du Toit *et al.*, 1987; Cockcroft *et al.*, 1989) although some conflicting data have been published (McWilliams *et al.*, 1984; Levene and McKenzie, 1986). Despite its bronchodilator and anti-inflammatory properties, theophylline's use in asthma therapy is limited by its pharmacokinetic properties and the frequency and potential severity of adverse reactions. At pharmacological concentrations, methylxanthines can exert pronounced effects in the central nervous system, kidney, cardiovascular system and gastrointestinal tract, which explains many of the side-effects seen in asthma therapy.

The demonstration of PDE isozymes has provided a foundation for the rational development of selective anti-inflammatory PDE inhibitors which is accompanied by the hope of finding potent compounds with minimal extrapulmonary actions. Inferentially, isozyme-selective PDE inhibitors may find use in other therapies and drugs are already being developed for various cardiovascular and CNS indications.

Are Theophylline's Anti-asthmatic Actions Mediated by PDE Inhibition?

The preceding discussion carries the assumption that theophylline's actions are mediated through inhibition of cyclic nucleotide PDEs. Although an effective PDE inhibitor, high concentrations (100–200 μM) are required to produce 50% inhibition of the enzyme *in vitro* (Bergstrand, 1980). A significant relaxation of isolated airway smooth muscle is, however, obtained already at low concentrations where no changes in intracellular cyclic nucleotide levels can be detected (Lohmann *et al.*, 1977; Kolbeck *et al.*, 1979). Furthermore, at therapeutic concentrations, theophylline is at best a weak inhibitor of PDE activity (Bergstrand, 1980; Nielson *et al.*, 1986).

Theophylline and other methylxanthines have been suggested to act via a number of other mechanisms, such as release of catecholamines, Ca^{2+} mobilization and adenosine receptor antagonism, which could potentially contribute to their pharmacological effects. For example, theophylline is 10–100 times more potent as an adenosine receptor antagonist than as a PDE inhibitor and it now seems likely that many of its extrapulmonary effects can be explained by this mechanism (e.g. Persson *et al.*, 1988). However, there is little evidence of adenosine being an asthma mediator and xanthines devoid of adenosine-antagonistic effects are still effective in asthma therapy (Pauwels *et al.*, 1985; Persson *et al.*, 1988). Hence, this particular action cannot account for their anti-inflammatory and bronchodilatory actions. The mechanism behind the desirable effects of the methylxanthines remains to be explained, but clinical trials in asthma patients with isozyme-selective and potent PDE inhibitors should throw some light as to the relative importance of this particular mechanism. Furthermore, a better insight into xanthine pharmacology may contribute to our understanding of asthma pathology.

Bronchodilator Effects of Novel Selective PDE Inhibitors

In human, bovine and canine airway smooth muscle at least five different PDE isozymes (types I, II, III, IV and V) have been demonstrated (Bergstrand, 1980; Torphy and Cieslinski, 1990; Shahid *et al.*, 1991; Giembycz and Dent, 1992). The physiological roles of various PDE isozymes in canine trachealis have been examined by correlating the functional responses (relaxation) of the tissue to isozyme-selective PDE inhibitors with cyclic nucleotide responses. PDE III and IV inhibitors act as functional antagonists, i.e. they relax the bronchial smooth muscle irrespective of the agent used to increase the tone. In canine trachealis, both siguazodan (SK&F 94836; PDE III inhibitor) and rolipram (PDE IV inhibitor) potentiated isoprenaline-induced relaxation and cAMP accumulation but did not influence responses to sodium nitroprusside, which stimulates cGMP synthesis. Conversely, zaprinast (PDE V inhibitor) potentiated sodium nitroprusside-induced relaxation and cGMP accumulation but did not affect responses to isoprenaline (Torphy *et al.*, 1988, 1991). These results demonstrate that PDE III and PDE IV hydrolyse cAMP in canine trachealis whereas PDE V hydrolyses cGMP. Bronchodilation is produced in the anaesthetized dog by non-selective PDE inhibitors as well as by inhibitors of PDE III and IV, but only PDE IV inhibitors are devoid of cardiovascular side-effects (Heaslip *et al.*, 1991) which tallies with functional data showing the importance of the PDE III isozyme in the cardiovasculature. Inhibitors of PDE III and/or IV also have been shown to inhibit bronchospasm in several other animal species including the guinea-pig, pig, cow, cat and mouse (Giembycz and Dent, 1992; Tomkinson *et al.*, 1993). A significant correlation has been demonstrated between relaxation of the guinea-pig trachea and inhibition of PDE III, but not PDE IV (Harris *et al.*, 1989). However, the correlation is significantly improved when relaxant actions are compared with high-affinity rolipram binding to brain membranes, indicating perhaps that such a binding site may also exist in the tracheobronchial smooth muscle and mediate relaxation. There is little data on a possible stereospecific interaction of rolipram in the airways (see below), but in a recent study Osborn *et al.* (1990) found (−)-rolipram to be two- to threefold more potent than the (+)-enantiomer at inhibiting ovalbumin-induced bronchospasm in the guinea-pig.

Although prominent isozymes in bronchial smooth muscle, the role of PDE I and II have yet to be elucidated, partly owing to the lack of potent and selective inhibitors of these two isozymes.

We have been particularly interested in the PDE IV isozyme since it seems to be involved in tracheobronchial smooth muscle relaxation and it has also been identified in a number of inflammatory cells (see below). A novel, potent and selective inhibitor of this isozyme has been synthesized, RP 73401 (3-cyclopentyloxy-*N*-(3,5-dichloropyridin-4-yl)-4-methoxybenzamide (Fig. 18.1; Ashton *et al.*, 1991). RP 73401 inhibits PDE IV isolated from pig aorta or guinea-pig eosinophils with an IC_{50} value of 1.0 nM, and is thus 30 to 3000 times more potent than the archetypal PDE IV inhibitor rolipram in these preparations (Table 18.2). RP 73401 is a potent relaxant of guinea-pig and bovine airway smooth muscle *in vitro*. In the unaesthetized guinea-pig and rat, RP 73401 dose-dependently inhibited histamine and antigen (ovalbumin)-induced bronchospasm and is consistently more potent than rolipram (unpublished data).

In human airway smooth muscle the functionally important PDE isozymes appear to be the PDEs III and IV. Studies in human isolated trachea *in vitro* have shown that inhibitors of PDEs III (SK&F 94120) and IV (rolipram, RP 73401) relax preparations with a spontaneous tone as well as those precontracted by different mediators (Giembycz *et al.*, 1992). Interestingly, in this study rolipram was able to relax methacholine-contracted tissues more effectively than those with a spontaneous tone

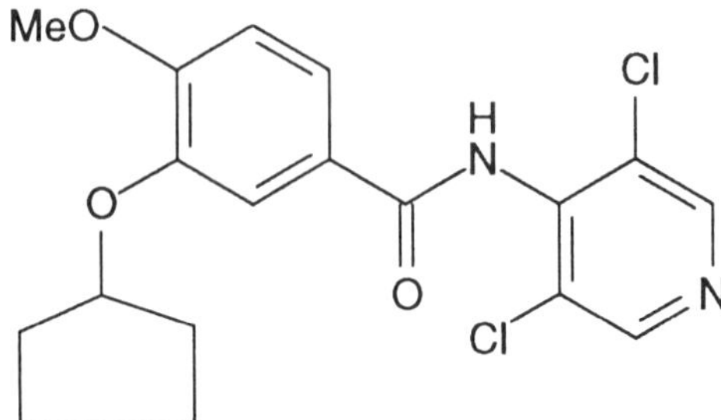

Fig. 18.1 Chemical structure of RP 73401.

Table 18.2
Phosphodiesterase isozyme selectivities of rolipram and RP 73401

	IC_{50} (μM)	
	Rolipram	RP 73401
Pig Aorta		
PDE I	> 1000	49 ± 1
PDE III	263 ± 13	267 ± 111
PDE IV	3 ± 0.7	0.001 ± 0.0001
PDE V	482 ± 53	19 ± 5
Eosinophil		
Bound PDE IV	0.20 ± 0.08	0.0007 ± 0.0002
Solubilized PDE IV	0.029 ± 0.004	0.0008 ± 0.0005

(Giembycz *et al.*, 1992). On the other hand, in a separate study rolipram was found to be consistently active in human bronchial preparations with both basal and induced tone (Advenier *et al.*, personal communication). Whether these apparent differences between RP 73401 and rolipram are due to these compounds having separate ways of interacting with the enzyme (see below) or whether the enzyme distribution varies with airway level is not yet known. Zardaverine, an inhibitor of both isozymes, also relaxes human bronchi *in vitro* (Rabe *et al.*, 1992).

Taken together, both *in vitro* and *in vivo*, data from animal experiments indicate an important role for PDE III and IV in relaxation of airway smooth muscle. Preliminary data in human airways *in vitro* seem to corroborate this view.

PDE Isozymes and Effects of Selective Inhibitors on Inflammatory Cells *in vitro*

PDE Isozymes in Inflammatory Cells

Inflammatory and immunocompetent cells have now been shown to have a varying repertoire of PDE isozymes (Table 18.1). The predominant isozyme is the cyclic AMP-specific PDE IV which is present in neutrophils (Wright *et al.*, 1990; Nielsen *et al.*, 1990), monocytes (White *et al.*, 1990), basophils (Peachell *et al.*, 1990), mast cells (Torphy and Undem, 1991) and lymphocytes (Robicsek *et al.*, 1989). PDE III is associated with lymphocytes (Robicsek *et al.*, 1989) and platelets (Simpson *et al.*, 1988).

Platelets also contain PDE V (Weishaar *et al.*, 1986). The PDE complement of endothelial cells from the airway microvasculature has not been established although aortic endothelial cells contain PDEs II and IV (Souness *et al.*, 1990; Lugnier and Schini, 1990). A recent paper (Kishi *et al.*, 1992) indicated the presence of PDE V in bovine aortic endothelial cells, although zaprinast does not exert a marked effect on cGMP accumulation in these cells (Souness *et al.*, 1990). PDE II is also found in T-lymphocytes (Robicsek *et al.*, 1989). Whether the presence of PDE II in endothelial cells and T-lymphocytes implies opposing actions of cAMP and cGMP, as has been demonstrated in other cells (MacFarland *et al.*, 1991) remains to be established. Several PDE isozymes have been demonstrated in murine peritoneal macrophages (Okonogi *et al.*, 1991), whereas the PDE IV seems to be the predominant PDE in guinea pig peritoneal macrophages (Burns and Souness, unpublished data).

The predominant and, perhaps only, PDE in guinea-pig eosinophils is PDE IV, which is almost exclusively tightly membrane bound (Souness *et al.*, 1991). This enzyme, like that of the neutrophil (Wright *et al.*, 1990), exhibits non-linear kinetics, suggesting the existence of two particulate PDE IV isozymes or one enzyme in more than one affinity state. No evidence for the presence of isozymes from other PDE families has been obtained to date. There is a poor correlation between the inhibitory activities of several inhibitors against bound, particulate PDE and their effects on whole cells (cAMP, superoxide release; Souness *et al.*, 1992). However, when the compounds were tested against cAMP PDE which had been solubilized with deoxycholate and NaCl, a very close relationship was obtained (Souness *et al.*, 1992). The main effect of solubilization seems to be an increase, by at least tenfold, in the inhibitory potencies of selective PDE IV inhibitors (rolipram, denbufylline and Ro-20-1724), whereas the activities of several non-selective inhibitors were not markedly altered. One possible explanation for these results is that solubilization exposes an inhibitory site at which PDE IV inhibitors potently interact. Incubation of freshly prepared eosinophil membranes with vanadate/glutathione complex (Souness *et al.*, 1985) activates cAMP PDE and also increases (> tenfold) the inhibitory potencies of selective PDE IV inhibitors, but not non-selective inhibitors such as dipyridamole and trequinsin (Souness *et al.*, 1992).

Only a small enantiomeric potency difference is observed in rolipram's inhibition of bound, particulate eosinophil cAMP PDE; however, against the solubilized or V/GSH-treated activities (−)-rolipram is about 15 times more potent than (+)-rolipram (Souness and Scott, 1992). Additionally, in intact cells, (−)-rolipram is 10-times as potent as its (+)-enantiomer in stimulating accumulation of cAMP. These studies lend further support to the existence of two sites on eosinophil PDE IV. Moreover, the strong correlation between stimulatory effects of several selective and non-selective inhibitors on cAMP-accumulation in intact cells and their inhibition of solubilized PDE as well as the stereospecificity of rolipram's actions on intact eosinophils suggest that the native enzyme may exist in a form similar to that produced by these particular treatments.

The (−)- and (+)-enantiomers of rolipram are equipotent against pig aortic PDE IV, suggesting either that the stereospecific site is not present in all PDE IVs or that it is concealed by the purification procedures. The latter contention is supported by reduced stereospecificity of the eosinophil solubilized cAMP PDE after anion-exchange chromatography (Souness and Scott, 1992). It is noteworthy that the (−)-enantiomer of rolipram is about 20 times more potent than the (+)-enantiomer in displacing [^{3}H]-rolipram from brain membranes (Schneider *et al.*, 1986). The similarities in the enantiomeric potency differences on eosinophil cAMP PDE, whole cell responses (cAMP) and competition for the brain rolipram binding site, tempts speculation that rolipram's actions on eosinophils may be via a closely related high-affinity site. Despite an inability to detect [^{3}H]-rolipram binding to eosinophil membranes, strong correlations were observed between the potencies of several PDE inhibitors on solubilized eosinophil cAMP PDE, cAMP accumulation in intact cells and in competition for the high-affinity rolipram binding site (Souness, unpublished data).

Interesting differences exist between the inhibitory actions of rolipram and RP 73401 on the eosinophil PDE. Whereas solubilization and V/GSH treatment increase the inhibitory potency of rolipram they do not influence the already potent inhibitory effect of RP 73401. Interestingly, whereas rolipram is a weak inhibitor of pig aortic PDE IV, RP 73401 exhibits similar potency against eosinophil and pig aorta enzymes (Table 18.2), suggesting either two distinct PDE IV isozymes or that different inhibitors can interact with PDE IV differently. Human monocyte PDE IV activity has been expressed in yeast cells (Torphy *et al.*, 1992). In these cells a high-affinity binding site for rolipram was found, although there was not a close correlation between binding and inhibition of PDE IV activity (Torphy *et al.*, 1992). Perhaps the eosinophil enzyme also has such a high-affinity site and that under certain conditions (V/GSH treatment, solubilization) it can mediate a change in enzyme activity. If rolipram interacts more potently at the high-affinity site than at the catalytic site, whereas RP 73401 does not discriminate between the two sites, this may explain the discrepant effects V/GSH or solubilization have on their respective potencies. If the high-affinity site is missing from partially purified pig aorta enzyme, this may explain why RP 73401 but not rolipram retains its potent inhibition of this activity.

Actions of PDE Inhibitors on Inflammatory Cells

Agents that elevate cAMP, including PDE inhibitors generally exert dampening effects on inflammatory cells. Inhibitors of PDE IV seem to have a particularly interesting spectrum of activities (Table 18.3) since this isozyme is present in many of these cells.

PDE IV inhibitors reduce antigen-induced mediator release from mast cells and basophils (Frossard *et al.*, 1981; Busse and Anderson, 1981; Torphy and Undem, 1991), cytokine release from monocytes (Maschler and Christensen, 1991; Pollock and Withnall, unpublished data) and lysosomal enzyme, superoxide, leukotriene B_4 (LTB_4) and platelet-activating factor (PAF) release from neutrophils (Nielsen *et al.*, 1990). Release of elastase from a human mixed granulocyte population is strongly inhibited by rolipram and RP 73401 (data unpublished). The

Table 18.3
In vitro actions of PDE IV inhibitors

1.	Bronchial smooth muscle	Relaxation
2.	Mast cells	Inhibition of antigen-induced mediator (histamine, LTC_4) release
3.	Basophils	Inhibition of antigen-induced mediator (histamine, LTC_4) release
4.	Neutrophils	Inhibition of: respiratory burst, degranulation, PAF, LTB_4 release
5.	Eosinophils	Inhibition of: respiratory burst, degranulation
6.	Endothelial cells	Reduction of permeability
7.	Macrophages	Inhibition of AA breakdown Inhibition of cytokine (TNF-α) release
8.	Monocytes	Inhibition of cytokine (TNF-α) release
9.	Lymphocytes	Inhibition of human cytotoxic T-lymphocyte activity Inhibition of IL-2 release from T-lymphocytes Inhibition of T-cell blastogenesis Inhibition of IgE production from lymphocytes of atopic subjects

respiratory burst in human neutrophils is reduced by PDE IV inhibitors, but not by PDE III or V inhibitors (Chilton *et al.*, 1989; Nielsen *et al.*, 1990).

In guinea-pig eosinophils, rolipram and RP 73401 dose-dependently inhibit spontaneous and opsonized zymosan-stimulated superoxide anion production (Fig. 18.2) in concentrations also suppressing PDE IV activity (Souness *et al.*, 1991; Dent *et al.*, 1991; unpublished data). Inhibitors of PDE types III (siguazodan) and V (zaprinast) are inactive (Fig. 18.3). fMLP-induced superoxide (Fig. 18.2) and ECP release from human granulocytes also is antagonized by rolipram and RP 73401, suggesting

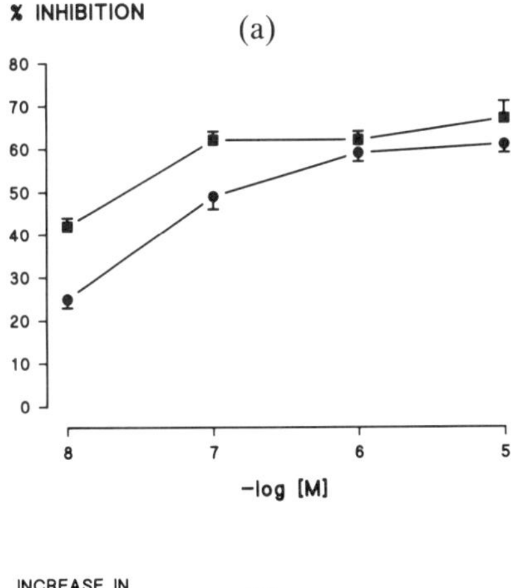

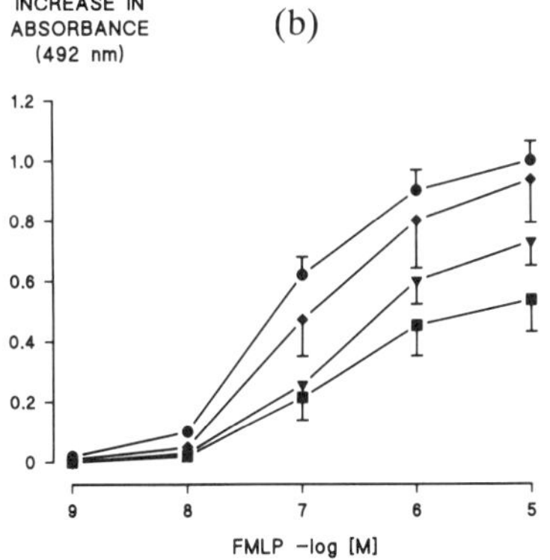

Fig. 18.2 (top) The effect of RP 73401 (■) and rolipram (●) on LTB_4-induced superoxide release from guinea-pig eosinophils *in vitro*. Mean ± S.E.M. data, $n = 9$–21. (bottom) The effect of RP 73401 on fMLP-induced superoxide release from human granulocytes *in vitro*: ●, vehicle control; ◆, RP 73401 0.1 nM; ▼ RP 73401 10 nM; ■ RP 73401 1μM. Mean ± S.E.M. data, $n = 5$–11.

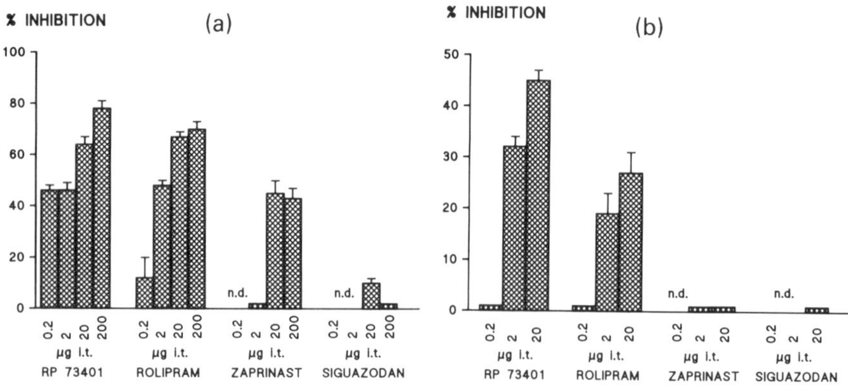

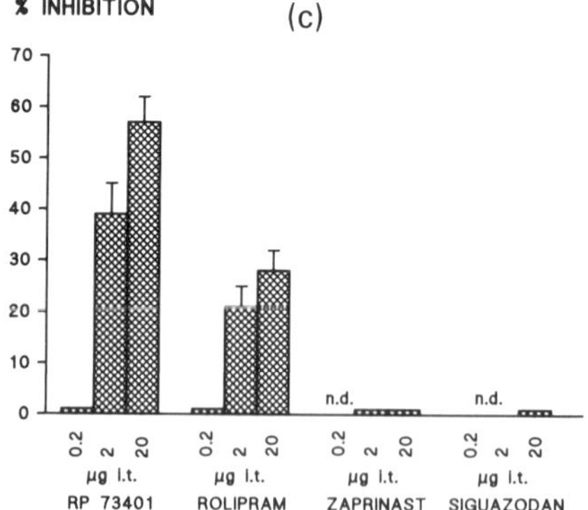

Fig. 18.3 The effect of RP 73401, rolipram, zaprinast and siguazodan on (a) antigen-induced bronchoconstriction, measured as increased in airway resistance, in the guinea-pig; (b) total cell population, recovered by BAL, 24 h after antigen challenge in the guinea-pig and (c) the eosinophil population, recovered by BAL, 24 h after antigen challenge in the guinea-pig. Mean ± S.E.M. data, n = 5–9.

that PDE IV is equally important in human eosinophils. Eosinophil-derived neurotoxin release from human cells has previously been shown to be inhibited by the non-selective inhibitors theophylline and IBMX (Kita *et al.*, 1991), which thus may have been through an interaction with PDE IV.

Immunoglobulin E (IgE) release from mononuclear leukocytes (B cells, derived from atopic subjects; Cooper *et al.*, 1985), the activity of cytotoxic T cells (Plaut *et al.*, 1983) and interleukin-2 release from human T-lymphocytes (Averill and Kammer, 1985) are also suppressed by inhibitors of PDE IV. The stimulation of human peripheral lymphocyte mitogenesis by phytohaemagglutinin (PHA) is accompanied by a marked increase in cAMP-PDE activity (Epstein and Hachisu, 1984). Since Ro-20-1724 blocks PHA-actions (Epstein and Hachisu, 1984), PDE IV may play a role in lymphocyte proliferation. Other cellular effects that have been described include a reduction of endothelial monolayer permeability by PDE III and IV inhibitors, which suggests that exudation of plasma proteins from the microvasculature could be reduced (Suttorp *et al.*, 1991).

PDE inhibitors potentiate the effects of agents that stimulate synthesis of cAMP in a number of inflammatory cells. This has potential therapeutic implications for asthma since amongst the mediators whose release from inflammatory cells is increased, would be several (such as prostaglandins of the E-series and certain peptides) which stimulate adenylate cyclase. It is therefore tempting to speculate that PDE inhibitors would be able to exert greater effects in the inflamed airway than in normal tissue because of this possible synergy.

Anti-inflammatory Effects of PDE Inhibitors *In Vivo*

It is well known from earlier studies that theophylline has demonstrable pulmonary and extrapulmonary anti-inflammatory effects in a number of animal species. For example, in mice, theophylline reduced bleomycin-induced pulmonary fibrosis (Lindenschmidt and Witschi, 1985) and PAF-induced mortality (Carlson *et al.*, 1987). Little is known about extrapulmonary anti-inflammatory effects of novel, selective PDE inhibitors, apart from studies showing that denbufylline inhibits arachidonic acid induced mouse ear oedema (Crummey *et al.*, 1987) and that rolipram reduces rat ear oedema (Klose *et al.*, 1986). No doubt, the increased availability of selective PDE inhibitors will unravel the role of cyclic nucleotides in various experimental inflammatory conditions.

Antigen-Induced Bronchospasm and Cell Infiltration

Antigen exposure of sensitized animals results in an acute airways obstruction and an influx of inflammatory cells into the bronchial mucosa and subsequently into the airway lumen. Aerosolized antigen produces an immediate bronchoconstriction in sensitized guinea-pigs, which has been reported to be followed by a late phase response 6–18 h later (Brattsand *et al.*, 1985; Iijima *et al.*, 1987; Hutson *et al.*, 1988). This late phase response is, however, not easily reproducible in all studies. When studied 24 h after challenge there is a two- to threefold increase in the number of inflammatory cells recovered in BAL fluid. Almost 50% of these cells are eosinophils, the remainder being predominantly macrophages with a small lymphocyte component. Infected animals, or those previously exposed to endotoxin, may have a high number of neutrophils.

Non-selective PDE inhibitors, such as theophylline, inhibit antigen- and PAF-induced bronchospasm and airway eosinophilia in guinea-pigs (Andersson and Bergstrand, 1981; Sanjar *et al.*, 1990a). AH 21-132, a mixed PDE III and IV inhibitor, also suppresses both bronchospasm and cell influx in this species (Sanjar *et al.*, 1990a,b). In these latter studies, the compounds were administered systemically for 6 days by use of osmotic minipumps and, thus, it remains to be shown whether AH 21-132 has similar effects after acute administration. Zardaverine, which has a similar profile to AH 21-132, has also been reported to have anti-inflammatory properties in guinea-pigs (Schudt *et al.*, 1991).

Airway anti-inflammatory effects of rolipram and other PDE IV inhibitors are emerging. When administered as a micronized dry powder directly into the airways both rolipram and RP 73401 almost completely inhibited the antigen-induced bronchospasm (Fig. 18.3). RP 73401 was more potent than rolipram as an inhibitor of the accompanying influx of inflammatory cells into the lavage fluid (Fig. 18.3). Interestingly, neither selective PDE III (siguazodan) nor PDE V (zaprinast) inhibitors reduced cell accumulation following antigen challenge (Fig. 18.3), suggesting that the efficacy of AH 21-132 and zardaverine rests with their ability to inhibit PDE IV.

PDE inhibitors may act at several levels to reduce cell trafficking into the airways. They have been shown to inhibit the generation of potent eosinophil chemoattractants such as PAF and complement C_2 (Lappin *et al.*, 1984). IL-2 has recently been identified as a particularly potent chemotactic agent for human eosinophils (Chapter 8), and IL-2 release from T-lymphocytes is suppressed by PDE IV inhibitors (Averill and Kammer, 1985). An alternative mechanism would be a diminished expression of select integrin adhesion molecules on either the capillary endothelium or the leukocyte itself. In apparent support of this latter possibility, increased levels of cAMP in neutrophils are associated with a decreased adhesiveness to endothelial layers (Riva *et al.*, 1989), although little is known about the role of this cyclic nucleotide in eosinophil adhesion. Elevation of cAMP directly reduces the expression of ELAM-1 and VCAM-1, but not ICAM-1, on the surface of endothelial cells (Pober *et al.*, 1992). Interestingly, PDE IV inhibitors inhibit release of tumour necrosis factor (TNF-α) from monocytes (Maschler and Christensen, 1991) and this cytokine is a potent inducer of ICAM-1 and ELAM-1 expression on endothelial cells (Wellicome *et al.*, 1990; Thornhill and Haskard, 1990), which thus could be an indirect means of regulating eosinophil migration.

In addition to acute effects on cell migration, we have observed that prolonged treatment (7 days) with rolipram decreases the number of circulating eosinophils (DeBrito *et al.*, 1991). The number of eosinophils in these parasite-infected mice was reduced by 39% ($P < 0.01$) and 34% ($P < 0.01$) in both the bone marrow and the peritoneal cavity, respectively. In this study rolipram had a glucocorticoid-like effect in that it inhibited the development of eosinophil progenitor cells. Although an attractive explanation, this effect seems unrelated to IL-5, since neither release from a murine T helper 2 clone, nor IL-5 stimulation of bone marrow cells were inhibited by rolipram (DeBrito *et al.*, 1991). Even if the acute inhibition of eosinophil migration cannot be accounted for by this mechanism, the ultimate consequence would obviously be a reduced number of circulating eosinophils.

Microvascular Leakage

Much attention has focused recently on the tracheobronchial microvasculature and its potential role in airway inflammation (Persson, 1986). The endothelium of post-capillary venules usually constitutes a tight barrier to circulating cells and macromolecules but in the inflammatory process gaps are formed between cells and large molecules such as plasma proteins can readily traverse these intercellular pathways. Proteins of, for example, the complement- and blood clotting-systems and their fragments have potent pro-inflammatory properties and together with other macromolecules these products can cause local tissue injury and fluid accumulation (oedema). Detection of proteins in BAL fluid and sputa from asthmatic patients has been argued as being a sign of an ongoing mucosal inflammation (Persson, 1986). Naclerio and co-workers (1988) have demonstrated that theophylline can reduce leakage of proteins into the nasal mucosa in rhinitis and sputum proteins are also reduced by therapeutic concentrations of this xanthine (Persson, 1986), supporting its clinical relevance. Theophylline has also been shown to inhibit PAF-induced leakage of a macromolecular tracer (FITC-dextran) in guinea-pig tracheobronchial tree and lavage fluid (Erjefält and Persson, 1991; Raeburn and Karlsson, 1992).

Adenylyl cyclase and guanylyl cyclase activities have been found in bovine and porcine aortic endothelial cells (Makarski, 1981; Martin *et al.*, 1988), together with type II and type IV PDE activities (Souness *et al.*, 1990; Lugnier and Schini, 1990). No direct demonstration of the

PDE isozyme present in the post-capillary venular endothelial cells, the site of active protein leakage, has been published. Agents elevating cAMP, including PDE III and IV inhibitors, reduce endothelial permeability *in vitro* (Suttorp *et al.*, 1991; Seibert *et al.*, 1992). Consistent with these data *in vitro*, we have demonstrated that rolipram and RP 73401 inhibit PAF-induced plasma extravasation in guinea-pig airways (Fig. 18.4; Raeburn and Karlsson, 1992). When administered as a dry powder into the airways 10 min before PAF challenge, both agents almost completely inhibited FITC-dextran leakage into the tracheobronchial tissue and airway lumen (Fig. 18.4). Interestingly, also topically administered zaprinast significantly inhibited plasma leakage (Fig. 18.4). Vinpocetine and siguazodan, however, were without effects (Raeburn and Karlsson, 1992). These data suggest a functional anti-leakage role for PDE types IV and V, but not I and III in the guinea-pig tracheobronchial microvascular endothelium.

Even though these compounds can be expected to act on the endothelial cell, an indirect effect on other cells in the airway mucosa to inhibit PAF-induced leakage cannot be wholly excluded from these experiments. Thus, endothelial cell contraction appears to be the major reason for gap formation although a direct relaxant effect of PDE inhibitors remains to be shown.

Bronchial Hyperresponsiveness

Mucosal inflammation is considered to be a major contributor to acute changes in bronchial hyperresponsiveness and drugs, such as glucocorticoids, which suppress this process also reduce the hyperrespon-

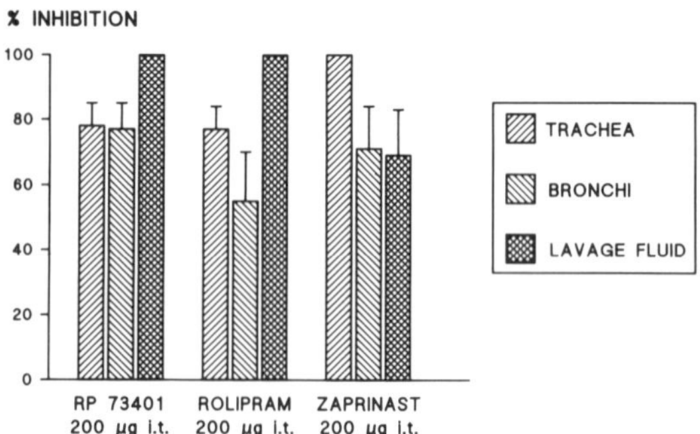

Fig. 18.4 The effect of RP 73401, rolipram and zaprinast on PAF-induced microvascular leakage of FITC-dextran in guinea-pig airways. Mean ± S.E.M. data, n = 4–8.

siveness. Animal models of airway hyperresponsiveness have been described, but with a few exceptions, the reactivity to a standard constrictor like histamine or acetylcholine is increased a modest two- to fourfold. Even with repeat antigen aerosol exposure in monkeys (Gundel *et al.*, 1989) and guinea-pigs (Ishida *et al.*, 1989) reactivity rarely increases more than tenfold. Exposure to aerosolized PAF is commonly used in studies of airway hyperresponsiveness in guinea-pigs and the degree of reactivity is examined by use of intravenous bombesin (e.g. Underwood *et al.*, 1992). Rolipram abolished the PAF-induced hyperresponsiveness to bombesin whereas theophylline only had a partial effect (Underwood *et al.*, 1992). In a recent study by Sanjar *et al.* (1990b), administration of the PDE III/IV inhibitor AH 21-132 or theophylline for up to a week did not significantly suppress antigen-induced hyperresponsiveness (although the eosinophilia was substantially reduced). These data suggest that the anti-inflammatory effects in the bronchi, the diminished influx of inflammatory cells and the suppression of mediator release, as well as the tightening of the microvascular endothelium may contribute to reduced hyperresponsiveness produced by PDE IV inhibitors.

Taken together, these data *in vivo* indicate that inhibitors of PDE IV exert a range of anti-inflammatory effects within the tracheobronchial tree. Although resident and migrating inflammatory cells contain a mixture of PDE isozyme activities, PDE IV appears to be of major importance in stabilizing the various cells contributing to the tracheobronchial mucosal inflammation.

Anti-asthmatic Effects of Novel Isozyme Selective PDE Inhibitors

cAMP PDE inhibitors such as 2,4-diamino-5-cyano-6-bromopyridine (Smith *et al.*, 1986), AH 21-132 (Small *et al.*, 1989) and zardaverine (Beume *et al.*, 1987) relax bronchial smooth muscle *in vitro* and the latter two compounds also act as bronchodilators *in vivo* (Beume *et al.*, 1987; Foster and Rakshi, 1990). In healthy subjects, AH 21-132 has been shown to reverse a methacholine-induced bronchoconstriction (Foster and Rakshi, 1990) and, when administered intravenously, to induce a small transient bronchodilation. Neither AH 21-132 nor zardaverine discriminate between PDE III and IV and it is therefore uncertain which isozyme contributes to their effects *in vivo*. Selective inhibitors of PDEs III, IV and V have attracted great interest for their potential anti-asthma effects. PDE III inhibitors are effective bronchodilators in a number of animal species (Torphy *et al.*, 1988): however, their effects on airways function are often accompanied by pronounced cardiovascular effects (Heaslip *et al.*, 1991). The PDE III inhibitor enoximone (MDL 17043) increases dynamic lung compliance and reduces specific airway resistance in subjects with chronic obstructive pulmonary disease (Leeman *et al.*, 1987). Zaprinast (M&B 22948), which emanates from a programme seeking to develop an orally active anti-allergic mast cell stabilizer, is widely used as an inhibitor of PDE V. It inhibits mediator release from rat but not human mast cells (Frossard *et al.*, 1981) and potently inhibits passive cutaneous anaphylaxis in the rat (Broughton *et al.*, 1975). Zaprinast is a weak bronchorelaxant but it potentiates sodium nitroprusside-induced relaxation and accumulation of cGMP in canine trachealis (Torphy *et al.*, 1991). In a placebo-controlled, double-blind crossover trial zaprinast (10 mg p.o.) reduced exercise-induced bronchoconstriction in adult asthmatics but did not inhibit histamine-induced bronchoconstriction, suggesting that it is not acting directly on the smooth muscle (Rudd *et al.*, 1983).

There is growing interest in the anti-asthma potential of selective PDE IV inhibitors. To date only one relatively weak PDE IV inhibitor, tibenelast (LY-186655), has been examined in asthmatics. At a single oral dose a slight, but non-significant improvement in FEV_1 was observed in asthmatics (Israel *et al.*, 1988). Owing to the weak PDE IV inhibitory activity of tibenelast, the role of this isozyme unfortunately remains unproven.

Conclusion

A wide range of PDE isozymes have been demonstrated in airway smooth muscle as well as in inflammatory and immunocompetent cells from various species, including man. The functional importance of cyclic nucleotides and these individual isozymes cannot be accurately assessed based on presence alone, since selective PDE inhibitors have markedly different effects. At least in preclinical experiments, inhibitors of PDE IV seem to have desirable anti-asthma characteristics: suppression of inflammatory cell activity, inhibition of microvascular leakage, reduction of airway hyperresponsiveness and relaxation of airway smooth muscle (Fig. 18.5). Some of these actions have been reproduced in human cells, for instance inhibition of mediator release from eosinophils, neutrophils, mast cells, basophils, monocytes and lymphocytes and relaxation of human bronchi. Preliminary studies in asthma patients with inhalation of combined PDE III/IV inhibitors have demonstrated bronchodilation. The compounds tested so far have been very weak inhibitors of the PDE IV

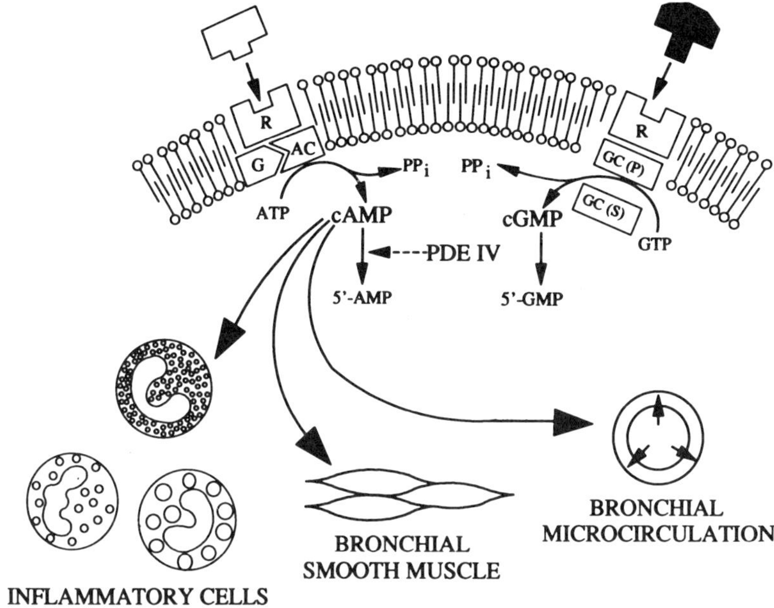

Fig. 18.5 Schematic drawing indicating intracellular cyclic nucleotide pathways of formation and degradation and the role of cAMP-dependent phosphodiesterase (PDE) in inflammatory cell activation.

compared with the new generation of inhibitors like RP 73401 which may thus display improved efficacy. Importantly, clinical studies with selective and more potent PDE inhibitors may also further our knowledge of the pathophysiology of the disease itself.

Acknowledgements

We would like to thank the following for their helpful contributions to the studies performed at RPR: C. Battram, F. DeBrito, S. Lewis, N.C. Turner, L. Wood, V. Woodman, A. Tomkinson and S. Underwood.

References

Ädelroth, E., Rosenhall, L., Johannson, S.-Å., Linden, M. and Venge, P. (1990). Inflammatory cells and eosinophil activity in asthmatics investigated by bronchoalveolar lavage. The effects of antiasthmatic treatment with budesonide or terbutaline. *Am. Rev. Respir. Dis.* **142**, 91–99.

Andersson, P. and Bergstrand, H. (1981). Antigen-induced bronchial anaphylaxis in actively sensitized guinea-pigs. Effect of long-term treatment with sodium cromoglycate and aminophylline. *Brit. J. Pharmacol.* **74**, 601–609.

Ashton, M.J., Cook, D.C., Fenton, G., Hills, S.J., McFarlane, I.M., Palfreyman, M.N., Ratcliffe, A.J. and Vicker, N. (1991). Rhône-Poulenc Rorer Patent; Benzamides; WO 921296-A1, 28 January.

Averill, L.E. and Kammer, G.M. (1985). Inhibition of interleukin-2 production is mediated by a cyclic adenosine monophosphate (cAMP)-dependent pathway. *Clin. Res.* **33**, 839A.

Beavo, J.A. and Reifsnyder, D.H. (1990). Primary sequence of cyclic nucleotide phosphodiesterase isozymes and the design of selective inhibitors. *Trends in Biochem. Sci.* **11**, 150–155.

Bergstrand, H. (1980). Phosphodiesterase inhibition and theophylline. *Eur. J. Respir. Dis.* **61** (suppl. 109), 37–44.

Beume, R., Eltze, M. and Kilian, U. (1987). Bronchodilatation due to inhibition of cAMP-PDE III; preclinical results on the pyridazinone derivative B842-90. *Naunyn-Schmiedeberg's Arch. Pharmacol.* **335**, R76.

Brattsand, R., Andersson, P., Wieslander, E., Linden, M., Axelsson, B. and Paulsson, I. (1985). Pathophysiological characteristics of a guinea-pig model for dual bronchial obstruction. In "Glucocorticoids, Inflammation and Bronchial hyperreactivity" (J.C. Hogg, R. Ellul-Micallef, R. Brattsand, eds), pp. 51–66. Excerpta Medica, Amsterdam.

Brenner, M., Berkowitz, R., Marshall, N. and Strunk, R.C. (1988). Need for theophylline in severe steroid-requiring asthmatics. *Clin. Allergy* **18**, 143–150.

Broughton, B.J., Chaplen, P., Knowles, P., Lunt, E., Marshall, S.M., Pain, D.L. and Wooldridge, K.R.H. (1975). Antiallergic activity of 2-phenyl-8-azapurin-6-ones. *J. Med. Chem.* **18**, 1117–1122.

Busse, W.W. and Anderson, V.I. (1981). The granulocyte response to the phosphodiesterase inhibitor Ro-20-1724 in asthma. *J. Allergy Clin. Immunol.* **67**, 70–74.

Butcher, R.W. and Sutherland, E.W. (1962). Adenosine 3′,5′-phosphate in biological materials. *J. Biol. Chem.* **237**, 1244–1250.

Carlson, R.P., O'Neill-Davis, L. and Chang, J. (1987). Pharmacologic modulation of PAF-induced mortality in mice. *Agents Actions* **21**, 379–381.

Chilton, F.H., Schmidt, D., Torphy, T.J., Goldman, D. and Undem, B. (1989). cAMP inhibits platelet activating factor (PAF) biosynthesis in the human neutrophil *FASEB J.* **3** (A308), abst. 474.

Cockcroft, D.W., Murdock, K.Y., Gore, B.P., O'Byrne, P.M. and Manning, P. (1989). Theophylline does not inhibit allergen-induced increase in airway responsiveness to methacholine. *J. Allergy Clin. Immunol.* **83**, 913–920.

Cooper, K.D., Kang, K., Chan, S.C. and Hanifin, J.M. (1985). Phosphodiesterase inhibition by Ro-20-1724 reduces hyper-IgE synthesis by atopic dermatitis cells *in vitro*. *J. Invest. Dermatol.* **84**, 477–482.

Crummey, A., Harper, G.P., Boyle, E.A. and Mangan, F.R. (1987). Inhibition of arachidonic acid-induced ear oedema as a model for assessing topical anti-inflammatory compounds. *Agents Actions* **20**, 69–76.

DeBrito, F.B., Ebsworth, K.E., and Lawrence, C.E. (1991). "Regulation of Eosinophilia by Cyclic AMP". Proceedings of the International Congress of Inflammation Meeting, 1991, Rome, Italy.

Dent, G., Giembycz, M.A., Rabe, K.F. and Barnes, P.J. (1991). Inhibition of eosinophil cyclic nucleotide PDE activity and opsonised zymosan-stimulated respiratory burst by type IV-selective PDE inhibitors. *Brit. J. Pharmacol.* **103**, 1339–1346.

Djukanovic, R., Roche, W.R., Wilson, J.W., Beasley, C.R.W., Twentyman, O.P., Howarth, P.H. and Holgate, S.T. (1990). Mucosal Inflammation in Asthma. *Am. Rev. Respir. Dis.* **142**, 434–457.

Du Toit, J.I., Salome, C.M. and Woolcock, A.J. (1987). Inhaled corticosteroids reduce the severity of bronchial hyperresponsiveness in asthma, but oral theophylline does not. *Am. Rev. Respir. Dis.* **136**, 1174–1178.

Epstein, P.M. and Hachisu, R. (1984). Cyclic Nucleotide phosphodiesterase in normal and leukemic human lymphocytes and lymphoblasts. *Adv. Cyclic Nucleotide Protein Phosphorylation Res.* **16** (303–324.

Erjefält, I. and Persson, C.G.A. (1991). Pharmacologic control of plasma exudation into tracheobronchial airways. *Am. Rev. Respir. Dis.* **143**, 1008–1014.

Finney, M.J.B., Karlsson, J.-A. and Persson, C.G.A. (1985). Effects of bronchoconstrictors and bronchodilators on a novel human small airways preparation. *Brit. J. Pharmacol.* **85**, 29–36.

Foster, R.W. and Rakshi, K. (1990). Bronchodilator potency, effectiveness and time course of inhaled nebulised AH-21-132 in normal human subject. *Brit. J. Pharmacol.* **99**, 193P.

Frossard, N., Landry, Y., Pauli, G. and Ruckstuhi, M. (1981). Effects of cyclic AMP- and cyclic GMP-phosphodiesterase inhibitors on immunological release of histamine and on lung contraction. *Brit. J. Pharmacol.* **73**, 933–938.

Giembycz, M.A. and Dent, G. (1992). Prospects for selective cyclic nucleotide phosphodiesterase inhibitors in the treatment of bronchial asthma. *Clin. Exp. Allergy* **22**, 337–344.

Giembycz, M.A., Belvisi, M.G., Miura, M., Peters, M.J., Yacoub, M. and Barnes, P.J. (1992). Cyclic nucleotide phosphodiesterases in human trachealis and the mechanical effect of isoenzyme-selective inhibitors. *Am. Rev. Respir. Dis.* **145**, A378.

Gundel, R.H., Gerritsen, M.E. and Wegner, C.D. (1989). Antigen-coated sepharose beads induce airway eosinophilia and airway hyperresponsiveness in cynomolgus monkeys. *Am. Rev. Respir. Dis.* **140**, 629–633.

Harris, A.L., Connell, M.J., Ferguson, E.W., Wallace, A.M., Gordon, R.J., Pagani, E.D. and Silver, P.J. (1989). Role of low Km cyclic AMP phosphodiesterase inhibition in tracheal relaxation and bronchodilation in the guinea-pig. *J. Pharmacol. Exp. Ther.* **251**, 199–206.

Heaslip, R.J., Buckley, S.K., Sickels, B.D. and Grimes, D. (1991). Bronchial vs. cardiovascular activities of selective phosphodiesterase inhibitors in the anaesthetized beta-blocked dog. *J. Pharmacol. Exp. Ther.* **257**, 741–747.

Hutson, P.A., Church, M.K., Clay, T.P., Miller, P. and Holgate, S.T. (1988). Early and late-phase bronchoconstriction after allergen challenge of nonanaesthetized guinea pigs. *Am. Rev. Respir. Dis.* **137**, 548–557.

Iijima, H., Ishii, M., Yamauchi, K., Chao, C.-L., Kimura, K., Shimura, S., Shindoh, Y., Inoue, H., Mue, S. and Takishima, T. (1987). Bronchoalveolar lavage and histologic characterization of late asthmatic response in guinea pigs. *Am. Rev. Respir. Dis.* **136**, 922–929.

Ishida, K., Kelly, L.J., Thomson, R.J., Beattie, L.L. and Schellenberg, R.R. (1989). Repeated antigen challenge induces airway hyperresponsiveness with tissue eosinophilia in guinea pigs. *J. Appl. Physiol.* **67**, 1133–1139.

Israel, E., Mathur, P.N., Tashkin, D. and Drazen, J.M. (1988). LY186655 prevents bronchospasm in asthma of moderate severity. *Chest* **91**, 71S.

Kishi, Y., Ashitaga, T. and Numano, F. (1992). Phosphodiesterases in vascular endothelial cells. *Adv. Second Messenger Phosphoprotein Res.* **25**, 201–213.

Kita, H., Abu-Ghazaleh, R.I., Gleich, G.J. and Abraham, R.T. (1991). Regulation of Ig-induced eosinophil degranulation by adenosine 3′,5′-cyclic monophosphate. *J. Immunol.* **146**, 2712–2718.

Klose, W., Kirsch, G., Huth, A., Frölich, W. and Laurent, H. (1986). Patent; Pharmazeutische Praeparate, DE 343 8839 A1.

Koëter, G.H., Kraan, J., Boorsma, M., Jonkman, J.H.G. and Van Der Mark, T.H.W. (1989). Effect of theophylline and enprofylline on bronchial hyperresponsiveness. *Thorax* **44**, 1022–1026.

Kolbeck, R.C., Speir, W.A. Jr., Carrier, G.O. and Bransome, E.D. Jr. (1979). Apparent irrelevance of cyclic nucleotides to the relaxation of tracheal smooth muscle induced by theophylline. *Lung* **156**, 173–183.

Lappin, D., Riches, D.W.H., Damerau, B. and Whaley, K. (1984). Cyclic nucleotides and their relationship to complement–component–C2 synthesis by human monocytes. *Biochem. J.* **222**, 477–486.

Leeman, M., Lejeune, P., Melot, C. and Naeije, R. (1987). Reduction in pulmonary hypertension and in airway resistance by enoximone (MDL 17043) in decompensated COPD. *Chest* **91**, 662–666.

Levene, S. and McKenzie, S.A. (1986). Protective effect of theophylline on histamine-induced bronchoconstriction in asthmatic children. *Brit. J. Clin. Pharmacol.* **21**, 445–449.

Lindenschmidt, R.C. and Witschi, H.P. (1985). Attenuation of pulmonary fibrosis in mice by aminophylline. *Biochem. Pharmacol.* **34**, 4269–4273.

Lohmann, S.M., Miech, R.P. and Butcher, F.R. (1977). Effects of isoproterenol, theophylline and carbachol on cyclic nucleotide levels and relaxation of bovine tracheal smooth muscle. *Biochim. Biophys. Acta* **499**, 238–250.

Lugnier, C. and Schini, V.B. (1990). Characterisation of cyclic nucleotide phosphodiesterases from cultured bovine aortic endothelial cells. *Biochem. Pharmacol.* **39**, 75–84.

MacFarland, R.T., Zelus, B.D. and Beavo, J.A. (1991). High concentrations of cGMP-stimulated phosphodiesterase mediate ANP-induced decreases in cAMP and steroidogenesis in adrenal glomerulosa cells. *J. Biol. Chem.* **266**, 136–142.

Makarski, J.S. (1981). Stimulation of cyclic AMP production by vasoactive agents in cultured bovine aortic and pulmonary artery endothelial cells. *In vitro* **17**, 450–458.

Martin, W., White, D.G. and Henderson, A.J. (1988). Endothelium-derived relaxing factor and atriopeptin II elevate cGMP levels in pig aortic endothelial cells. *Brit. J. Pharmacol.* **93**, 229–239.

Maschler, H. and Christensen, S.B. (1991). International Patent Application; Novel derivatives of phenylcycloalkanes and -cycloalkenes; WO 91 15451.

McWilliams, B.C., Menendez, R., Kelly, H.W. and Howick, J. (1984). Effects of theophylline on inhaled methacholine and histamine in asthmatic children. *Am. Rev. Respir. Dis.* **130**, 193–197.

Naclerio, R.M., Bartenfelder, D., Proud, D. *et al.* (1988). Theophylline reduces histamine release during pollen-induced rhinitis. *J. Allergy Clin. Immunol.* **78**, 874–879.

Nielson, C.P., Crowley, J.J., Cusack, B.J. and Vestal, R.E. (1986). Therapeutic concentrations of theophylline and enprofylline potentiate catecholamine effects and inhibit leukocyte activation. *J. Allergy Clin. Immunol.* **78**, 660–667.

Nielson, C.P., Crowley, J.J., Vestal, R.E., Sturm, R.J. and Heaslip, R. (1990). Effects of selective phosphodiesterase inhibitors on the polymorphonuclear leukocyte respiratory burst. *J. Allergy Clin. Immunol.* **86**, 801–808.

Okonogi, K., Gettys, T.W., Uhing, R.J., Tarry, W.C., Adams, D.O. and Pipic, V. (1991). Inhibition of prostaglandin E_2-stimulated cAMP accumulation by lipopolysaccharide in murine peritoneal macrophages. *J. Biol. Chem.* **266**, 10305–10312.

Osborn, R.R., Ferracone, J.D., Novak, L.B. and Hand, J.M. (1990). Effects of rolipram enantiomers on *in vitro* and *in vivo* guinea pig pulmonary models. *FASEB J.* **4**, A615.

Pauwels, R., Van Reuterghem, D., Van Der Straeten, D., Johannesson, N. and Persson, C.G.A. (1985). The effect of theophylline and enprofylline on allergen induced bronchoconstriction. *J. Allergy Clin. Immunol.* **76**, 583–589.

Peachell, P.T., Undem, B.J., Schleimer, R.P., Lichtenstein, L.M. and Torphy, T.J. (1990). Action of isozyme-selective phosphodiesterase (PDE) inhibitors on human basophils *FASEB J.* **4**, A639 (abst.).

Persson, C.G.A. (1985). On the medical history of xanthines and other remedies for asthma: a tribute to HH Salter. *Thorax* **40**, 881–886.

Persson, C.G.A. (1986). Role of plasma exudation in asthmatic airways. *Lancet* **2**, 1126–1128.

Persson, C.G.A. and Karlsson, J.-A. (1987). *In vitro* responses to bronchodilator drugs. In "Drug Therapy for Asthma: Research and Clinical Practice" (J.W. Jenne, S. Murphy, eds), pp. 129–176. Marcel Dekker, New York.

Persson, C.G.A., Erjefält, I. and Gustafsson, B. (1988). Xanthines – symptomatic or prophylactic in asthma? *Agents Actions* suppl. 23, 137–155.

Plaut, M., Marone, G. and Gillespie, E. (1983). The role of cyclic AMP in modulating cytotoxic T-lymphocytes II. Sequential changes during culture in responsiveness of cytotoxic lymphocytes to cyclic AMP-active agents. *J. Immunol.* **131**, 2945–2952.

Pober, J.S., Slowik, M., Deluca, L. and Ritchie, A.J. (1992). Elevated cAMP inhibits endothelial expression of ELAM-1 and VCAM-1 but not ICAM-1. *FASEB J.* **6**, A1592.

Rabe, K.F., Bodtke, K., Liebig, S. and Magnussen, H. (1992). Modulation of inherent tone of human airways *in vitro*. *Am. Rev. Respir. Dis.* **145**, A378.

Raeburn, D. and Karlsson, J.-A. (1992). Comparison of the effects of isoenzyme selective phosphodiesterase inhibitors and theophylline on PAF-induced plasma leak in the guinea-pig airways *in vivo*. *Am. Rev. Respir. Dis.* (in press). **145**, A612.

Riva, C.M., Morganroth, M.L., Marks, R.M., Toddy, R.F. III., Ward, P.A. and Boxer, L.A. (1989). Iloprost inhibits activated human neutrophil (PMN) adherence to endothelial cells via increased cyclic AMP. *Clin. Res.* **37**, 949A.

Robicsek, S.A., Krzanowski, J.J., Szentivanyi, A. and Polson, J.B. (1989). High pressure liquid chromatography of cyclic nucleotide phosphodiesterase from purified human T-lymphocytes. *Biochem. Biophys. Res. Commun.* **163**, 554–560.

Rudd, R.M., Gellert, A.R., Studdy, P.R. and Geddes, D.M. (1983). Inhibition of exercise-induced asthma by an orally absorbed mast cell stabilizer (M&B 22948). *Brit. J. Dis. Chest* **77**, 78–86.

Sanjar, S., Aoki, S., Boubeckeur, K., Chapman, I.D., Smith, D., Kings, M.A. and Morley, J. (1990a). Eosinophil accumulation in pulmonary airways of guinea-pigs induced by exposure to an aerosol of platelet activating factor: effect of anti-asthma drugs. *Brit. J. Pharmacol.* **99**, 267–272.

Sanjar, S., Aoki, S., Kritersson, A., Smith, D. and Morley, J. (1990b). Antigen challenge induces pulmonary airway eosinophil accumulation and airway hyperreactivity in sensitized guinea-pigs: the effect of anti-asthma drugs. *Brit. J. Pharmacol.* **99**, 679–686.

Schneider, H.H., Schmiechen, R., Brezinski, M. and Seidler, J. (1986). Stereospecific binding of the antidepressant rolipram to brain protein structures. *Eur. J. Pharmacol.* **127**, 105–115.

Schudt, C., Winder, S., Litze, M., Kilian, U. and Beume, R. (1991). Zardaverine: A cyclic AMP specific PDE III/IV inhibitors. *Agents Actions* **34**, 161–177.

Seibert, A.F., Thompson, W.J., Taylor, A., Wilborn, W.H., Barnard, J. and Haynes, J. (1992). Reversal of increased microvascular permeability associated with ischemia-reperfusion: role of cAMP. *J. Appl. Physiol.* **72**, 389–395.

Shahid, M., van Amsterdam, R.G.M., de Boer, J., ten Berge, R.E., Nicholson, C.D. and Zaagsma, J. (1991). The presence of five cyclic nucleotide phosphodiesterase isoenzyme activities in bovine tracheal smooth muscle and the functional effects of selective inhibitors. *Brit. J. Pharmacol.* **104**, 471–477.

Simpson, A.W.M., Reeves, M.L. and Rink, T.J. (1988). Effects of SK&F 94120, on inhibitor of cyclic nucleotide phosphodiesterase type III, on human platelets. *Biochem. Pharmacol.* **37**, 2315–2320.

Small, R.C., Boyle, J.P., Duty, S., Elliot, K.R.F., Foster, R.W. and Watt, A.J. (1989). Analysis of the relaxant effects of AH-21-132 in guinea-pig isolated trachealis. *Br. J. Pharmacol.* **97**, 1165–1173.

Smith, P.F., Thompson, W.J., de Haen, C., Halonen, M., Palmer, J.D. and Johnson, D.G. (1986). Bronchodilator activity of a non-xanthine phosphodiesterase inhibitor: 2,4-diamino-5-cyano-6-bromopyridine (compound 1). *J. Pharmacol. Exp. Ther.* **237**, 114–119.

Souness, J.E. and Scott, C.L. (1992). Stereospecificity of rolipram (R) actions on eosinophil (E) cAMP phosphodiesterase. *FASEB J.* **6**, A1847.

Souness, J.E., Thompson, W.J. and Strada, S.J. (1985). Adipocyte cyclic nucleotide phosphodiesterase activation by vanadate. *J. Cyclic Nucleotide Protein Phosphorylation Res.* **10**, 383–396.

Souness, J.E., Diocee, B.K., Martin, W. and Moodie, S.A. (1990). Pig aortic endothelial-cell cyclic nucleotide phosphodiesterases. Use of phosphodiesterase inhibitors to evaluate their roles in regulating cyclic nucleotide levels in intact cells. *Biochem. J.* **226**, 127–132.

Souness, J.E., Carter, C.M., Diocee, B.K., Hassall, G.A., Wood, L.J. and Turner, N.C. (1991). Characterization of guinea-pig eosinophil phosphodiesterase activity. Assessment of its involvement in regulating superoxide generation. *Biochem. Pharmacol.* **42**, 937–945.

Souness, J.E., Maslen, C. and Scott, C.L. (1992). Effects of solubilization and vanadate/glutathione complex on inhibitor potencies against eosinophil cyclic AMP-specific phosphodiesterase. *FEBS Letts.* **302**, 181–184.

Suttorp, N., Welsch, T., Weber, U., Richter, U. and Schudt, C. (1991). Activation of cAMP-dependent protein kinase blocks hydrogen peroxide-induced enhanced endothelial permeability *in vitro*. *Am. Rev. Respir. Dis.* **143**, A572.

Thompson, W.J. (1991). Cyclic nucleotide phosphodiesterases: Pharmacology, Biochemistry and Function. *Pharmac. Ther.* **51**, 13–33.
Thornhill, M.H. and Haskard, D.O. (1990). IL-4 regulates endothelial cell activation by IL-1, tumor necrosis factor, or IFN-gamma. *J. Immunol.* **145**, 865–872.
Tomkinson, A., Karlsson, J.-A. and Raeburn, D. (1993). Comparison of the effects of rolipram and siguazodan, selective inhibitors of phosphodiesterase type IV and type III, in airway smooth muscle preparations with differing β-adrenoceptor subtype populations. *Brit. J. Pharmacol.* **108**, 57–61.
Torphy, T.J. and Cieslinski, L.B. (1990). Characterisation and selective inhibition of cyclic nucleotide phosphodiesterase isozymes in canine tracheal smooth muscle. *Molec. Pharmacol.* **37**, 206–214.
Torphy, T.J. and Undem, B.J. (1991). Phosphodiesterase inhibitors: new opportunities for the treatment of asthma. *Thorax* **46**, 512–523.
Torphy, T.J., Burman, M., Huang, L.B.F. and Tucker, S.S. (1988). Inhibition of the low Km cyclic AMP phosphodiesterase in intact canine trachealis by SK&F 94836: mechanical and biochemical responses. *J. Pharmacol. Exp. Ther.* **246**, 843–850.
Torphy, T.J., Zhou, H.-L., Burnham, M. and Huang, L.B.F. (1991). Role of cyclic nucleotide phosphodiesterase isoenzymes in intact canine trachealis. *Molec. Pharmacol.* **39**, 376–384.
Torphy, T.J., Stadel, J.M., Burman, M., Cieslinski, L.B., McLaughlin, M.M., White, J.R. and Levi, G.P. (1992). Coexpression of human cAMP-specific phosphodiesterase activity and high affinity rolipram binding in yeast. *J. Biol. Chem.* **267**, 1798–1804.
Underwood, S.L., Lewis, S.A. and Raeburn, D. (1992). RP 59227, a novel PAF receptor antagonist: effects in guinea pig models of airway hyperreactivity. *Eur. J. Pharmacol.* **210**, 97–102.
Weishaar, R.E., Burrows, S.D., Kobylarz, D.C., Quade, M.M. and Evans, D.B. (1986). Multiple molecular forms of cyclic nucleotide phosphodiesterase in cardiac and smooth muscle and in platelets. *Biochem. Pharmacol.* **35**, 787–800.
Wellicome, S.M., Thornhill, M.H., Pitzalis, C., Thomas, D.S., Lanchbury, J.S., Panayi, G.S. and Haskard, D.O. (1990). A monoclonal antibody that detects a novel antigen on endothelial cells that is induced by tumor necrosis factor, IL-1, or lipopolysaccharide. *J. Immunol.* **144**, 2558–2565.
White, J.R., Torphy, T.J., Christensen, S.B. IV, Lee, J.A. and Mong, S. (1990). Partial purification of the rolipram sensitive phosphodiesterase from human monocytes. *FASEB J.* **4**, A1987 (abst.).
Wright, C.D., Kuipers, P.J., Kobylarz-Singer, D., Devall, L.J., Klinkefus, B.A. and Weishaar, R.E. (1990). Differential inhibition of human neutrophil functions: role of cyclic AMP-specific, cyclic GMP-insensitive phosphodiesterase. *Biochem. Pharmacol.* **40**, 699–707.

Discussion

G.J. Laurent

Obviously, these inhibitors can exert a lot of effects. How many of the effects observed do you think are related to changes in cyclic-AMP or cyclic-GMP? Are those levels assessed in some of the biological assays?

J.-A. Karlsson

The levels have not been regularly assessed in our systems, but we have looked at cyclic-AMP accumulation in isolated cells. There is a very good correlation between the accumulation and the function of the cell. *In vivo*, it is very difficult to state conclusively that it is the exact mechanism of action, although I think there is quite good *in vitro* evidence for this being the case.

G.J. Laurent

Secondly, obviously other parts of those transduction pathways are susceptible to manipulation. Have any of those been investigated, and how do you think the inhibitors you are looking at would stand in comparison to what might be used at other points in that pathway?

J.-A. Karlsson

There are a number of intracellular signalling pathways which researchers have taken interest in, such as inhibition of protein kinase C and tyrosine kinase. There is a lot of *in vitro* data, but I think there is generally a lack of *in vivo* information in inflammatory systems. It is not really possible, therefore, to compare the relative importance and potential efficacy of these different classes of compounds.

B.B. Vargaftig

I wonder about the correlation that might be found between the activity of the substance you have been discussing and leukotriene (LT) C_4 formation on one side, and basically phospholipase A_2 – not only because of the obvious relevance of LTC_4 coming from the eosinophils and modulated by the drugs, but because of some observations we have on phospholipase A_2 from guinea-pig eosinophils which is secreted during their activation.

How could these drugs be used in order better to understand the interaction between phospholipase A_2 and the leukotrienes as a system, and have you measured LTC_4?

J.-A. Karlsson

No, we have not done that. We have been able only to look at a few specific things as I mentioned in my talk, and of course we don't know whether other aspects of cell function are also inhibited or downregulated.

On the other hand, if we look at the effect LTC_4, for example, on airways smooth muscle, I think we would expect it to be blocked by this type of functional inhibitor.

A.R. Leff
The β-agonists prevent vascular leak during challenge if they are given prior to the challenge but not if given afterwards. Have you found with your PDE IV inhibitor that vascular leak can be reversed once the process starts or must the inhibitor be given before the challenge?

J.-A. Karlsson
We have only studied the effect of pretreatment with RP 73401.

A.R. Leff
I would expect that the same effect would be observed as with β-agonists, which means that the vascular leak effectiveness would be confined to having the drugs given well in advance of the challenge or stimulus – which may not be a problem for maintenance medication.

C. Page
Over the last 10–15 years there has been a lot of literature about theophylline and lymphocytes. There is evidence that it can be immunosuppressive and affect transplantation. Has there been a chance to look at your compound in models of transplantation?

J.-A. Karlsson
We have found that rolipram, a PDE IV inhibitor, suppresses activity in a murine T helper cell. We have not looked at RP 73401 in transplantation models, but it would be very interesting to do that.

C. Page
Theophylline has been demonstrated to synergize with cyclosporin A in terms of organ transplantation.

R. Dahl
The β-agonists can usually do what theophyllines can in all these respects of vascular leakage, inhibition of mediator release and quite a lot of other things. The concern about β-agonists is that in many cases there can be tachyphylaxis to these effects during exposure for a longer period. Was this looked for?

J.-A. Karlsson
We have dosed for a week with high doses of RP 73401, and then looked at function, for example, bronchodilatation. There is no difference in the efficacy of the drug over that time period. It is a question that

probably has to be addressed in much longer studies, which has not yet been done.

R. Dahl
I guess this drug could – or would – be used as an oral preparation, or do you think it could be given as an inhaled preparation? There are quite marked differences between the protective and bronchodilator effects of oral and inhaled forms.

J.-A. Karlsson
If we look at the cells on which this drug is expected to act, we might think that the oral route would probably be better, to have it available to the entire circulation and hence systemic exposure. On the other hand, surprisingly perhaps, in all these animal models there is very good activity with airway administration of the compound. I think this will be the intended route.

S.T. Holgate
Recent studies have shown the presence of type IV PDE in the human bronchial epithelial cell, in particular in tissue culture. I am aware of some studies showing that this class of compound, particularly rolipram, is cytoprotective; in other words, if animals are pretreated and endotoxin is then presented to the airways, the effect can be overcome to a much greater degree than without the drug. Cytoprotection is one area that would be worth pursuing with this class of compound.

Secondly, Dr Dahl has just raised the subject of the form of delivery of the drug. With theophylline, the drug goes straight through into the circulation and there is a transient effect. Fairly early in the developmental plan of such compounds, I think it would be worthwhile looking at the pharmacokinetics of a drug to see whether its absorption limits its kinetics or whether its prolonged duration of action relates purely to its very strong affinity for the binding site on the enzyme. Have you any comments about the kinetics of inhaled compound?

J.-A. Karlsson
We have done some preliminary studies on the appearance of the compound in blood after oral and inhaled administration. It seems that it is retained in the airways for an unexpectedly long period of time – which is very different, as you mentioned, to theophylline which goes straight through. This is an encouraging finding. Equally, by oral dosing, there appears to be a limited absorption, and very low amounts of the intact drug can be detected in plasma.

S.T. Holgate
The problem with this class of compounds given by the oral route is the vomiting that many patients have. Clearly, it would be very good if this can be circumvented.

M.K. Church
To expand a little on Professor Holgate's question, the two factors that are needed from a new drug are, first, efficacy and, secondly, safety (perhaps they should sometimes be in the reverse order). Potentially, these drugs would appear to have toxic problems at high doses because they work on so many tissues inhibiting cyclic-AMP. Could you tell us something about the systemic effects unrelated to the asthma area that may be expected, particularly in high dosage, or overuse of a drug?

J.-A. Karlsson
It is very difficult to speculate on this because it depends very much on the pharmacodynamics and the pharmacokinetics of the individual compound.

Compounds like rolipram can be detected in plasma, we know it passes very rapidly over the gastrointestinal mucosa and then exerts effects in the central nervous system (CNS). Denbufylline and rolipram have been developed for CNS disorders. If large amounts of these compounds are present in the CNS, of course, it would be expected that they will be active in inhibiting type IV PDE activity. However, it is worth mentioning that rolipram failed as an antidepressant in clinical testing which may be due either to its pharmacodynamic or pharmacokinetic properties that were not foreseeable from animal studies.

The problem of vomiting has been mentioned, but I think this has also been related to an effect directly in the CNS.

19

Concluding Remarks – Possibilities for Future Therapies

S.T. HOLGATE

Immunopharmacology Group, Southampton General Hospital, Tremona Road, Southampton SO9 4XY, UK

At the end of a long meeting like this, in which we have seen so much new and interesting material, it is hard to know where to start pulling together items relating to pharmacology and the development of new drugs. We have already heard about a large number of new possibilities. To begin with, I think we can learn a lot from the current drugs that are available for treating human allergic diseases, and see what opportunities these teach us about potentially new avenues for intercepting the inflammatory process.

I want to deal briefly with five topics:

1) Bronchodilators. In particular, the relationship of bronchodilatation to any other activities that these drugs may have in relation to clinical efficacy.
2) Corticosteroids and their mechanism of action.
3) The opportunities created through the recognition of leukocyte endothelial adhesion modules (LECAMs).
4) The contribution of cytokines as signalling molecules in allergic inflammation.
5) A few comments relating to the bronchial epithelium, as the origin and target for the inflammatory response in asthma.

The changes that can be seen in a bronchial biopsy taken from a young asthmatic patient who was not receiving any prophylactic treatment highlights the various aspects of the pathology that have been addressed

T-Lymphocyte and Inflammatory Cell Research in Asthma
ISBN 0-12-388170-6

during this meeting. Attention has focused on eosinophils, lymphocytes and macrophages as important effector cells of the asthmatic with the bronchial epithelium being a target for this immunological attack. It is recognizing that there are steps at which one can intervene in this inflammatory response that provides both industry and academics with a feeling of optimism about the future for new drug development.

It will be recalled that in the UK and elsewhere the commonest drugs currently prescribed for asthma are the inhaled β_2-agonists. Worldwide, they account for 80% of the prescriptions for anti-asthma treatments. Thus, to ignore this class of drug when considering asthma management would be to neglect a major therapeutic area.

In considering the way that bronchodilator drugs work, the target for their development has been focused on reversing the effects of bronchospastic mediators, such as histamine, prostaglandin D_2 and the sulphidopeptide leukotrienes, that are released by mast cells and eosinophils – and, in this respect, serve as functional antagonists on both smooth muscle and possibly vascular responses.

However, from what has already been said, it appears that there is relatively little interest in developing better bronchodilator agents essentially in the face of the newly introduced long-acting inhaled β_2-agonists. With the recognition of the importance of inflammation in asthma more emphasis is now being placed on understanding and hopefully controlling the disordered immune response whether at the level of the T cell or on the recognition and processing of antigens by cells in the epithelium. The development of long-acting β_2-agonists at a time when there is increasing concern over the way the drugs are used to treat asthma has aroused considerable interest both in clinical and industrial circles. It will be recalled that in the mid-1960s and early 1970s the selectivity of the inhaled β-agonists was improved by the development of agents such as salbutamol and terbutaline. More recently, the duration of action of long-acting bronchodilator drugs has been greatly improved by the introduction of salmeterol (Glaxo) and formoterol (Ciba-Geigy). When given by inhalation both of these drugs produced bronchodilatation of duration in excess of 12 h and as such represent a tremendous advance in bronchodilator therapy. Data in guinea pigs and *in vitro* studies on human lung have demonstrated clear inhibitory effects on mast cell- and eosinophil-mediated early and late phase allergen responses respectively. While we are able to confirm salmeterol's protective efficacy against the allergen-induced early and late responses and acquired increase in airways responsiveness in asthma, it was not possible to say whether this was due to β_2-mediated bronchodilatation or acute anti-inflammatory activities as suggested by the animal studies. In positioning this drug and formoterol in the clinical armamentarium this differentation of mechanisms is clearly important. It is because of this dilemma that we progressed to a formal placebo-controlled clinical study of 6 weeks of regular salmeterol treatment.

Two groups of matched patients were treated twice daily with inhaled salmeterol (50 μg) or matched placebo and indices of clinical efficacy followed. As many others have shown with this drug, there was a very impressive clinical response, which when compared with placebo, produced a highly significant reduction in both night-time and day-time symptoms, a reduction in the use of escape medication in the form of inhaled salbutamol and improvement in bronchial responsiveness, assessed by a reduction in diurnal variation of PEF and, 4–6 h after dosing, a three- to fivefold increase in PC_{20} methacholine. An additional component of this study was bronchoscopy with mucosal biopsy and lavage before and at the end of a 6-week treatment period. Bronchial inflammation relevant to the asthma process was assessed by the number of mast cells and eosinophils present in the mucosa, the number and activation status of T cells and the concentration of mast cells and eosinophils and their mediators in bronchoalveolar lavage (BAL). Despite an excellent clinical response, salmeterol failed to influence any of these indices of airway inflammation, leading us to the conclusion that a substantial proportion (if not all) the beneficial effect observed with this drug related to its bronchodilator property.

This does not diminish the relevance of the clinical findings with salmeterol in relation to efficacy, but because of concerns over the use of symptomatic treatment for asthma alone with a drug of this type, it does influence the clinical indications. It remains possible that long-acting β_2-agonists could modify the relatively acute airway events of the allergen-provoked early response, but not late response; if this is the case, then one has to question the value of these test systems for assessing the activity of drugs such as salmeterol against chronic inflammation.

Both national and international management strategies for asthma are being directed towards treating airway inflammation rather than relying on symptom relief alone, and as a consequence drugs such as sodium cromoglycate, nedocromil sodium and topical corticosteroids are assuming the position of first-line therapies. For over 20 years clinicians have recognized the valuable role that inhaled corticosteroids have in treating chronic asthma but the scientific rationale for their use has, until recently, not become available, although it has long been known that these drugs influence the asthma process by mechanisms other than by simple smooth muscle relaxation.

To address this problem we have applied the same trial protocol as used in the salmeterol study, but this time replacing salmeterol with beclomethasone dipropionate (BDP), given twice daily for 6 weeks (2000 μg/day for 2 weeks and 1000 μg/day for 4 weeks). Mucosal biopsy and lavage samples were obtained from the airways before and after the 6-week treatment period. The observed clinical response with BDP was almost identical to that achieved with salmeterol – a 60–70% reduction in symptom scores, a rise in morning PEF to near normal levels and a fivefold reduction in bronchial responsiveness to methacholine challenge. However, the biopsy and lavage data differed markedly from those observed with salmeterol. When the mast cells were enumerated by their content of granule tryptase, the inhaled BDP produced a two- to fourfold reduction in their numbers both in the epithelium and in the submucosa. An even more dramatic reduction was seen in the number of eosinophils (identified by their granule content of cationic protein (ECP)), colonizing the airway wall. These data clearly indicate that this topical corticosteroid, while achieving similar clinical efficacy to salmeterol, works in an entirely different way – in this case reducing the cells known to be important in the inflammatory response. Loss of mast cells and eosinophils was paralleled by a reduction in the lavage content of the mediators histamine and tryptase from mast cells and eosinophils and ECP from eosinophils, mediators that are considered to contribute to the disordered airway function in asthma.

Using a monoclonal antibody directed against lipocortin 1β, we were able to show the presence of this steroid-induced protein in epithelial cells and mononuclear cells. In the same study in which biopsies were obtained from patients who had been treated with inhaled beclomethasone dipropionate, we also looked at the number and activation status of T-lymphocytes in BAL. There was no significant difference in the total number of T cells or the CD4 and CD8 subtypes after the steroid treatment. However, for signals of cell activation, the α-chain of the interleukin-2 (IL-2) receptor (CD25) and the major histocompatibility complex (MHC) class II molecule, HLA-DR, the inhaled corticosteroid treatment produced a highly significant reduction. These findings may be interpreted as corticosteroids downregulating the activity of a subpopulation of T cells (TH_2) which are probably important in propagating the inflammatory response. Such a mechanism involving reduced release of pro-inflammatory cytokines could explain why mast cell and eosinophil populations in the airways are greatly reduced during this form of treatment.

Looking at the inflammatory response from another perspective, it seems at least theoretically possible to block the influx of leukocytes into the airway wall by interfering with the leukocyte–vascular interaction. If bronchial biopsies are taken from clinically active asthmatic patients there is a greatly increased number of eosinophils and mononuclear cells in close association with post-capillary endothelial cells within the submucosal blood vessels. Looking carefully at these cells, the endothelium appears and contains submembrane vesicles. These observations, together with the presence of pseudopods from the leukocyte to the endothelial cells indicates a specific adhesion process. In a collaborative study with Professor Tak Lee and Dr Dorian Haskard we have looked at the expression of cell adhesion molecules involved in the endothelium and on the leukocyte as part of this recruitment process. One of these molecules is the intercellular adhesion molecule-I (ICAM-I), which is a member of the superimmunoglobulin family and is involved in the recruitment of eosinophils and T cells in to the inflammatory zone. The expression of this molecule was investigated in bronchial biopsies of asthmatics both before and 4 h after local segmental (per bronchoscopic) allergen challenge. When compared with the saline-challenged site, allergen caused a marked increase in immunostaining of vessels for ICAM-I. The E-selectin (endothelial leukocyte adhesion molecule-I (ELAM-I)) was also upregulated but at 4 h no difference was seen in vascular cell adhesion molecule-I (VCAM-I).

One of the most important ligands for ICAM-I is the integrin LFA-1 (CD11a/CD18) which is expressed on most leukocytes. Four hours after allergen but not saline challenge, large numbers of LFA-1^+ leukocytes are observed infiltrating the airway wall. Using monoclonal antibodies to individual cell markers, these largely comprise neutrophils and eosinophils, although some increase in T cells and, surprisingly, mast cells was also seen.

While studies such as this demonstrate that leukocyte–endothelial adhesion is important in the relatively acute situation of allergen challenge, the important question is whether similar events occur naturally. In studying perennial rhinitis, we have recently shown that ICAM-I and VCAM-I are chronically upregulated, accounting for the prominence of eosinophils in active phases of the disease by using their complementary ligands LFA-1 and VLA-4 for recruitment.

In considering the recruitment of eosinophils and the upregulation of mast cells involving IgE, we have heard a lot at this conference about the potential of cytokines to affect such mechanisms. Presentation of processed antigens to T cells results in a change in the T cell phenotype to that expressing the cytokines involved in mast cell- and eosinophil-mediated inflammation. This subtype of $CD4^+$ lymphocyte has been designated the TH_2-lymphocyte. The reason for so much interest in this cell is because it appears to elaborate the messages and the cytokines involved in the replication, priming and migration of eosinophils, mast cells and basophils and, through IL-4, to trigger switching of B-lymphocytes to the synthesis of IgE. On the other hand, the TH_1 subtype elaborates cytokines (predominantly interferon-γ (IFN-γ)) that downregulate the TH_2 cell and switch off IgE synthesis. During this symposium we have heard evidence for the participation of this particular type of T cell in the inflammatory response characteristic of asthma. In considering IL-3, IL-4 and IL-5 as effector cytokines of the mast cell, eosinophil and IgE in allergic inflammation, the question that arises is whether there is evidence that these cytokines are present in the diseased tissue itself? Using thin glycolmethacrylate sections of bronchial biopsies stained with monoclonal antibody to IL-4 (provided by Dr C. Heusser, Ciba-Geigy) we can clearly show cells staining positively for IL-4, which in adjacent sections did not stain for the T cell receptor. We were intrigued by this observation, and in a collaborative study with our colleagues at Ciba-Geigy we attempted to identify the cellular provenance of the IL-4 immunostaining. In both normal airways and in those of mild–moderate asthmatics IL-4 was localized to tryptase-containing cells, namely mast cells. Eighty per cent of the IL-4 product was mast cell-associated, while 80–100% of mast cells stained for IL-4. We have now progressed this observation by studying purified human mast cells taking advantage of the expression of *c-kit* as an antigen marker on the surface of mast cells and magnetic beads liganded to the anti-c-kit, TB5 B8 monoclonal. In > 98% of purified mast cell populations either from lung or skin IL-4 immunoreactivity was again shown. In further collaborative studies with Dr Heusser, we have successfully shown IgE-dependent release of IL-4 when the cytokine was assayed in an antigen capture ELISA. This suggested strongly that not only is IL-4 stored within mast cells but that there is a secretory mechanism involving IgE that can release it into the microenvironment, and that this cell is indeed an important source of this mediator. Subsequently, immunohistochemistry has been used to study a number of other cytokines. We have been able to show that 30–80% of mast cells in the airways stain for IL-5, IL-6 and TNF-α. Thus, in addition to being involved in the upregulation of endothelial adhesion molecules (IL-4, IL-5 and TNF-α), the mast cell cytokines may play a pivotal role in maintaining the inflammatory response through recruitment and activation of eosinophils (TNF-α, IL-5) and the maintenance of the TH_2 cell population (IL-4).

The IgE-related release of cytokines from mast cells also provides a unique mechanism to explain how drugs like sodium cromoglycate and nedocromil sodium interfere with the late reaction. It is difficult to consider that the late response, which reaches maximum 4–6 h post-allergen challenge, relates to cytokine production by T cells because this takes ~ 4 h to reach reasonable levels. By contrast an explosive release of cytokines from mast cells to initiate the late response, is a step which could be sensitive to the inhibitory effects of drugs acting on the mast cell. This would be of special interest if the cellular biochemical pathways for cytokine secretion differed from that for the classical mediators. Such a pathway (if it exists) might provide a further opportunity for looking at the way that new mast cell stabilizing drugs could interfere with cytokine release, as opposed to looking only at their effects on preformed histamine and eicosanoid release alone.

In creating a scenario, it seems that in genetically susceptible individuals, macrophages and dendritic cells process specific antigens and through the secretion of amplification cytokines, such as IL-1 and IL-6, expand the antigen-specific T cells comprising largely the TH_2 subtype. These TH_2 cells are able to elaborate the cytokines, IL-3, IL-4, IL-9, IL-10 and GM-CSF, that may well be involved in promoting the priming and supporting the growth of basophils and mast cells, the upregulation of eosinophils, and the isotype switching of B cells to IgE synthesis. In allergen-sensitized subjects the whole process could be started by an initiating stimulus provided by the mast cell through the release of TNF-α, IL-4 and IL-5 and amplified by IL-6.

Finally, not to miss an opportunity to come back to the point raised both by Professor Lee and by a number of others during their presentations, namely the role of the epithelium, recent studies have suggested that the epithelium is a primary focus for the inflammatory response in asthma. When comparing biopsies from asthmatic and normal subjects stained with monoclonal antibodies to a number of heat-shock proteins (HSP 92 and HSP 30), increased expression of these stress proteins in the epithelium can be shown. The epithelium can respond to a site-directed inflammatory attack in a number of ways. It could be destroyed, thus destroying all of its functions. Alternatively, when provoked, epithelial cells may switch on genes that make important pharmacologically active substances. It appears that in asthma there is enhanced epithelium expression of endothelin-1, the inducible form of nitric oxide synthase, IL-1β, GM-CSF and IL-8. This indicates a very dynamic role for the epithelium in maintaining and possibly augmenting the inflammatory response.

When reviewed by transmission electron microscopy, some remarkable changes can be seen in the epithelium of asthmatics. In addition to eosinophils interfacing with endothelial cells, leukocytes are seen to be present within the perivascular space and migrating up to the epithelium, which itself appear oedematous. There is clear separation of columnar cells from the basal cells that form the pseudo-stratified structure. This is likely to be a consequence of a breakdown in the integrity of adhesion molecules which secure the columnar cells to the basal cells. In disconnecting the epithelium, its permeability is likely to increase, a feature well described after allergen challenge and with exacerbations of asthma.

Using a panel on monoclonal antibodies to different adhesion molecules, a picture can be built up of the classes of adhesion molecules which are important in maintaining the integrity of the normal bronchial epithelium. The bronchial epithelium in asthmatics and normals is attached to the basement membrane by hemidesmosomal proteins largely comprising the integrin $\alpha_6\beta_4$. In addition, there are hemidesmosomal attachments in the sub-mucosal microvasculature. The epithelium cells that comprise the columnar layer-ciliated cells, Clara and the goblet cells do not express hemidesmosomal proteins. From both bronchoalveolar lavage and biopsy studies in asthmatics epithelial disruption presents itself as cleavage just above the basal layer. With little trauma the columnar cells will have a tendency to shear off into the airway lumen. Using immunohistochemical procedures three adhesion structures appear important in maintaining the structural integrity of the normal epithelium: tight junctions at the apices, intermediate junctions containing uvomorulin just beneath these and, most important of all, many desmosomes located along the lateral, basolateral and basal borders of the columnar cells. We believe it is these latter structures that become damaged in asthma.

From our recent studies with Dr Clive Robinson, on the way that activated eosinophils interact with the epithelium *in vitro*, we believe that weakening of desmosomal links occurs following a cognate interaction between the eosinophil and epithelial cell (possibly involving ICAM-1) with subsequent induction of epithelial-derived proenzymes of the metalloendoproteases such as collagenase type IV.

Clearly much further work needs to be undertaken to investigate the ways in which the epithelium becomes both stimulated and changed in asthma and how this may contribute towards the chronicity of the inflammatory response. However, cytoprotection provides another possible opportunity for protecting the airways in asthma and possibly reduces some of the chronic components of the inflammatory response.

Index

Tables in **bold**, Figures in *italic*.